Real-Time 3D Echocardiography for Congenital Heart Disease

From Fetus to Adult

Real-Time 3D Echocardiography for Congenital Heart Disease

From Fetus to Adult

Shuping Ge, MD, FACC, FASE

Department of Pediatrics
Section of Cardiology
St. Christopher's Hospital for Children
Drexel University College of Medicine
Philadelphia, Pennsylvania
Department of Pediatrics
Deborah Heart and Lung Center
Browns Mills, New Jersey

2014
People's Medical Publishing House—USA
Shelton, Connecticut

People's Medical Publishing House-USA
2 Enterprise Drive, Suite 509
Shelton, CT 06484
Tel: 203-402-0646
Fax: 203-402-0854
E-mail: info@pmph-usa.com

PMPH-USA

14 15 16 17/**King**/9 8 7 6 5 4 3 2 1

ISBN-13 978-1-60795-155-1
ISBN-10 1-60795-155-X
eISBN-13 978-1-60795-265-7

Printed in the United States of America by **King Printing Company, Inc.**
Editor: Linda H. Mehta; Copyeditor/Typesetter: diacriTech; Cover designer: Mary McKeon

Library of Congress Cataloging-in-Publication Data
Real-time 3D echocardiography for congenital heart disease : from fetus to adult / [edited by] Shuping Ge.
p. ; cm.
Includes bibliographical references and index.
ISBN 978-1-60795-155-1 — ISBN 1-60795-155-X — ISBN 978-1-60795-265-7 (eISBN)
I. Ge, Shuping, editor.
[DNLM: 1. Echocardiography, Three-Dimensional. 2. Heart Defects, Congenital—diagnosis. WG 141.5.E2]
RC683.5.U5

616.1'207543—dc23

2014007055

Sales and Distribution

Canada
McGraw-Hill Ryerson Education
Customer Care
300 Water St
Whitby, Ontario L1N 9B6
Canada
Tel: 1-800-565-5758
Fax: 1-800-463-5885
www.mcgrawhill.ca

Foreign Rights
John Scott & Company
International Publisher's Agency
P.O. Box 878
Kimberton, PA 19442
USA
Tel: 610-827-1640
Fax: 610-827-1671

Japan
United Publishers Services Limited
1-32-5 Higashi-Shinagawa
Shinagawa-ku, Tokyo 140-0002
Japan
Tel: 03-5479-7251
Fax: 03-5479-7307
Email: kakimoto@ups.co.jp

United Kingdom, Europe, Middle East, Africa
McGraw Hill Education
Shoppenhangers Road
Maidenhead
Berkshire, SL6 2QL
England
Tel: 44-0-1628-502500
Fax: 44-0-1628-635895
www.mcgraw-hill.co.uk

Singapore, Thailand, Philippines, Indonesia, Vietnam, Pacific Rim, Korea
McGraw-Hill Education
60 Tuas Basin Link
Singapore 638775
Tel: 65-6863-1580
Fax: 65-6862-3354
www.mcgraw-hill.com.sg

Australia, New Zealand
Elsevier Australia
Locked Bag 7500
Chatswood DC NSW 2067
Australia
Tel: 161 (2) 9422-8500
Fax: 161 (2) 9422-8562
www.elsevier.com.au

Brazil
SuperPedido Tecmedd
Beatriz Alves, Foreign Trade Department
R. Sansao Alves dos Santos, 102 | 7th floor
Brooklin Novo
Sao Pãulo 04571-090
Brazil
Tel: 55-16-3512-5539
www.superpedidotecmedd.com.br

India, Bangladesh, Pakistan, Sri Lanka, Malaysia
CBS Publishers
4819/X1 Prahlad Street 24
Ansari Road, Darya Ganj,
New Delhi-110002
India
Tel: 91-11-23266861/67
Fax: 91-11-23266818
Email: cbspubs@vsnl.com

People's Republic of China
People's Medical Publishing House
International Trade Department
No. 19, Pan Jia Yuan Nan Li
Chaoyang District
Beijing 100021
P.R. China
Tel: 8610-67653342
Fax: 8610-67691034
www.pmph.com/en/

Dedication

To my wife Rose, daughter Joy, and son Andrew for their understanding, support, and love.

Contents

List of Contributors

Robert H. Anderson, BSc, MD [1, 7]
Division of Pediatric Cardiology
Department of Pediatrics
Medical University of South Carolina
Charleston, South Carolina

Rula Balluz, MD, MPH [5]
Section of Pediatric Cardiology
Drexel University College of Medicine
Heart Center for Children
St. Christopher's Hospital for Children
Philadelphia, Pennsylvania

Sonal Chandra, MD [2, 16]
Health System Clinician in Medicine–Cardiology
Department of Medicine
Division of Cardiology
Northwestern Universiy
Feinberg School of Medicine
Chicago, Illinois

Greggory R. DeVore, MD [14]
Director, Fetal Diagnostic Center
Pasadena, California

Shuping Ge, MD [4, 5]
Department of Pediatrics
Chief, Section of Cardiology
St. Christopher's Hospital for Children
Drexel University College of Medicine
Philadelphia, Pennsylvania
Acting Chair, Department of Pediatrics
Deborah Heart and Lung Center
Browns Mills, New Jersey

Fadi G. Hage, MD [3, 15]
Division of Cardiovascular Diseases
University of Alabama at Birmingham
Section of Cardiology
Birmingham Veterans Affairs Medical Center
Birmingham, Alabama

Anthony M. Hlavacek, MD [1, 7]
Division of Pediatric Cardiology
Department of Pediatrics
Medical University of South Carolina
Charleston, South Carolina

Leng Jiang, MD [9]
Professor of Medicine
Tufts University School of Medicine
Boston, Massachusetts
Visiting Professor
Shanghai Institute of Cardiovascular Diseases
ZhongShan Hospital
Fudan University
Shanghai, China

Navin C. Nanda, MD [3, 15]
Division of Cardiovascular Diseases
University of Alabama at Birmingham
Birmingham, Alabama

CuiZhen Pan, MD [9]
Professor of Medicine
Shanghai Institute of Cardiovascular Diseases
ZhongShan Hospital
Fudan University
Shanghai, China

David A. Roberson, MD [6, 10, 11]
Associate Professor of Pediatrics
Chicago Medical School
Chicago, Illinois
Director of Pediatric Echocardiography
The Heart Institute for Children
Hope Children's Hospital
Oak Lawn, Illinois

Jeffrey F. Smallhorn, MBBS [8, 12, 13]
Professor of Pediatrics
University of Alberta
Division of Pediatric Cardiology
Stollery Children's Hospital
Edmonton, Alberta, Canada

Lissa Sugeng, MD, MPH [2, 16]
Associate Professor of Medicine
Department of Internal Medicine (Cardiology)
Section of Cardiovascular Medicine
Yale University School of Medicine
New Haven, Connecticut

Vivian Wei Cui, MD [6, 10]
Imaging Research Coordinator
The Heart Institute for Children
Hope Children's Hospital
Oak Lawn, Illinois

Sinai C. Zyblewski [7]
Division of Cardiology
Children's Hospital
Medical University of South Carolina
Charleston, South Carolina

Preface

Over the last four decades, 3D echocardiography (3DE) has evolved from a blurry and bizarre static image to a series of dynamic gray-scale and Doppler color images available at the push of a button. It has become an integrated, innovative, and promising technology in echocardiography, the most commonly used imaging technology for cardiovascular diseases. As 3DE technology is available in almost all of the standard and some of the portable systems and as the literature and evidence become increasingly available, there is a growing need to learn, re-learn, and apply this technology for those of us who take care of fetuses, children, and adults with congenital heart disease.

I have been fortunate enough to be able to assemble a team of internationally renowned contributors with significant experience and expertise in 3DE as related to congenital heart disease to write a textbook addressing this special need. I have arranged the chapters into three groups: Chapters 1 to 5 present general concepts and considerations of 3DE for congenital heart diseases, including 3DE sequential segmental analysis, 3DE instrumentation, 3DE normal views, 3D color Doppler, and 3D quantification of volumes, mass and function for left and right and single ventricles. Chapters 6 to 13 relate to 3DE for major congenital heart diseases, both simple and complex. Finally, Chapters 14 to 16 discuss special use of 3DE in fetuses and adults as well as the use of transesophageal 3DE.

This textbook would not have been possible without the enthusiasm, professionalism, and perseverance of many dedicated individuals, including but not limited to Mr. Jason Malley, previously from PMPH-USA, who first approached me with his vision for a book of this type; Diana Winter from Academic Publishing Services at Drexel University College of Medicine for organizing, editing, and proofing many of the materials; and finally Linda Mehta from PMPH-USA for her professionalism and efficiency in bringing this project to fruition.

I am also indebted to my colleagues at the Heart Center at St. Christopher's Hospital for Children, Drexel University College of Medicine, and the Department of Pediatrics at Deborah Heart and Lung Center for their enthusiastic support of this project and for covering my clinical, educational, and administrative responsibilities when needed, so that I could concentrate on the project.

Last, but not least—I believe I can say this on behalf of all of the contributors—that our trainees and, more importantly, our patients are always sources of inspiration for our work every day.

Shuping Ge, MD, FACC, FASE
Philadelphia, Pennsylvania and Browns Mill, New Jersey

Foreword

This text is the first book dedicated to real-time 3D echocardiography (RT3DE) for congenital heart disease (CHD) from fetuses to adults. It is an evidence-based, high-quality, extremely well-illustrated, comprehensive, multi-author publication on applications of real-time 3-dimensional echocardiography for congenital heart disease. Comprehensive text and high-quality illustrations abound, from an international group of experts in anatomy of congenital heart disease and imaging of congenital heart disease.

Contents include: Chapter 1, a review of a 3D echocardiographic approach to sequential segmental analysis of congenital heart disease by Drs. Robert Anderson and Anthony Hlavacek; Chapter 2, on instrumentation for RT3DE by Drs. Lissa Sugeng and Sonal Chandra; Chapter 3, on normal views by Drs. Fadi Hage and Navin Nanda; Chapter 4, on volumetric real-time Doppler flow by Dr. Shuping Ge; and Chapter 5, on measurement of volumes, mass and function of the atria and ventricles by Drs. Rula Balluz and Shuping Ge.

The following eight chapters consist of a series of 3D anatomically oriented treatises dealing with anatomy of various defects as assessed by RT3DE: Chapter 6, atrial septal defects (Drs. Roberson and Cui); Chapter 7, ventricular septal defects (Drs. Zyblewski, Hlavacek, and Anderson); Chapter 8, atrioventricular septal defects (Dr. Jeffrey Smallhorn); Chapter 9, left heart obstructive defects (Drs. Jiang and Pan); Chapter 10, complex outflow tract defects (Drs. Roberson and Cui); Chapter 11, Univentricular heart defects (Dr. Roberson); Chapter 12, mitral valve defects (Dr. Smallhorn); and Chapter 13, tricuspid valve defects (Dr. Smallhorn).

The final chapters of the book focus on other types of RT3DE applications: Chapter 14 on 3D fetal echocardiography by Dr. Greggory DeVore; Chapter 15 on adults with CHD by Drs. Hage and Nanda, and finally Chapter 16 on 3D matrix transesophageal 3D by Drs. Sugeng and Chandra.

For those of us who take care of fetuses, children, and adults with CHD, we are intrigued by the powerful tool of RT3DE not only by the ability it gives us to "hold the malformed hearts in our hands to examine them in 3D and in motion," but also by the ability to measure size, volume, flow, and function in such a direct, qualitative, and quantitative manner that has never before been possible with any previous technology. It is our hope that this new technology and its widespread application will enable us to improve our understanding, care, and outcome of CHD. Already we have seen a growing body of evidence in the established and emerging clinical applications of RT3DE in CHD; evidence that has led to the need for such a text to enable more widespread use of RT3DE for CHD care.

In summary, this book is evidence-based, comprehensive, well-referenced, and *extremely* well-illustrated. It is sure to be an important addition to the libraries of pediatric cardiologists, adult congenital heart disease specialists, OB perinatologists, and fetal echocardiographers, as well as general cardiac imaging specialists with an interest in congenital heart disease.

— David J. Sahn, MD
Professor of Pediatrics, Diagnostic Radiology,
OB/GYN and Biomedical Engineering
Division of Pediatric Cardiology
Oregon Health & Science University
Portland, Oregon

CHAPTER

1

THE THREE-DIMENSIONAL ECHOCARDIOGRAPHIC APPROACH TO SEQUENTIAL SEGMENTAL ANALYSIS OF THE CONGENITALLY MALFORMED HEART

Robert H. Anderson, BSc, MD, FRCPath;
Anthony M. Hlavacek, MD

ABSTRACT

It was the introduction of segmental analysis that revolutionized the analysis and description of the congenitally malformed heart. The segmental approach then evolved into sequential segmental analysis, initially with the impression gained by some that there were fundamental differences in the approaches. The perceived differences are more apparent than real, as now demonstrated by interrogation using three-dimensional echocardiography (3DE). The resolution currently available using this technique now permits morphology to be displayed with as much, if not more, accuracy during life as when we hold the autopsied hearts in our hands. We have chosen still images to illustrate the salient points of analysis. The chosen images show the principles of sequential segmental analysis. We presume that the techniques used to demonstrate them using 3DE will be illustrated in much greater detail within the chapters that follow to form the body of this book.

INTRODUCTION

The advent of segmental analysis[1] revolutionized the analysis and description of the congenitally malformed heart. As the system evolved, major differences seemingly emerged in the approach to description and in the terms used to describe the various arrangements. In reality, these differences were more apparent than real. The resolution currently available using three-dimensional echocardiography (3DE) now permits morphology to be displayed with as much, if not more, accuracy during life as when we hold the autopsied hearts in our hands. This has permitted clarification of many previous controversies. In this chapter, we summarize the evolution of sequential segmental analysis,[2] emphasizing how the system has adapted in the light of the newly developed technologies. We make no attempt to be all-inclusive in our choice of illustrations, but rather we have chosen images to illustrate the salient points of analysis. It is well accepted that still frame images do not show the morphology with nearly the same detail as that obtained with moving data sets. We hope, nonetheless, that our images show the principles of sequential segmental analysis. The techniques used to demonstrate them using 3DE are illustrated in much greater detail within the chapters that follow to form the body of this book.

THE BASIS OF SEQUENTIAL SEGMENTAL ANALYSIS

As with the normal heart, the congenitally malformed heart retains the scaffold of three major components, namely, the atrial chambers, the ventricular mass, and the arterial trunks (Fig. 1-1). There is limited potential for variation in each of these so-called cardiac segments. There are also very limited ways in which the segments can be joined together. It was the emergence of cross-sectional echocardiography that made it possible to detect in life the potential anatomic variations across the junctions between the cardiac building blocks. Junctional connections, nonetheless, cannot be established without knowledge of the morphology of the individual segments, so the arrangements within the segments remain as the starting point for analysis.[1] It remains popular to describe the junctional arrangements themselves in terms of concordance and discordance. It is less well appreciated, however, that when first introduced, these terms were used to define harmony between the topological arrangements of the segments, rather than the way in which the components were joined together. Thus, concordance described the association of "situs solitus" with right-hand ventricular topology (d-looping) or "situs inversus" with left hand ventricular topology (l-looping), irrespective of how the atrial chambers were or were not connected to the underlying ventricles.[1] When we suggested that the segmental approach should incorporate descriptions of junctional morphology, naming our version sequential segmental analysis,[2] we used the terms "concordance" and "discordance" to describe specific connections between the atria and the ventricles. This created unnecessary confusion and disagreement. Nowadays, therefore, we describe concordant or discordant atrioventricular connections, rather than concordance and discordance. In this and other ways, sequential segmental analysis has evolved with the passage of time.[3,4] Despite the changes in terminology introduced during this evolution, it continues to follow its initial basic and simple rules. Morphology, junctional union or nonunion, and relationships of the segmental components are recognized as three individual facets of the cardiac make-up. Each can now be determined with exquisite accuracy using 3DE. We retain our belief that, when describing these features, clarity is more important than brevity. It has been the desire to achieve optimal clarity that has led to the changes in descriptions made during the process of evolution of sequential segmental analysis. We make no apologies for these changes,[5] which have eradicated initially illogical points from the system to its advantage.

The importance of the morphological method

Segmental analysis[1] depends on the ability to distinguish the morphology of the individual atrial and ventricular chambers and to recognize the nature of the arterial trunks originating from the ventricular mass. When the heart is congenitally malformed, these chambers, or the arterial trunks, may lack some of the morphologic features that most obviously characterize them in the normal heart. For example, the most obvious feature of the normal morphologically left atrium is its connection to the pulmonary veins. The left atrium can be recognized in hearts with totally anomalous pulmonary venous connection, nonetheless, even though the pulmonary veins are connected to extracardiac sites. Recognition of such facts prompted the sensible suggestion that structures within the heart should be defined in terms of their intrinsic morphology, rather than on the basis of other structures that themselves were variable. This concept spawned the establishment of the so-called morphological method.[6,7] It is the application of the method to sequential segmental analysis that has removed its initially illogical suggestions.[5]

When we look at how the concept has been used to define the morphology of the atrial chambers, then it follows that the connections of the great veins are ruled out as markers of morphological rightness or leftness, simply because they do not always connect to their anticipated atrial chamber. Septal morphology is also of little help, since the septum can be absent, while the atrial vestibules are disqualified as markers, being comparable morphologically in the two atriums. It is the appendage that is most constant when the atrial chambers are congenitally malformed. The structure of the appendages, furthermore, when judged on the extent of their contained pectinate muscles, always distinguishes between morphological rightness and leftness.[8] These features, along with the distinctive differences in shape and junctional morphology, can now be distinguished using 3DE (Fig. 1-2). It is also a fact that the coronary sinus occupies the morphologically left atrioventricular junction, a collecting venous channel being absent from the morphologically right junction. This anatomic feature, along with the extent of the pectinate muscles, and the shape of the appendages, should now permit atrial rightness and leftness always to be established during life by using 3DE interrogation.

Figure 1-1

Figure showing the basic building blocks of the normal and congenitally malformed heart, emphasizing how knowledge of the connections between the so-called segments is dependent on analysis of their own components.

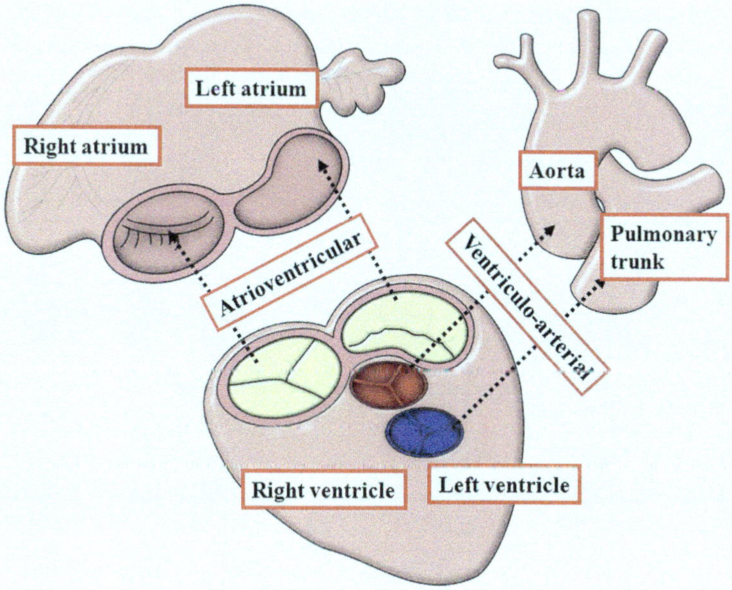

Figure 1-2A and B

3DE images comparing the blunt triangular appearance of the morphologically right atrial appendage, its broad junction with the remainder of the atrial chamber, and the extent of the pectinate muscles within the atrium relative to the atrioventricular junction, *A*, relative to the tubular nature of the morphologically left atrial appendage and its narrow junction with the body of the left atrium, *B*.

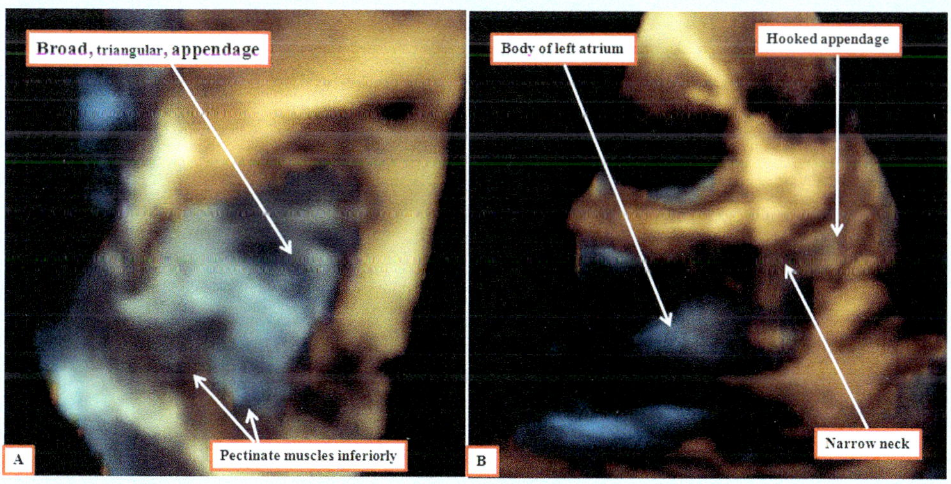

Figure 1-3A and B

A, A heart that has been dissected to show how the normal morphologically right ventricle possesses inlet, apical trabecular, and outlet components. Such components are also readily recognized in the morphologically left ventricle. *B*, This figure shows how it is the palmar surface of only the right hand that can be placed on the septal surface of the ventricle with the thumb in the tricuspid valve and the fingers in the infundibulum. This is the essence of so-called right-hand ventricular topology.

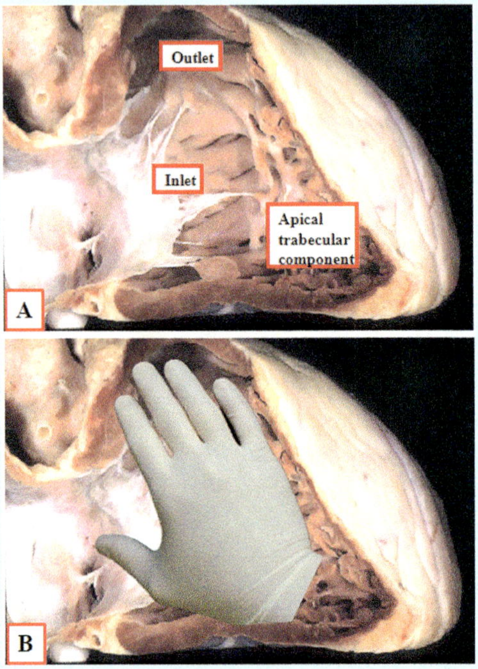

3DE also comes to the fore when assessing the value of the morphologic method as applied to the ventricular mass. The ventricles extend from the atrioventricular to the ventriculoarterial junctions. Within the ventricular mass, as thus defined, there are almost always two ventricles. Such ventricles, no matter how malformed they may be, are best analyzed in tripartite fashion, recognizing the inlet, apical trabecular, and outlet components (Fig. 1-3A). Of these three components, it is the apical trabecular component that is most universally present in normal, malformed, and incomplete ventricles. It is then the pattern of the apical trabeculations that best differentiates the morphologically right from the left ventricle. It is these apical components that form the basis of incomplete ventricles, which lack either an inlet or an outlet component, or sometimes both of these components. When the morphology of individual ventricles is identified according to the apical myocardium, all hearts with two ventricles can readily be analyzed according to the way that the inlet and outlet components are shared between the apical trabecular components. When describing the overall ventricular mass, it is also necessary to describe the way that the two ventricles themselves are related to each other. The two patterns, which are mirror images of each other, can be conceptualized in terms of the way that, figuratively speaking, the palmar surface of the hands can be placed on the septal surface of the morphologically right ventricle. In the morphologically right ventricle of the normal heart, irrespective of its position in space, it is the palmar surface of the right hand that can be placed on the septal surface such that the thumb occupies the inlet and the fingers fit into the outlet (Fig. 1-3B). The palmar surface of the left hand then fits in comparable fashion within the morphologically left ventricle, but it is the right hand that is taken as the arbiter for the purposes of categorization. The usual pattern, therefore, can be described as right-hand ventricular topology. The mirror-imaged pattern, described as left-hand topology, is found in the mirror-imaged normal heart, or in the variant of congenitally corrected transposition found with usual atrial

Figure 1-4A and B

As shown in panels A and B, the essence of right-hand ventricular topology is readily demonstrated using 3DE.

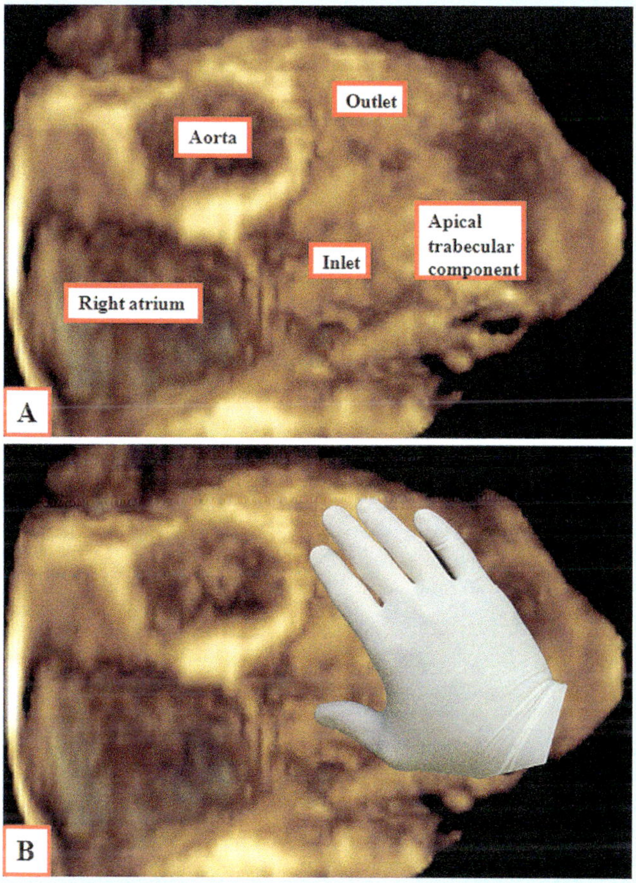

arrangement. With this pattern, it is the palmar surface of the left hand that fits on the septal surface of the morphologically right ventricle with the thumb in the inlet and the fingers in the outlet. These features are readily visualized using 3DE (Fig. 1-4).

When determining the identity of the arterial trunks, there are no intrinsic features that enable an aorta to be distinguished from a pulmonary trunk, or from a common or solitary arterial trunk, but the patterns of branching of the trunks are usually sufficiently characteristic to permit the necessary distinctions (Fig. 1-5). The aorta gives rise to at least one coronary artery, along with the bulk of the systemic arteries. The pulmonary trunk gives rise directly to both, or one or other, of the pulmonary arteries. A common trunk directly supplies the coronary, systemic, and pulmonary arteries. In the absence of the intrapericardial pulmonary arteries, it cannot be stated with certainty whether the arterial trunk present within the pericardial cavity is common or aortic. Hence, it is best described as being solitary. It should now be possible to distinguish all these patterns using 3DE.

Basic sequential segmental analysis

The first step in sequential analysis is to establish the arrangement of the atrial chambers, a feature often described in terms of atrial situs. Attention is then concentrated on how the atrial myocardium is joined to the ventricular myocardial mass around the orifices of the atrioventricular valves or valve. Most often there are two

Figure 1-5

Figure showing features of the different anatomic arterial trunks.

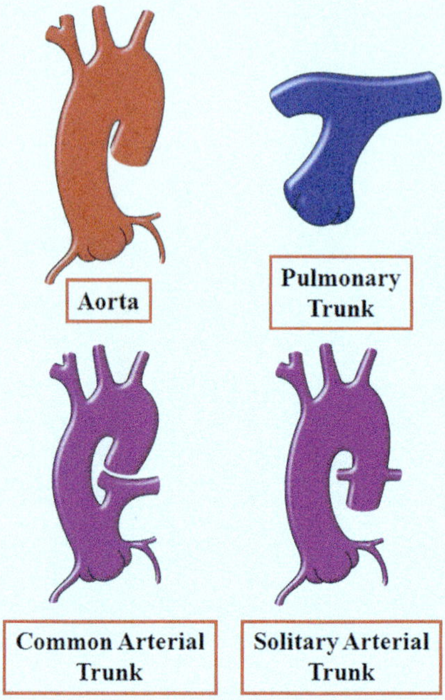

atrioventricular junctions, although they can be present in common format. 3DE is an ideal tool for identifying these anatomic connections across the atrioventricular junctional regions and permits separate analysis of the valve or valves that guard the junctions. Thus, the technique shows how, in the normally constructed heart, there are two atrioventricular valves, each guarding a separate atrioventricular junction (Fig. 1-6A). Such interrogation also reveals how the junction can be a common structure, guarded by a common valve (Fig. 1-6B). The presence of the common junction does not change the overall fashion in which the atrial myocardium is connected to the ventricular mass. In some circumstances, such as when the atrial appendages are isomeric, full description of the junctional arrangement also requires description of ventricular topology, while the relationships of the chambers within the ventricular mass should be described when they deviate from the expected.

Interrogation then moves to the ventriculoarterial junctions. These should be analyzed in terms of the connections of the ventricles with the arterial trunks, the morphology of the arterial valves guarding them, the morphology of the outflow tracts, and the relationships of the great arterial trunks.

Clinical diagnosis then requires a catalogue to be made of all associated cardiac and, when pertinent, noncardiac malformations. This should include features such as the location of the heart and the arrangement of the other thoracic and abdominal organs. Although features such as bronchial anatomy are not readily shown using 3DE, other 3D techniques are now available to reveal these features with exquisite accuracy (Fig. 1-7). When each system of organs is analyzed in its own right, and not designated according to changes observed in other systems, then there is no such thing as "situs ambiguus."

Atrial arrangement

When the great veins drain to their morphologically appropriate atrial chambers, then almost always this finding signifies the presence of either usual or mirror-imaged atrial arrangement. The presence of markedly abnormal venous connections is an indicator of the likely presence of so-called visceral heterotaxy. In this setting, it is a mistake to seek to use the venoatrial connections as a marker of atrial arrangement, since this would be a direct abrogation of the morphologic method. In the current era, it should now be possible to determine clinically the

Figure 1-6A and B

3D images showing how two atrioventricular junctions can be guarded by separate atrioventricular valves, *A*, or a common valve, *B*. The presence of the common junction does not disguise the fact that the atrial chambers join in concordant fashion to the underlying ventricles.

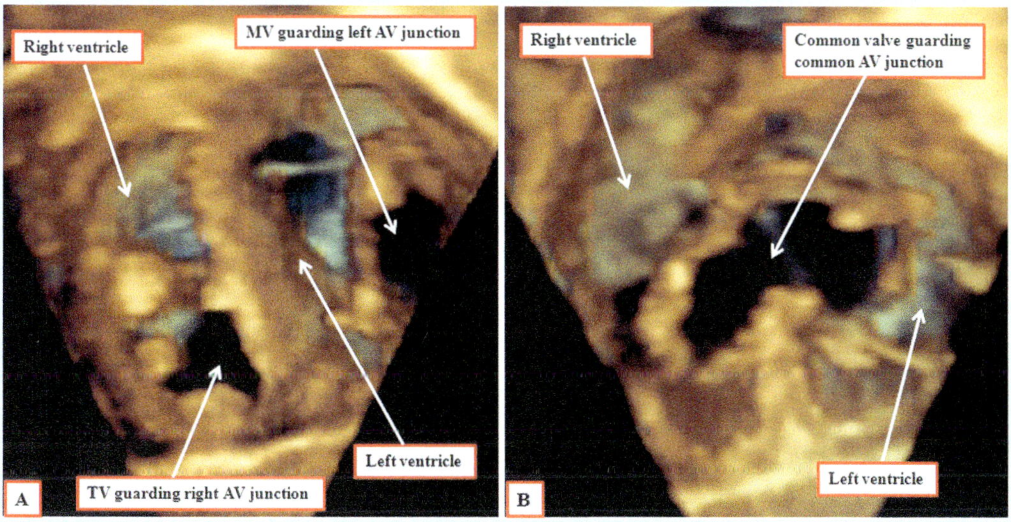

Figure 1-7

Computed tomographic image showing how bronchial anatomy is readily distinguished, revealing how the morphologically left bronchus is significantly longer than its morphologically right partner.

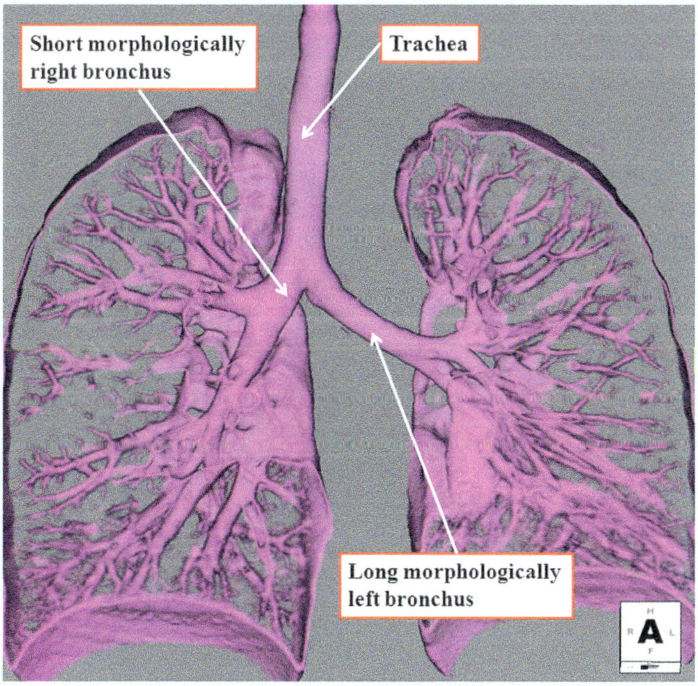

Figure 1-8

Figure showing the four possible arrangements of the atrial appendages. Recognition of atrial arrangement on the basis of the morphology of the appendages is the initial step in sequential segmental analysis.

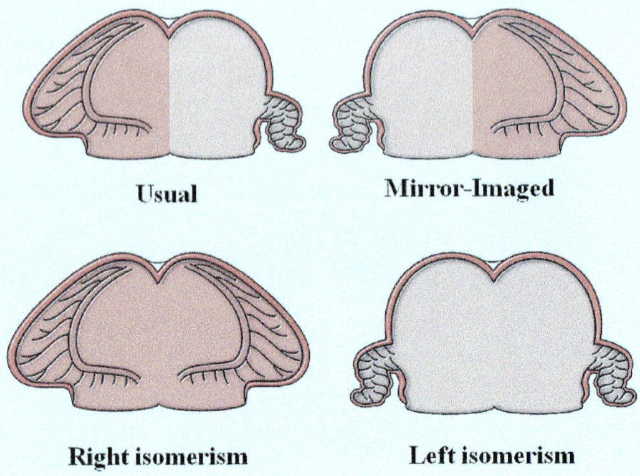

morphology of the atrial appendages. Since all hearts have two such appendages, each of which can only be of morphologically right or left type, there are only four possible patterns (Fig. 1-8). With the usual and mirror-imaged arrangements, the morphologically right appendage is on one side of the heart and the morphologically left appendage on the other. The two other arrangements show isomerism, the appendages having the same morphology on both sides of the heart. Direct identification of these patterns, for the skilled interrogator, should now be possible using 3DE. In most clinical situations, however, it is rarely necessary to rely on direct identification. This is because, almost always in the setting of so-called heterotaxy, the morphology of the appendages is in harmony with the arrangements of the lungs and bronchi. Thus, in the setting of heterotaxy, the lungs and bronchial tree are almost always symmetrical. When heterotaxy is suspected, therefore, presence or absence of isomerism of the atrial appendages can almost always be inferred from the bronchial anatomy, which is shown to best advantage by computed tomography. Inferences similar to those provided by bronchial arrangement can also usually be obtained noninvasively when cross-sectional ultrasonography is used to image the abdominal great vessels,[8] albeit with less accuracy than that provided by establishment of bronchial anatomy. When the atrial appendages are lateralized, the inferior caval vein and aorta lie on opposite sides of the spine, with the caval vein on the side of the morphologically right appendage. In the setting of right isomerism, the great vessels usually lie to the same side of the spine, with the caval vein anterior. An azygos vein carrying the inferior caval venous blood, lying on the same side and posterior to the abdominal aorta, is almost always an indicator of left isomerism. Interruption of the inferior caval vein can sometimes be found in the settings of either usual or mirror-imaged arrangement, but in these latter circumstances, the intracardiac anatomy tends to be normal, so there should be little room for confusion. Generally speaking, right isomerism is also associated with absence of the spleen, whereas left isomerism is typically associated with multiple spleens. The association between atrial morphology and splenic arrangement, nonetheless, is far from constant.[8–10] It is less useful clinically, therefore, to subclassify heterotaxy on the basis of splenic morphology. It is much better to describe both the state of the spleen and the morphology of the appendages, the latter feature then concentrating attention on the heart, and setting the scene for ongoing sequential analysis.

The atrioventricular junctions

In the normal heart, the atrial myocardium is contiguous with the ventricular myocardium around the orifices of both the mitral and tricuspid valves (Fig. 1-6), albeit separated electrically by the insulating tissues of the atrioventricular junctions. In abnormal hearts, so as to analyze the morphology of the atrioventricular junctions accurately, it is necessary first to know the atrial arrangement and then to relate this to the morphology of the chambers in the ventricular mass. In every heart, because there are two atrial chambers, the potential exists

Figure 1-9

3D image showing how, in the commonest variant of tricuspid atresia, the muscular floor of the morphologically right atrium is separated from the base of the ventricular mass by the fibrofatty tissues of the right atrioventricular groove. This is absence of the right atrioventricular connection (RAVC). The right ventricle is then incomplete, because it lacks its inlet component.

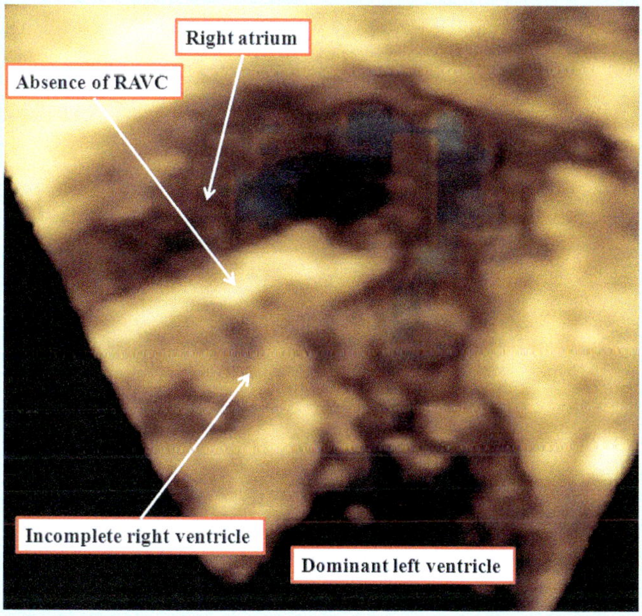

for formation of two atrioventricular connections. As we have already seen, two junctions, if present, can be guarded by a common valve rather than separate right and left atrioventricular valves (Fig. 1-6B). One of two atrioventricular connections may be blocked by an imperforate valve, but such an arrangement will not disguise the presence of two recognizable atrioventricular connections. In some patients, however, one or other of the atrioventricular connections can be completely absent, the myocardium of one of the atriums then having no direct connection with the underlying ventricular myocardium, being separated entirely from the ventricular mass by the fibrofatty tissues of the atrioventricular groove. It is this arrangement that produces the most common form of atrioventricular valvar atresia (Fig. 1-9).

In terms of overall morphology of the atrioventricular junctions, all patients will fall into one of three groups. In the first group, by far the most common, each atrial chamber is connected actually or potentially, but separately, to an underlying ventricle. In the second group, the atrial chambers are connected to only one ventricle, although in this situation two ventricles are almost always present, the second being incomplete and rudimentary. In the third, and rarest, group, one atrioventricular connection is absent, the solitary atrioventricular junction being connected to two ventricles by a straddling valve. This arrangement is uniatrial but biventricular.[11]

In patients with biventricular atrioventricular connections, the pattern produced can be concordant, discordant, or biventricular and mixed. Concordant connections, with each atrium connected to a morphologically appropriate ventricle, are by far the commonest pattern. Discordant connections are found most frequently in the setting of congenitally corrected transposition. The mixed pattern is found in patients with right or left isomerism. Because of the isomeric nature of the appendages, the arrangement cannot be concordant or discordant, since, of necessity, half of the heart is concordantly connected and the other half discordantly connected, irrespective of the type of isomerism or the topological pattern of the ventricular mass. The mixed variant, therefore, requires specification of both atrial arrangement and ventricular topology to make the description complete. Previously described as being ambiguous, any potential ambiguity is removed when details are provided of both the type of isomerism and the pattern of ventricular topology.

Figure 1-10

3D image in short axis showing double-inlet left ventricle through two separate atrioventricular valves. The right ventricle, which has no connection with the atrial chambers, is again incomplete, and in this instance grossly hypoplastic because of the presence of pulmonary atresia. The aorta arises from the dominant left ventricle.

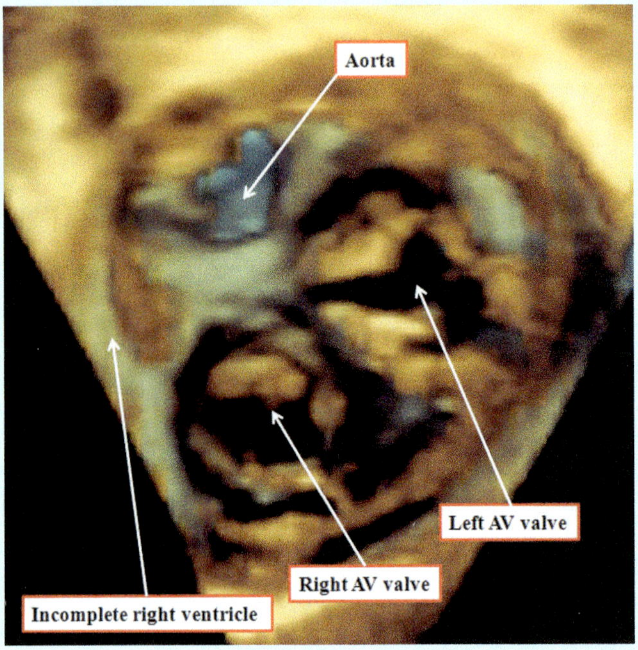

Three possible junctional arrangements are possible in the patients having univentricular atrioventricular connections. The first is double-inlet atrioventricular connection, irrespective of whether the right-sided and left-sided atrioventricular junctions are guarded by two atrioventricular valves (Fig. 1-10) or by a common valve. The other two arrangements are absence of either the right-sided (Fig. 1-9) or left-sided atrioventricular connection. Patients with any of the univentricular atrioventricular connections can have usually arranged, mirror-imaged, or isomeric atrial appendages. Each type of connection can be found when the atrial chambers are connected to a dominant left ventricle, a dominant right ventricle, or very rarely to a solitary and morphologically indeterminate ventricle. Ventricular morphology should always be determined and described in patients with any of the univentricular atrioventricular connections, since the same connection can exist with different ventricular morphologies.[8] For the morphologist, this can be achieved by taking note of the apical trabecular patterns of the ventricles. For the clinician, the relationships between dominant and incomplete ventricles are almost always sufficiently constant to provide the necessary information. Incomplete right ventricles, whether they are positioned to the right or left side, are always carried on the shoulders of the ventricular mass, in anterosuperior location. This finding, therefore, indicates that the dominant ventricle is of left morphology. In contrast, incomplete left ventricles are positioned posteroinferiorly, most usually in left-sided position but sometimes on the right side, indicating that the dominant ventricle is morphologically right. Only very rarely will hearts be found with a solitary ventricular chamber of indeterminate morphology. In clinical practice, however, it can be difficult to distinguish the truly solitary ventricle from apparently solitary left or right ventricles in which the incomplete ventricle is too small to be demonstrated.

The morphology of the valves guarding the overall atrioventricular junctional area, within the constraints imposed by the connections themselves, is an independent feature of patients with congenitally malformed hearts. When the cavities of both atrial chambers communicate directly to the ventricular mass, the right-sided and left-sided atrioventricular connections may be guarded by two patent valves, by one patent valve and one imperforate valve, by a common valve, or by straddling and overriding valves. These arrangements can all be found with concordant, discordant, mixed, or double-inlet connections. Either the right-sided or left-sided valve may be imperforate, producing atresia, but in the setting of a potential as opposed to an absent atrioventricular connection. A common valve (Fig. 1-6B) guards both right-sided and left-sided atrioventricular connections, irrespective of its morphology. A valve straddles when its tension apparatus is attached to both sides of a septum within the ventricular mass. It overrides when its annulus is connected to ventricles on both sides of a septal structure. A right-sided valve, a left-sided valve, or a common valve can straddle, can override, or can straddle and override (Fig. 1-11). When one atrioventricular connection is absent, the possible modes of connection are greatly reduced. The solitary atrioventricular valve is usually committed in its entirety to one ventricle, but may straddle, override, or straddle and override. It is these latter patterns that produce the extremely rare group of uniatrial but biventricular connections.[11]

Presence of an overriding atrioventricular valve has an additional influence on description, since the degree of commitment of the overriding atrioventricular junction determines the precise nature of the atrioventricular connections. Hearts with overriding valves are anatomically intermediate between those with, on the one hand, biventricular and, on the other hand, univentricular atrioventricular connections. 3DE is the ideal technique with which to divide this spectrum. When most of an overriding junction is connected to a ventricle that already receives the other atrioventricular connection, then the connection is double inlet. If the overriding junction is connected mostly to a ventricle not itself connected to the other atrium, each atrium is categorized as though connected to its own ventricle (Fig. 1-11).

Figure 1-11

3D image, in short axis, showing overriding and straddling of the right atrioventricular valve. The overriding describes the sharing of the atrioventricular junction between the ventricles, whereas the straddling is defined on the basis of the location of the valvar tension apparatus within both ventricles. The *star* shows the muscular ventricular septum. In this patient, most of the overriding junction remains connected to the right ventricle, so that the atrioventricular connections are concordant.

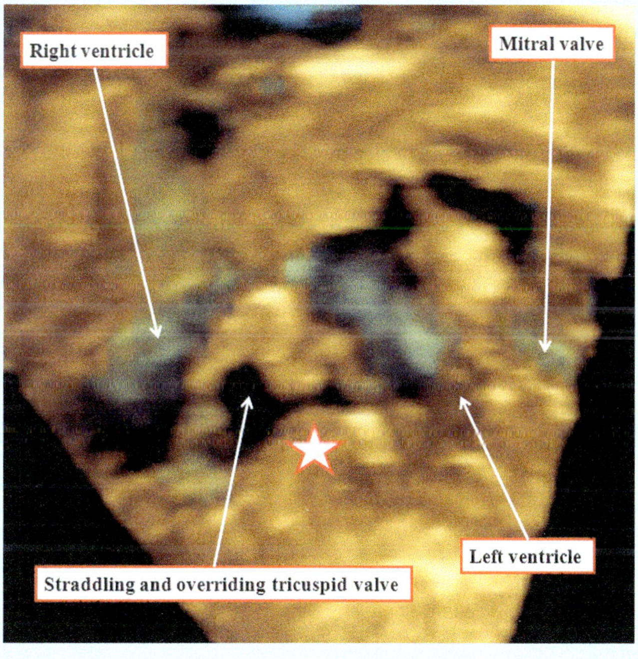

Figure 1-12

3D image, in short axis, showing the trifoliate nature of the left atrioventricular valve in the setting of atrioventricular septal defect and common atrioventricular valve. In this patient, there are separate right and left valvar orifices within the common junction, but the left-sided orifice retains its trifoliate configuration.

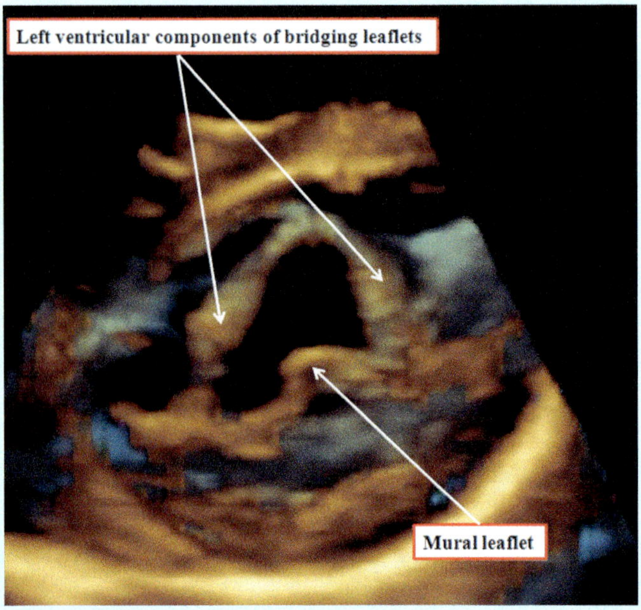

When describing the atrioventricular valves, the adjectives "mitral" and "tricuspid" are having biventricular atrioventricular connections and separate atrioventricular junctions, each guarded by its own valve. The tricuspid valve is then always found in the morphologically right ventricle and the mitral valve in the morphologically left ventricle. In hearts with biventricular atrioventricular connections but with a common junction, in contrast, the common valve lacks mitral and tricuspid components, even when it is divided into right and left components. The left-sided component of the common junction in this setting is guarded by a valve with three leaflets (Fig. 1-12), in contrast to the bifoliate configuration of the leaflets guarding the normal mitral valvar orifice. In hearts with double-inlet connection, two valves, if present, are again better considered right-sided and left-sided (Fig. 1-10), rather than mitral or tricuspid. Similarly, when one connection is absent, although it is usually possible to deduce the presumed nature of the remaining solitary valve from concepts of morphogenesis, this is not always practical or helpful. The valve can always accurately be described as being right-sided or left-sided.

Ventricular relationships

Topological arrangements can be modified by rotation or twisting, accounting for so-called criss-cross and upstairs-downstairs hearts. When describing such unexpected ventricular relationships, it may be necessary to account for right-left, anterior-posterior, and superior-inferior coordinates. 3DE makes it possible to analyze the position of the ventricular components relative to each other. The position and relationships of incomplete ventricles to dominant ventricles should also be described in patients with univentricular atrioventricular connections. In this setting, the relationships are independent of both the connections and the ventricular morphology. For example, while the incomplete right ventricle is usually anterior and right-sided in classical tricuspid atresia, it can be anterior and left-sided without markedly altering the clinical presentation and hemodynamic findings. Similarly, in hearts with double-inlet ventricle, the position of the incomplete ventricle plays only a minor role in determining the clinical presentation. When accounting for the position of incomplete ventricles, note should be taken of their location relative to the dominant ventricle in terms of right-left, anterior-posterior, and superior-inferior coordinates. The finding of an anterosuperiorly located incomplete ventricle identifies it as being of right morphology, whereas posteroinferiorly located incomplete ventricles are always of left morphology. When using 3DE, therefore, it is easier for the clinician to use these relationships to identify the morphology of the dominant ventricle rather than to rely on recognition of the pattern of the apical ventricular trabeculations.

The ventriculoarterial junctions

When analyzing the ventriculoarterial junctions, attention should be directed separately to the way the arterial trunks arise from the ventricles, their relationships to each other, and the infundibular morphology. Such an approach minimizes ongoing controversies such as the role of the "bilateral conus" in the diagnosis of double-outlet right ventricle. If connections, infundibular morphology, and arterial relationships are described independently, with mutually exclusive terms, then there is no room for confusion.

The ventriculoarterial connections can be concordant, discordant, double outlet, or single outlet. Single outlet itself may take one of four forms. A common trunk is found when both ventricles are connected by a common arterial valve (Fig. 1-13) to one trunk that gives rise directly to the coronary arteries, at least one pulmonary artery, and the majority of the systemic circulation. A solitary arterial trunk exists when it is not possible to identify any remnant of an atretic pulmonary trunk within the pericardial cavity. The other forms of single outlet, namely, single pulmonary trunk with aortic atresia, and single aortic trunk with pulmonary atresia,

Figure 1-13

3D image, in short axis, showing a common ventriculoarterial junction, which is the phenotypic feature of a common arterial trunk. Analysis in long axis showed that the trunk directly supplied the coronary arterial, systemic, and pulmonary circulations. Note the fibrous continuity between the leaflets of the truncal and mitral valves, and that the trunk arises predominantly from the right ventricle.

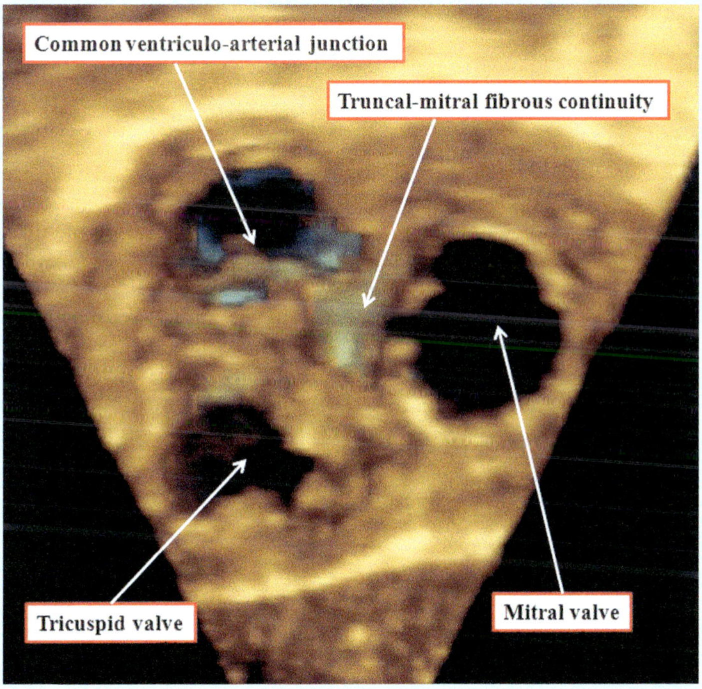

are described only when, using clinical techniques, it is not possible to establish the precise connection of an atretic arterial trunk to an underlying ventricular cavity. If its connection can be established, but is found to be imperforate, the appropriate connection is described, and the imperforate valve is then categorized separately.

There are fewer modes of connection at the ventriculoarterial than at the atrioventricular junctions. A common arterial valve (Fig. 1-13) exists only when there is also a common arterial trunk. Straddling of an arterial valve is impossible, since arterial valves have no tension apparatus. Thus, the potentially variable modes of connection are for there to be two perforate valves, one or both of which may override, or one perforate and one imperforate valve. The degree of override of an arterial valve determines the precise ventriculoarterial connections. As with the atrioventricular junctions, the advent of 3DE now makes it possible to allocate an overriding valve to the ventricle supporting the greater part of its circumference. If more than half of an overriding aortic valve is shown to be connected to the left ventricle, the pulmonary trunk being connected to the right ventricle, then the ventriculoarterial connections are appropriately described as being concordant (Fig. 1-14). In contrast, if more than half of the overriding aortic valve is shown to be connected to the right ventricle in this situation, then the effective ventriculoarterial connection is double outlet. Arbitration is made on the basis of the ventricular short axis, determining the proportions of the overriding junction supported by the right as opposed to the left ventricle.

Three-dimensional echocardiography also permits the infundibular regions to be recognized as the outlet components of the ventricular mass. When analyzed in this fashion, they create no problems in recognition and description. The morphology of the ventricular outlet portions is variable for any heart. Potentially, each ventricle can possess a complete muscular funnel as its outlet portion, and thus each arterial valve can be

Figure 1-14

In this patient, with the image shown in short axis, the orifice of the aortic valve is overriding the crest of the muscular ventricular septum. The infundibular morphology permits the diagnosis of tetralogy of Fallot. When the attachments of the aortic valvar leaflets are assessed in short axis, the majority of the aortic root is supported above the left ventricle (*red dotted line*). The effective ventriculoarterial connections, therefore, are concordant.

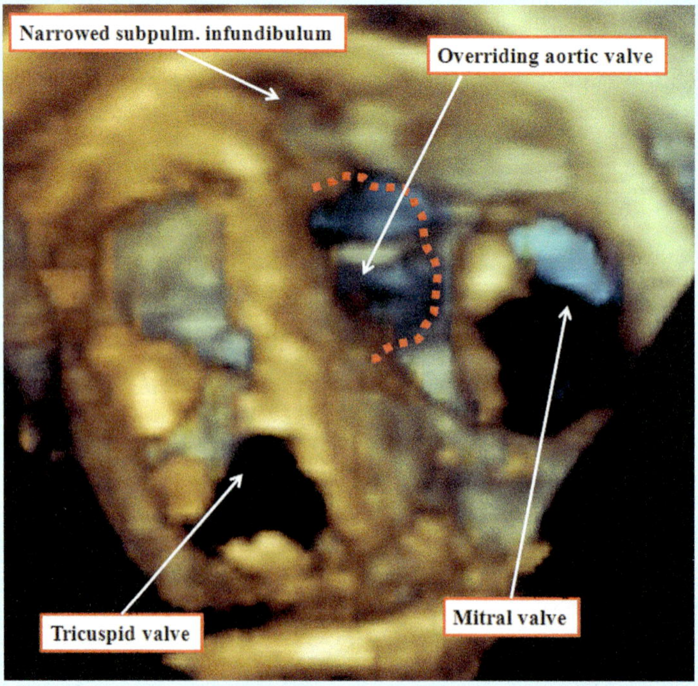

Figure 1-15

3D data set, in subcostal oblique orientation, showing both arterial trunks arising from the morphologically right ventricle. The inner heart curvature, or ventriculoinfundibular fold (*double-headed arrow*), interposes between the leaflets of the aortic and mitral valves, and the pulmonary valve is also supported by a complete muscular infundibulum. In this instance, therefore, the patient has bilateral conuses. Both arterial trunks, nonetheless, can still arise unequivocally from the morphologically right ventricle when there is fibrous continuity between the leaflets of the aortic and mitral valves. If identified, this feature would not detract from the fact that the ventriculoarterial connection remained one of double outlet.

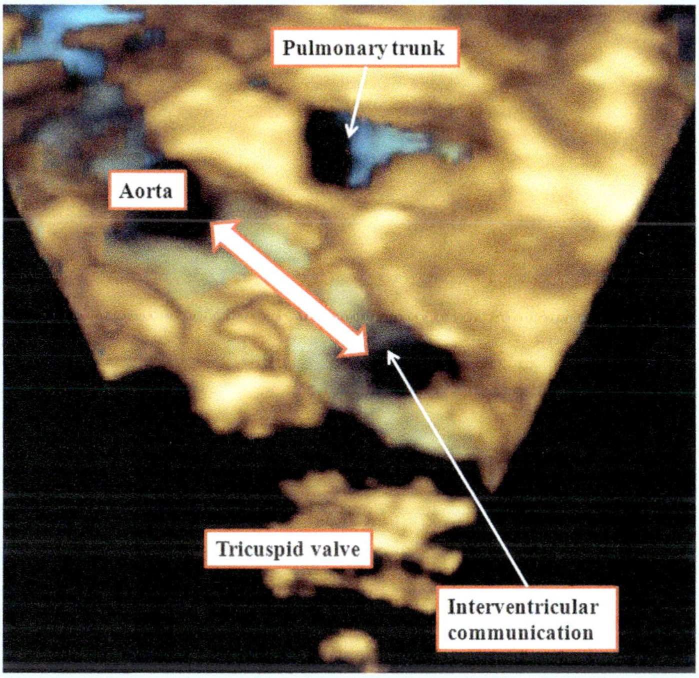

supported by a complete infundibulum. In most hearts, some part of the infundibular musculature is effaced so that there is fibrous continuity between the leaflets of one of the arterial valves and the atrioventricular valves. Most frequently, it is the morphologically left ventricular part of the ventriculoinfundibular fold, or inner heart curvature, that is attenuated, so there is fibrous continuity between the leaflets of the mitral valve and the arterial valve supported by the left ventricle. When both arterial trunks are connected to the morphologically right ventricle, the ventriculoinfundibular fold often persists in its entirety, and there is bilateral atrioventricular-arterial valvar discontinuity (Fig. 1-15). Many hearts in which both arterial valves are connected unequivocally to the right ventricle, nonetheless, have atrioventricular-arterial valvar continuity. Such hearts unequivocally possess a double outlet ventriculoarterial connection. The ventriculoinfundibular fold, therefore, does not need to be intact bilaterally to justify the diagnosis of double-outlet right ventricle.

The final feature of the ventriculoarterial junctions is the relationships of the great arteries and their valves. Valvar relationships are best described in terms of right-left and anterior-posterior coordinates. Note should also be taken of the arrangement of the arterial trunks. Either the pulmonary trunk spirals around the aorta as it ascends or else the two trunks ascend in parallel fashion. Spiraling trunks are usually associated with concordant ventriculoarterial connections, and parallel trunks with discordant or double-outlet connections, but there is no predictive value in these relationships. The rare conditions of "anatomically corrected malposition" and "isolated ventricular discordance" are greatly simplified when it is realized that these arcane terms are used to describe patients with concordant ventriculoarterial connections, but with parallel rather than spiraling arterial trunks.[12] 3DE also shows the sidedness of the aortic arch, which can pass either to the right or left of the trachea, and permits the position of the descending aorta to be defined relative to the vertebral column.

ASSOCIATED MALFORMATIONS

Most patients with congenitally malformed hearts have normal intersegmental connections, together with normal morphology and relations. In such settings, it is the associated malformations that will be the major anomalies. The specific morphologic and clinical features of these anomalies are described in the remaining chapters of this book, along with the techniques required by the 3D echocardiographer to illustrate their morphological features. Consideration must also be given to the position within the chest of the heart itself, and of the cardiac apex, or for that matter, identification of a heart positioned outside the thoracic cavity, so-called ectopia cordis. An abnormal position of the heart within the chest is best considered as an associated malformation, since the cardiac malposition should not be promoted as a prime diagnosis. This is not to decry the importance of cardiac malposition, if only to interpret an electrocardiogram, but knowing that the heart is malpositioned gives no information concerning its internal architecture. Full sequential segmental analysis is needed to determine these features.

CONCLUSIONS

Machines now available for 3DE interrogation are now so sophisticated that all the features of normal and abnormal cardiac anatomy should be seen with just as much facility during life as in the autopsy room, with the added advantage that serial studies during life will now permit establishment of the natural and unnatural history of the various lesions. The moving data sets produced by the machines provide far more information than the still images we have selected to show the principles of sequential segmental analysis. The lessons being learned from the use of this new technique, nonetheless, should now resolve the unhelpful controversies with regard to nomenclature that have bedeviled clinicians over recent decades.

REFERENCES

1. Van Praagh R. The segmental approach to diagnosis in congenital heart disease. *Birth Defects Orig Artic Series.* 1972;8:4–23.
2. Shinebourne EA, Macartney FJ, Anderson RH. Sequential chamber localization—logical approach to diagnosis in congenital heart disease. *Br Heart J.* 1976;38(4):327–340.
3. Anderson RH, Ho SY. Sequential segmental analysis—description and categorization for the millenium. *Cardiol Young.* 1997;7:98.
4. Anderson RH, Shirali G. Sequential segmental analysis. *Ann Pediatr Cardiol.* 2009;2(1):24–35.
5. Jacobs ML, Anderson RH. Nomenclature of the functionally univentricular heart. *Cardiol Young.* 2006;16(suppl 1):3–8.
6. Lev M. Pathologic diagnosis of positional variations in cardiac chambers in congenital heart disease. *Lab Invest.* 1954;3(1):71–82.
7. Van Praagh R, David I, Wright GB, Van Praagh S. Large RV plus small LV is not single LV. *Circulation.* 1980;61(5):1057–1059.
8. Huhta JC, Smallhorn JF, Macartney FJ. Two dimensional echocardiographic diagnosis of situs. *Br Heart J.* 1982;48(2):97–108.
9. Anderson C, Devine WA, Anderson RH, et al. Abnormalities of the spleen in relation to congenital malformations of the heart: A survey of necropsy findings in children. *Br Heart J.* 1990;63(2):122–128.
10. Uemura H, Ho SY, Devine WA, Anderson RH. Analysis of visceral heterotaxy according to splenic status, appendage morphology, or both. *Am J Cardiol.* 1995;76(11):846–849.
11. Anderson RH, Rigby ML. The morphologic heterogeneity of "tricuspid atresia" [editorial note]. *Int J Cardiol.* 1987;16:67.
12. Cavalle-Garrido T, Bernasconi A, Perrin D, Anderson RH. Hearts with concordant ventriculoarterial connections but parallel arterial trunks. *Heart.* 2007;93(1):100–106.

CHAPTER

2

INSTRUMENTATION FOR REAL-TIME THREE-DIMENSIONAL ECHOCARDIOGRAPHY

Lissa Sugeng, MD, MPH; Sonal Chandra, MD

ABSTRACT

This chapter encompasses the historical development of three-dimensional echocardiographic (3DE) methods to their current iterations, from nonsequential and sequential two-dimensional (2D) gated acquisition and the first volumetric real-time 3D probes to the development of the current fully sampled matrix-array technology. Major strides in 3DE have been attributed to improved ultrasound crystal technology, more efficient electronics, and more powerful computing capabilities. Acquisition modes (narrow angled, zoom, and wide angled, and recently one-beat, full-volume data acquisition); image display (volume rendering, wireframe and surface rendering, cut-planes, orientation, and multiplanar reconstruction); and quantitative analysis are discussed.

INTRODUCTION

Echocardiography has undergone a major transformation from ice-pick-like signals to a "life-like" approximation of true cardiac anatomy in three dimensions. Some may even add time as the "fourth" dimension. Three-dimensional echocardiography (3DE) was conceived at about the time that two-dimensional echocardiography (2DE) was established as a clinical modality. The evolution of echocardiography from two to three dimensions is a natural progression, enabled by a combination of advancements in ultrasound technology, computer hardware, and electronics. This chapter encompasses the historical development of 3D methods to their current iterations.

HISTORICAL PERSPECTIVE

Nonsequential 2D gated acquisition

The concept of 3D imaging initially involved multiple 2D images, which were acquired from several acoustic windows using either an acoustic locator (spark gap method) or a magnetic field to determine spatial location while being gated to an electrocardiograph (ECG).[1–5] Images were then reformatted in time and space in a Cartesian format. Although this method resulted primarily in wireframe casts, this approach established a broad base of evidence demonstrating the superior accuracy of 3DE compared with 2DE in estimating left ventricular volumes and function. Using this method, investigators validated left and right ventricular volumes in vivo and in vitro and demonstrated the superiority of 3DE compared with traditional 2DE. Wireframe images were a typical manner of display because endocardial tracings were performed during analysis. Unfortunately, the method proved nonviable for clinical use because the acquisition of images was time-consuming, the equipment was not portable, and the postprocessing time and analyses were lengthy. In subsequent efforts, Levine et al.[2] used this technique to study the anatomy of the mitral valve, proving that it was not a flat annular plane but rather a saddle-shaped annulus located higher in the anteroposterior aspect than in the lateromedial planes.

Sequential 2D gated acquisition

An alternative method of data collection eventually emerged requiring placement of a probe at a single acoustic window in order to obtain multiple 2D images sequentially gated to the ECG and respiration.[6,7] This approach initially used a free-hand scanning method that required the user to move the device slowly over the region of interest (Fig. 2-1). An electromagnetic locator attached to the probe tracked the position of the image during the acquisition phase. Commercially available transthoracic and transesophageal probes were mounted on a mechanical device and images were acquired by the coordinated incremental movement of the probe over a certain distance (parallel scanning) while angulating (fan-like scanning) or rotating over 180° (rotational scanning), as shown in Figures 2-2A–C. The parallel scanning method was not feasible when used transthoracically; rather, its use was limited to transesophageal windows. A large transesophageal

Figure 2-1

Electromagnetic tracking method.

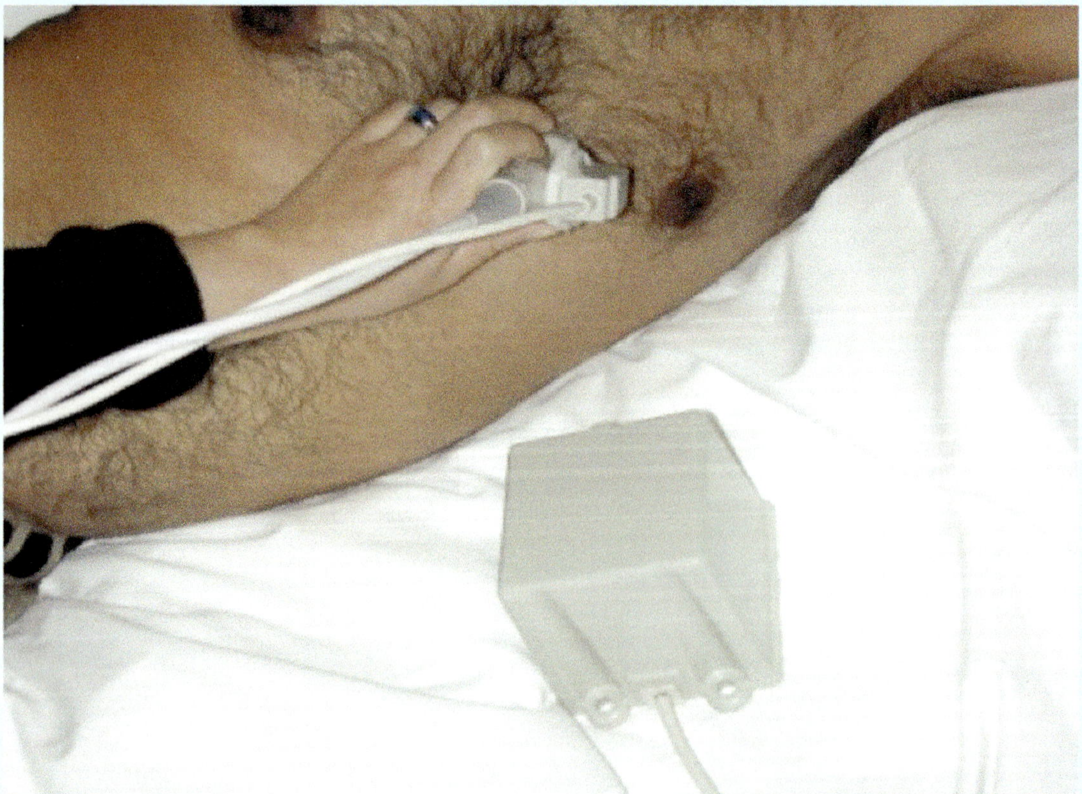

probe was invented that obtained data in a parallel mode using a phased-array ultrasound probe that moved on a "track." Although the probe allowed high-resolution transesophageal echocardiographic imaging for 3D reconstruction online, it was not widely popular owing to the size and inflexibility of the transducer.

In the mid-1990s, one of the first solutions obviating a mechanical device emerged as a commercially available transesophageal probe enabling electronic rotation of the imaging plane over 180°, stopping every 3° to 5° to obtain 2D images while gated to ECG and respiration. The transthoracic probe was similarly designed (Fig. 2-2D). These images were then arranged in time and space in a Cartesian format to allow further image manipulation and quantitation. This process too was eventually adapted for a transthoracic probe. The technique enabled visualization of anatomic information as well as quantitative volumetric data, permitting simple 2D measurements derived from the 3D data set. Overall, a sequential 2D gated method of acquisition was a more workable solution to 3D imaging than the previous method, but it still required an ultrasound machine and a separate computer for data acquisition, image processing, and display. An electronically driven acquisition process reduced dependency on the computer to coordinate acquisition, thereby facilitating portability and efficiency in setup; however, it did not help with the issue of the lengthy acquisition time. This method continued to require offline image processing and analysis; therefore it was not truly in real time. Additionally, with increased respiration, arrhythmias, and minor operator movement, artifacts were common with this type of data collection.

Figure 2-2A, B, C, and D

Multiple 2D gated sequential method. Data acquisition was performed at one acoustic window either with a probe attached to a motorized device in a parallel method *A*, a fan-like mode *B*, or in a rotational method *C*. Further advances in this method used an electronically driven rotational method *D*.

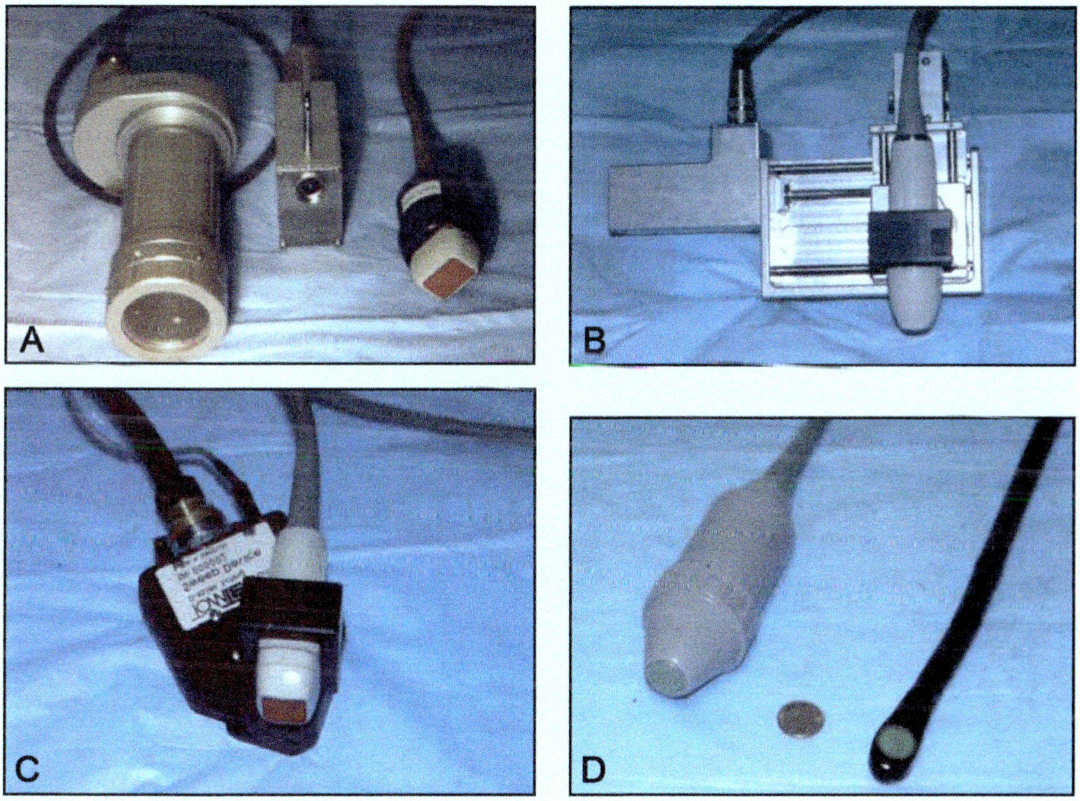

Volumetric acquisition

Given the limitations of multislice gated data collection, another approach to 3D imaging was to image a larger volume with a matrix-array probe. This first-generation volumetric real-time 3D probe consisted of approximately 256 elements that allowed imaging in simultaneous orthogonal planes, which permitted display of several short-axis planes (sparse matrix array). Using this technology, investigators proved that 3DE not only provided accurate left and right ventricular volumes and function but also offered an alternative method of stress imaging with simultaneous orthogonal and "C" scan planes.[8] Although further offline image processing was necessary to produce a 3D reconstruction, the concept was a major innovation in echocardiography that led to further efforts in the development of the current probe-based technology.

CURRENT REAL-TIME 3D ECHOCARDIOGRAPHY

Three-dimensional echocardiography is now more evident in clinical practice because of its true real-time nature. The ability to display 3D images immediately on an ultrasound machine obviates the time-consuming reconstruction (minutes to hours) required by earlier 3D methods. Moreover, the ability to perform 2D and 3D imaging with the same probe, the improved image quality, and the availability of quantitative analysis packages on-cart have had the most impact on its current ubiquitous use. These major strides in 3DE have been attributed to improved ultrasound crystal technology, more efficient electronics, and more powerful computing capabilities.

Three-dimensional echocardiographic imaging is performed using a fully sampled matrix-array transducer that, in contrast to the sparse array probe, consists of thousands of elements (up to 3000, depending on the vendor), which allows traditional 2DE, pulsed-wave, continuous-wave, and color Doppler in addition to 3D imaging (Fig. 2-3A).[9]

Since the first transthoracic matrix-array probe became commercially available in 2003, development has accelerated and other probes have been introduced into the market with varied methods of acquisition, display, and software for quantitative analysis. To date, transesophageal fully sampled matrix-array transducer (Fig. 2-3B) offering real-time 3D imaging has become available. Acquisition of 3D volume data is typically ECG gated with or without a breath-hold or based on time set on the machine. Images can be viewed, manipulated in their orientation or display, and analyzed with quantitative software online. Volume data are stored as DICOM (Digital Imaging and Communications in Medicine) native data, which can then be postprocessed, and images are displayed as movie clips.

Figure 2-3A and B

A, Fully sampled matrix-array transthoracic probes. *B*, Transesophageal probes.

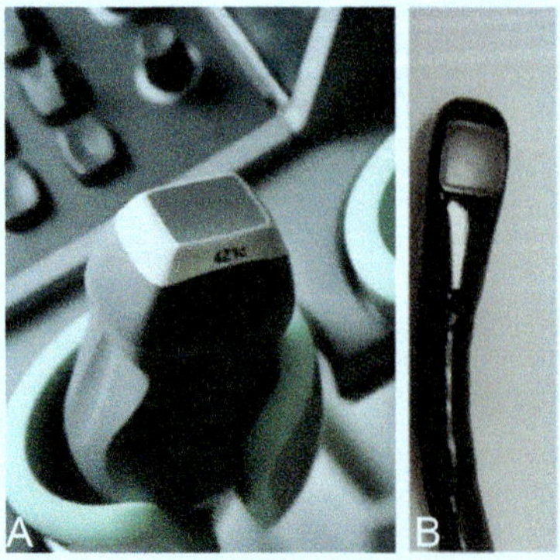

Regardless of vendor, common steps are required to perform 3DE: acquisition, image display (rendering, cut-planes, and orientation), and quantitative analysis.

Acquisition modes

There are three modes of acquisition: narrow angled (live 3D), zoom, and wide angled (full volume). All three modes of acquisition are true real-time 3D imaging acquired in one beat as shown in Figure 2-4.

Narrow-angled mode.

Narrow-angled (live 3D) acquisition is useful to view the preliminary 3D image in order to determine appropriate window and gain settings. The likelihood of gaining additional information when switching from 2D to the live 3D mode (Fig. 2-4A–C) is decreased.

Zoom mode.

The zoom mode is valuable when one needs to focus on a defined region of interest such as a valve, a mass, an aneurysm, or another focal abnormality. The advantages of both narrow-angled and zoom modes, other than being real time, are that in both, the sector limits serve to autosegment the area of interest, and the number of artifacts is decreased from one-beat acquisition. One-beat acquisition is particularly helpful in patients with atrial fibrillation or ventricular bigeminy (Fig. 2-4D-F).

Wide-angled (full-volume) mode.

Wide-angled (full-volume) mode is commonly used to obtain a large region of interest such as cardiac chambers or structural elements such as valves, which require higher frame rates. ECG gating is commonly used with or without a breath-hold (Fig. 2-4G–I). The acquisition time increases as the volume data set increases in size. The number of cardiac cycles requires a range between two and seven beats for gray scale and between 7 and 14 beats for color 3D acquisition. The most frequent issue with this type of data collection is a linear artifact that is evident between subvolumes called a "stitch artifact" occurring from increased or irregular respiratory cycles, arrhythmias, or operator movement resulting in subvolume misalignment. Currently, the stitch artifact is avoided with the use of one-beat, full-volume mode, and, although the higher temporal resolution is preserved, it is at the expense of spatial resolution. Hence, users must weigh their options: a multi-beat acquisition with higher spatial resolution, equal or lower temporal resolution, and possible artifacts against a single-beat solution.

As discussed in the section on "Wide-angled mode," one can choose the size of the volume data set in each acquisition mode; this option is known as "density" or "volume size." The size of the volume data set is inversely related to the line density: the smaller the volume, the higher the line density; conversely, the larger the volume, the lower the line density. Choice of size can depend on the region of interest. For example, when imaging the aortic valve, a small volume with high line density is preferable; in patients with a dilated aortic root, a medium or large volume is chosen to fit the object of interest into the sector.

To further enhance 3D rendering, algorithms called "vision" controls (visions A--H, available on iE33, Philips Healthcare, Andover, MA) provide the operator with a choice of the types of 3D appearances. Visions F through H are highest in resolution, with vision H as the preferred choice because of the blue shading that further augments the three-dimensionality of the image. Similar controls are available on other systems. Most controls for rendering, which include gain, compression, smoothing, and gray-scale correction (gamma), can be manipulated after acquisition. Nevertheless, gain settings are important when one wants to optimize image quality during acquisition. The two controls that are not enabled postacquisition are time gain compensation and lateral-gain compensation.

One concept in 3D imaging that is key to data acquisition by either the transthoracic or the transesophageal approach is to keep the region of interest in the middle of the sector because line density is highest in the middle. Off-axis imaging or foreshortening may lead to poor image quality or even exclusion of the apex in a full-volume mode when imaging the left ventricle. Another important point in 3DE is that 3D image quality is heavily dependent on 2D image quality. In addition, a 2D image artifact becomes a 3D image artifact.

Figure 2-4A, B, C, D, E, F, G, H, and I

Acquisition mode. There are three acquisition modes: narrow-angled or live 3D acquisition *A–C*; zoom acquisition *D–F*; and wide-angled or full-volume acquisition *G–I*. Panels B, E, and H are transthoracic images and panels C, F, and I are transesophageal images.

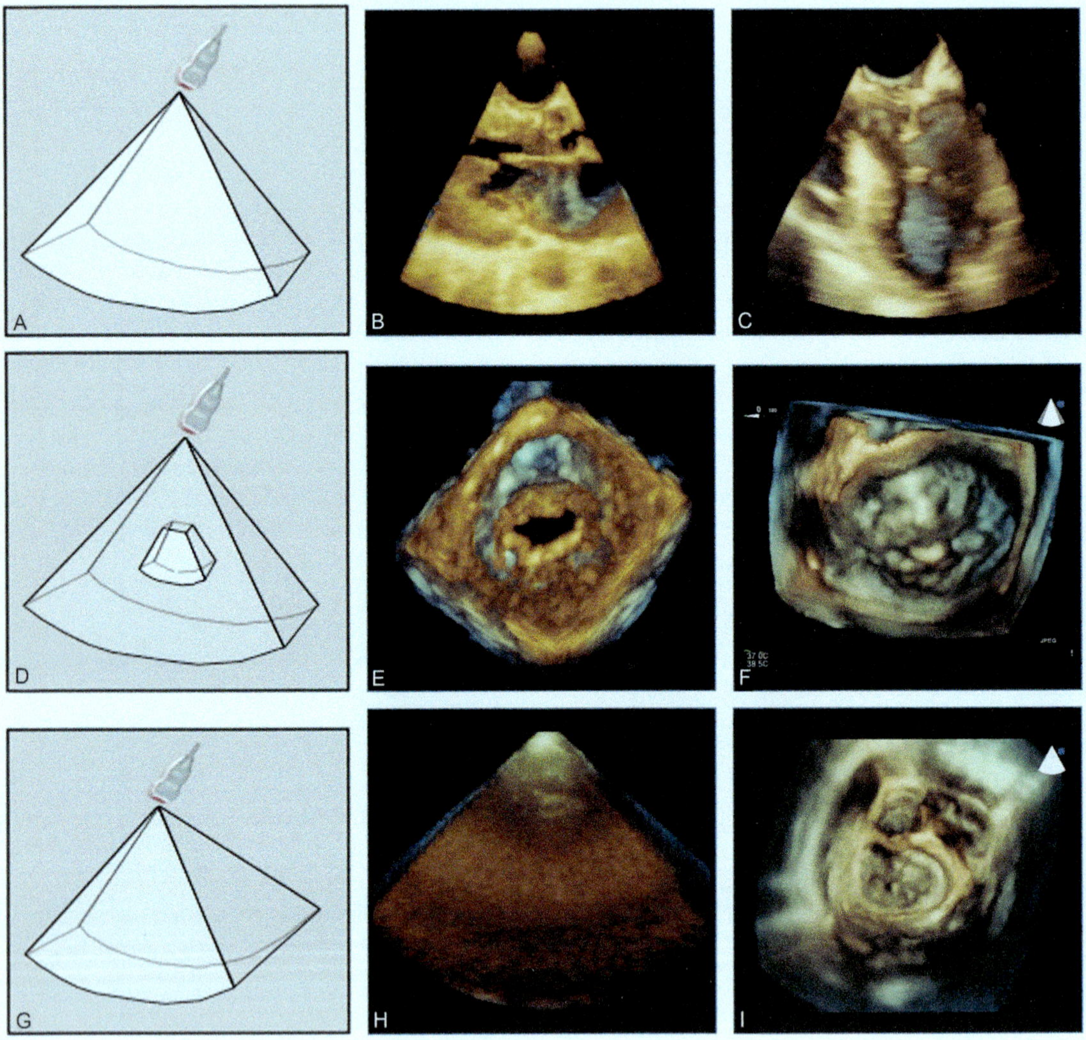

Display

Once a 3D volume is obtained, several methods of display are available for 3D information: volume rendered; wireframe and surface rendered; and multiplanar reconstruction (MPR) (Figs. 2-4I and 2-5A–C). The volume-rendered 3D display mode is used to demonstrate anatomic and pathological images with all voxel information. Volume-rendered image display can encompass several postprocessing functions including rendering, cut-planes, and orientation. Rendering involves setting thresholds to determine which voxels become cardiac structures. Values that are under the set threshold become part of the cavity. This function uses gain controls to increase or decrease thresholds. As stated in the preceding section, gains should be adjusted during the time of acquisition particularly during the live 3D mode. The gains should not be too low or too high because such gains will limit the range after acquisition. Optimal settings are difficult to define but should not be set too high in order to avoid cavity cluttering nor too low to avoid dropout. Opacification determines transparency of cardiac structures; it is adjusted through the compress knob. Smoothing can be applied to the edges to improve appearance.

Other algorithms specific to the ultrasound vendor may enhance the three-dimensionality of a 3D image. Cut-planes may be necessary if the region of interest is within a larger volume data set, especially when acquired using a full-volume mode. There are different approaches to cut-planes depending on the vendor. Orientation and standard display of a 3D image is important; however, there is no consensus to date. In general, the orientation based on the surgeon's point of view has been used specifically for viewing diseased valves.

In contrast to the previous mode, surface rendering is a result of endocardial border tracings or tracking of valve leaflets. Rather than demonstrating the anatomic information, more quantitative parameters are derived such as volume, function, dimensions, angle, and area. A wireframe image is the initial display after borders are tracked (Fig. 2-5A). If a surface or covering is placed over the wireframe reconstruction, it becomes a surface-rendered 3D display (Fig. 2-5B).

Multiplanar reconstruction

Lastly, 3D volume data are displayed in 2D slices either in a parallel fashion such as a short-axis stack or in a triplane fashion along the left ventricular long axis (Fig. 2-5C). This MPR view is typically shown as

Figure 2-5A, B, and C

Additional display methods of 3D images. *A*, Wireframe image. *B*, Surface-rendered image. *C*, Multiplanar reconstructions allow a 2D analysis of a 3D volume.

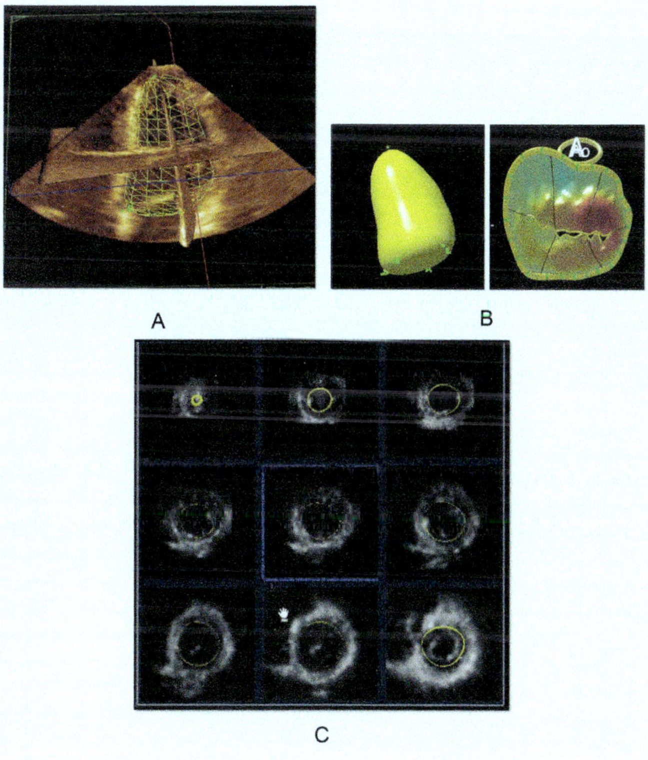

two orthogonal planes and one short axis. Two-dimensional measurements can be made on MPR views; for instance, the mitral valve area can be measured in mitral stenosis.

Quantitative analysis

Multiple packages are now available on-cart to enable simple 2D measurements such as distance, area, angle, and perimeter and 3D analysis of left or right ventricular volume, function, and 3D strain. Mitral valve analysis, although currently in static mode, can quantify a long list of parameters of the mitral apparatus and aortic mitral angle.

As an integral component of 3DE, quantitative analysis of these measurements will be discussed in detail in the related chapters of this textbook for interested readers.

REFERENCES

1. King DL, King DL Jr, Shao MY. Three-dimensional spatial registration and interactive display of position and orientation of real-time ultrasound images. *J Ultrasound Med.* 1990;9:525–532.
2. Levine RA, Handschumacher MD, Sanfilippo AJ, et al. Three-dimensional echocardiographic reconstruction of the mitral valve, with implications for the diagnosis of mitral valve prolapse. *Circulation.* 1989;80:589–598.
3. Nixon JV, Saffer SI, Lipscomb K, Blomqvist CG. Three-dimensional echoventriculography. *Am Heart J.* 1983;106:435–443.
4. Geiser EA, Ariet M, Conetta DA, et al. Dynamic three-dimensional echocardiographic reconstruction of the intact human left ventricle: technique and initial observations in patients. *Am Heart J.* 1982;103:1056–1065.
5. Linker DT, Moritz WE, Pearlman AS. A new three-dimensional echocardiographic method of right ventricular volume measurement: In vitro validation. *J Am Coll Cardiol.* 1986;8:101–106.
6. Delabays A, Pandian NG, Cao QL, et al. Transthoracic real-time three-dimensional echocardiography using a fan-like scanning approach for data acquisition: methods, strengths, problems, and initial clinical experience. *Echocardiography.* 1995;12:49–59.
7. Flachskampf FA, Franke A, Job FP, et al. Three-dimensional reconstruction of cardiac structures from transesophageal echocardiography. *Am J Card Imaging.* 1995;9:141–147.
8. Sheikh K, Smith SW, von Ramm O, Kisslo J. Real-time, three-dimensional echocardiography: feasibility and initial use. *Echocardiography.* 1991;8:119–125.
9. Sugeng L, Weinert L, Thiele K, Lang RM. Real-time three-dimensional echocardiography using a novel matrix array transducer. *Echocardiography.* 2003;20:623–635.

CHAPTER

3

NORMAL REAL-TIME THREE-DIMENSIONAL ECHOCARDIOGRAPHIC VIEWS OF THE CARDIOVASCULAR SYSTEM: A SYSTEMATIC APPROACH

Fadi G. Hage, MD; Navin C. Nanda, MD

ABSTRACT

This chapter describes a simplified and standard approach for three-dimensional transthoracic echocardiography (3DTTE) that depends on the familiar two-dimensional (2D) views and on anatomic orientation standards in order to consistently display cardiac structures and interpret cardiac pathology. The 3D examination uses the same acquisition windows that are used in the 2D echocardiographic examination (left parasternal long-axis, apical, suprasternal, supraclavicular, right parasternal, and subcostal) acquired from the standard transducer positions that are familiar to echocardiographers. After the acquisition of a full-volume pyramidal dataset, sagittal, coronal, and transverse cropping planes are used to dissect the heart.

INTRODUCTION

The development of live real-time three-dimensional transthoracic echocardiography (3DTTE) has revolutionized the practice of echocardiography.[1] The current echocardiographic technology is the result of a succession of innovations from M-mode to two-dimensional echocardiography (2DE) followed by Doppler and color Doppler, transesophageal echocardiography (TEE), contrast and tissue Doppler, and 3D echocardiography. 3DTTE can provide beneficial information on top of traditional 2DTTE and 2DTEE and allow for a more anatomically realistic perspective of cardiac structures. In order to fully exploit the potential value of 3DE, use of a systematic approach is important.

IMAGING PRINCIPLES

Current 3D phased-array transducers allow for instantaneous 3D volume-rendered, color Doppler, and harmonic imaging.[2] The transducer is composed of thousands of small elements, each of which is capable of producing an ultrasonic wave beam. By controlling the firing time of the elements, the phase of the wave beams can be changed and the direction of the wave front can be altered. In this manner, the ultrasound beam scans the X-axis from one point to another. This scanning line then performs azimuth steering along the Y-axis to form a 2D sector image and elevation steering along the Z-axis to form the pyramidal 3D dataset containing imaging data along all three perpendicular coordinate axes (Fig. 3-1).[2]

Therefore, imaging in real time can provide a pyramidal dataset with a wide region of interest that can include the entire heart in pediatric patients without moving the transducer. Because this image is acquired over several heartbeats, it is desirable although not mandatory if the subject can hold his or her breath to minimize the moving artifact associated with respiration.

Figure 3-1

The scanning beam performs azimuth steering along the Y-axis in a phased array manner and produces 2D sector images. The 2D sector image performs elevation steering along the Z-axis and finally produces a pyramidal 3D dataset. Courtesy of Philips Medical Systems, Bothell, WA. (Reproduced with permission from Wang et al.[2] [Fig. 2].)

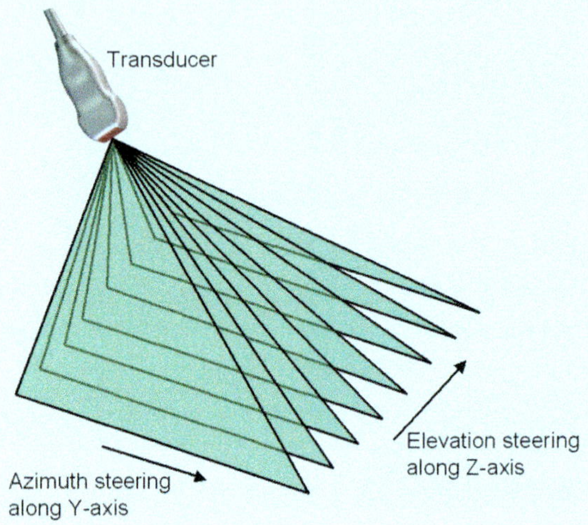

3D EXAMINATION PROTOCOL

With 3DTTE, heart structures are imaged in a realistic manner that does not require mental reconstruction from the echocardiographer. However, because the images can be viewed from any perspective, the challenge is to methodically and systematically image the various cardiac structures without overlooking significant findings. In order to perform this within a reasonable timeframe, understanding that there are limitless imaging displays that can be used, some have proposed a simplified and standard approach for 3DTTE imaging that depends on the familiar 2DTTE views and on anatomic orientation standards in order to consistently display cardiac structures and interpret cardiac pathology.[3]

Unlike other imaging modalities such as computed tomography and magnetic resonance imaging, which display images in relation to the standard anatomic position of the human body, echocardiography has traditionally displayed images in relation to the left ventricle. The reason for this distinction is that echocardiographers are interested in imaging the left ventricle in true long and short axes. This is particularly important because the axis of the human body is at an angle with the axis of the heart. Using the axis of the body would result in foreshortening of the left ventricle (Fig. 3-2). Thus, the parasternal short-axis view displays the true short axis of the left ventricle; the apical four-chamber view displays the horizontal long axis of the left ventricle; and the apical two-chamber view displays the vertical long axis of the left ventricle.

The 3D examination uses the same acquisition windows that are used in the 2D echocardiographic examination: the left parasternal, apical, suprasternal, supraclavicular, right parasternal, and subcostal using the standard transducer positions that are familiar to echocardiographers (Fig. 3-3). The display assumes that the patient is standing upright and facing the observer.

After the acquisition of a full-volume pyramidal dataset, cropping planes are used to dissect the heart. This can be performed at the bedside or at a later time if more convenient, because the dataset can be stored. We have found that this can be of great value to the person who is reading the images but not performing the examination because visualizing a particular structure does not depend on the views captured by the echocardiographer. The dissection allows for the visualization of 3D structures using a 2D screen. For this purpose, the dissection planes are also oriented with relation to the heart rather than to the heart's orientation to the body. These planes, which are usually color coded, are perpendicular to each other (Figs. 3-2 and 3-4).[3]

Figure 3-2

Cropping planes used for 3DE. The long axis of the heart is at an angle to the body axis. The planes of the heart are in reference to the heart itself and not the body axis. (Reproduced with permission from Nanda et al.[3] [Fig. 2].)

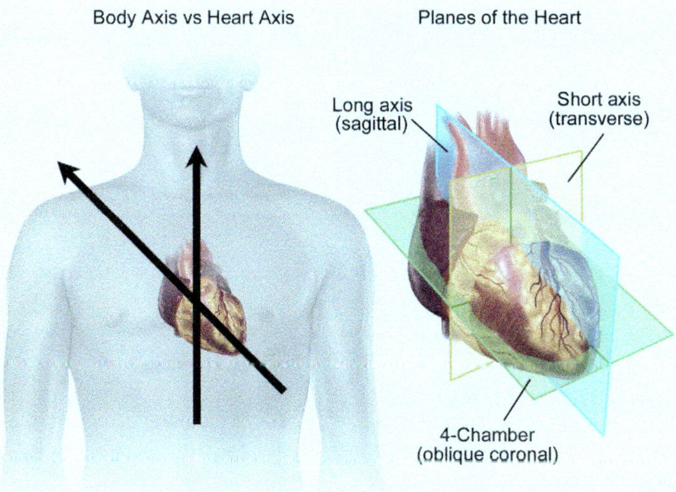

Figure 3-3

Transducer positions for live 3DE standard examination used to acquire a full-volume dataset of the heart. (Reproduced with permission from Nanda et al.[3] [Fig. 1].)

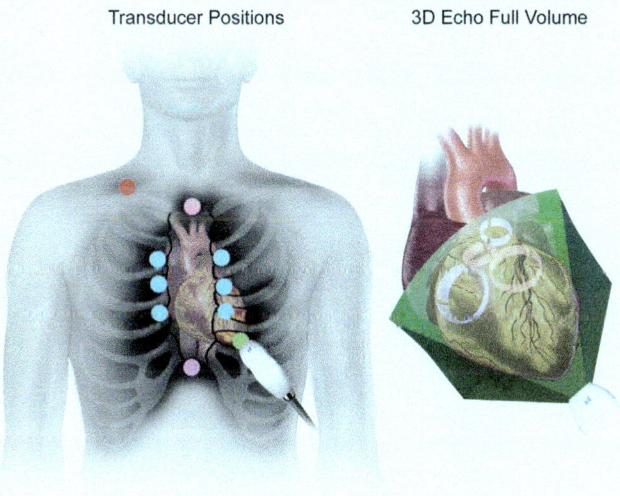

Figure 3-4

The use of anatomic planes to describe live 3DE images results in six different cardiac perspectives for any cardiac structure. These may be described using two terms, the plane and the viewing perspective. (Reproduced with permission from Nanda et al.[3] [Fig. 3].)

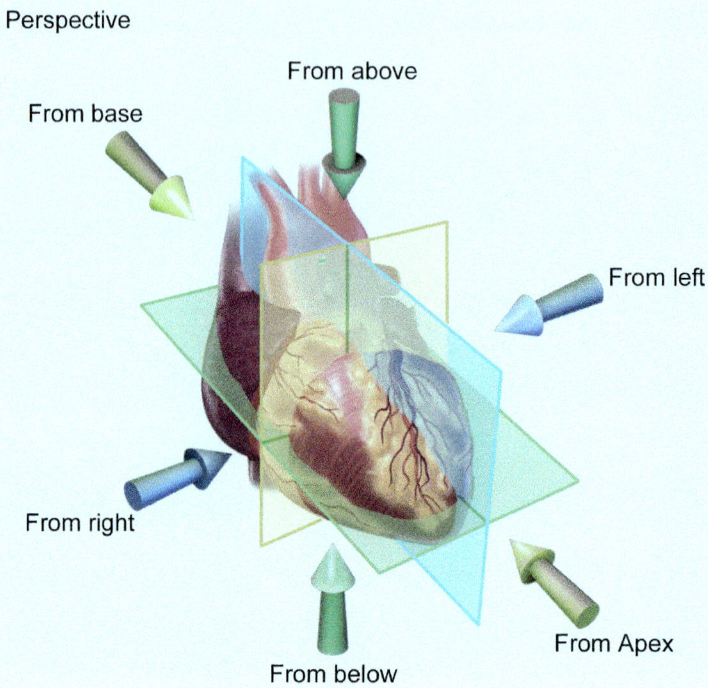

Sagittal plane: The sagittal plane is a longitudinal, long-axis, vertical plane that divides the heart into right and left portions. This can be visualized as a left-to-right or lateral control. A parasternal long-axis view is seen by using a sagittal plane.
Coronal plane: The coronal plane is another vertical plane that divides the heart into anterior and posterior portions. This is top-to-bottom or elevation control. An apical four-chamber view is seen by using a coronal plane.
Transverse plane: The transverse plane is a short-axis plane that dissects the heart into superior and inferior portions. This is front-to-back or depth control. A parasternal short-axis view of the heart is seen by using a transverse plane.

The use of these dissection planes results in six different perspectives from which any cardiac structure can be visualized (Fig. 3-4). These dissection or cropping planes can be more easily understood as an analogy to the anatomic dissection of the heart but with the ability to maneuver seamlessly from one view to another.[3] Therefore, the heart can be sectioned and these sections displayed consecutively like viewing pages in a book. With the apex displayed downward, the heart can be dissected using sagittal sections (Fig. 3-5), coronal sections (Fig. 3-6), or transverse sections (Fig. 3-7). In addition, software is available that allows for dissection along oblique planes that do not correspond to any of the above perpendicular planes if the need arises to view a cardiac structure from a different perspective in order to complete a comprehensive examination.

Figure 3-5

Sagittal (long-axis or longitudinal) section viewed from left side or right side as used in live 3DE. (Reproduced with permission from Nanda et al.[3] [Fig. 4].)

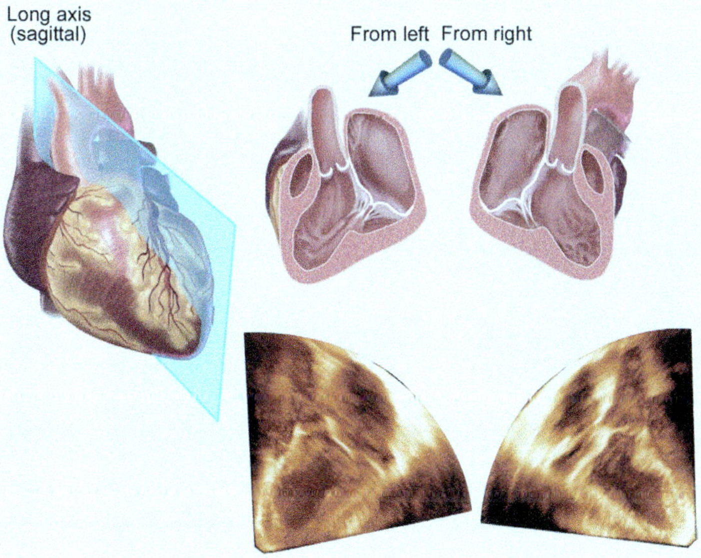

Figure 3-6

Oblique coronal (frontal) section viewed from above and below as used in live 3DE. (Reproduced with permission from Nanda et al.[3] [Fig. 5].)

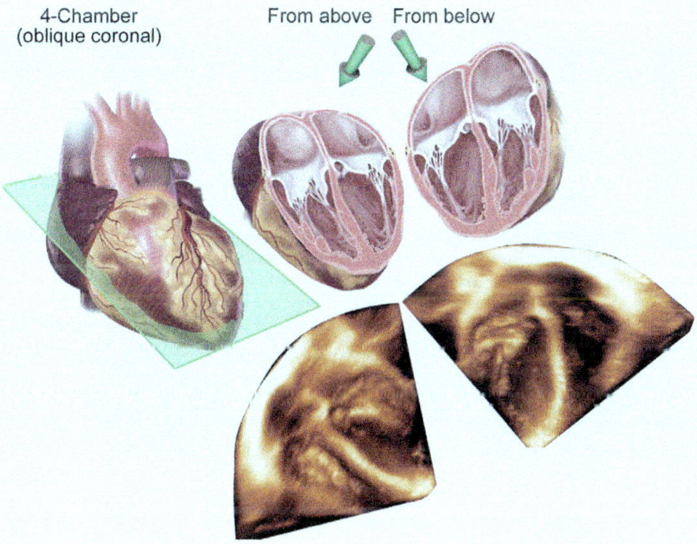

Figure 3-7

Transverse (short-axis) section viewed from base or apex as used in live 3DE. (Reproduced with permission from Nanda et al.[3] [Fig. 6].)

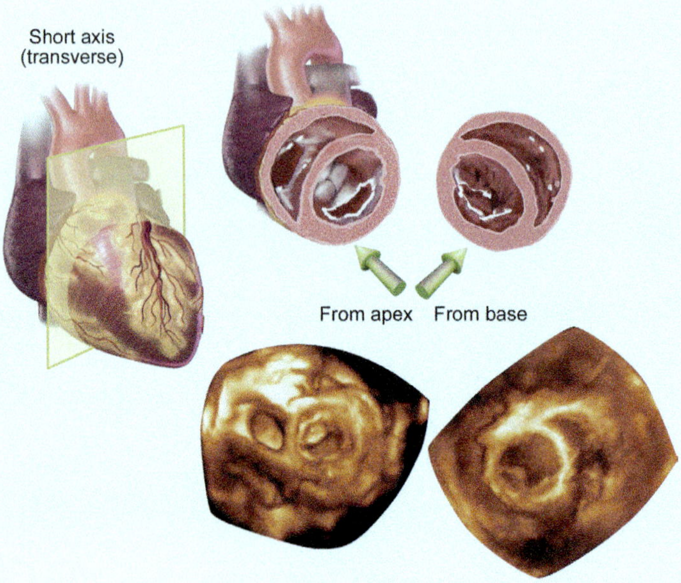

STANDARD VIEWS

The standard views used with 3DTTE correspond to their counterparts with 2DTTE that are familiar to all echocardiographers. Once one of these views is captured in 3D, the dataset can then be sectioned as detailed above to obtain a wealth of information by visualizing the cardiac structures from different perspectives and at any depth.[2] As with the 2D examination, visualizing some structures may necessitate deviation from these standard views especially for congenital heart defects and this should be encouraged.

Left parasternal long-axis view

The left parasternal long-axis view can be used for visualization of the mitral valve, the left atrium, and the interventricular septum. It is suitable for the assessment of mitral stenosis (Fig. 3-8) and ventricular septal defects (Fig. 3-9).[4,5] It can be very helpful for the visualization of patches used for ventricular septal defect repair (Fig. 3-10).[2] This approach can also be used to identify normal structures and differentiate them from pathologic entities. For example, the echo-free space posterior to the proximal ascending aorta in this view has been traditionally described as the right pulmonary artery, but we have shown using 3DTTE that in the majority of cases this space corresponds to the superior vena cava (Fig. 3-11). Some individuals have two echo-free spaces that correspond to the superior vena cava and the right pulmonary artery, and in a minority of patients the space actually represents the right pulmonary artery.[6]

Apical views

From the apex, the entire left ventricle can be captured in order to measure end-systolic and end-diastolic volumes and calculate the left ventricular ejection fraction (Fig. 3-12).[2] This approach has been shown to provide accurate and rapid assessment of left ventricular volumes and ejection fraction with good correlation to magnetic resonance imaging without geometric assumptions, thus overcoming many of the shortcomings of 2DTTE.[7–9] An advantage of 3DTTE is its ability to tell whether the left ventricle is foreshortened, a particularly common limitation of 2DTTE. Furthermore, the two-, three-, four-, and five-chamber apical

Figure 3-8

Live 3DE in mitral stenosis. A live 3D image from the long-axis view of the left side of the heart in diastole. The left atrium (LA) is enlarged and there is restricted opening of the mitral orifice (*arrow*). (Reproduced with permission from Wang et al.[2] [Fig. 9B].)

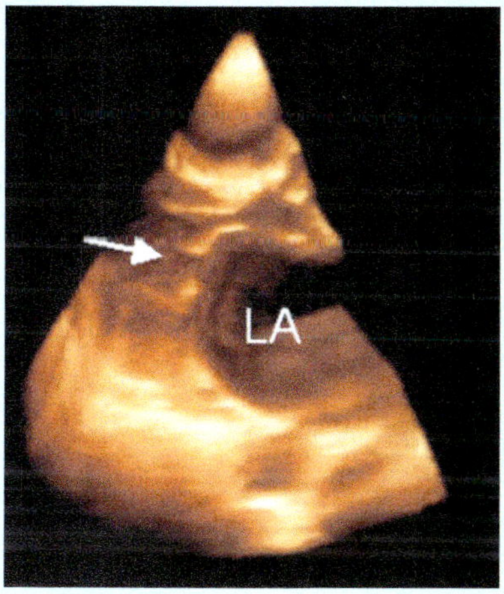

Figure 3-9

Live 3DE using narrow-angle display in a patient with a ventricular septal defect. The defect is visualized clearly (*arrow*). LA, left atrium; LV, left ventricle; RV, right ventricle. (Reproduced with permission from Wang et al.[2] [Fig. 7A].)

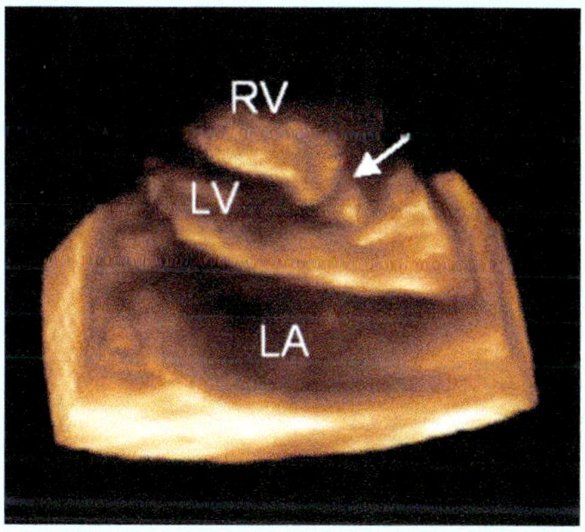

Figure 3-10 A and B

Live/real-time 3D TTE images of an interventricular septal defect that was repaired with a patch (*arrow*) from two perspectives. (A) Long-axis view of the left side of the heart viewed from the superior aspect. (B) The echo of the chest wall was removed and the patch appears separating the right and left ventricles (RV and LV). (Reproduced with permission from Wang et al.[2] [Fig. 11].)

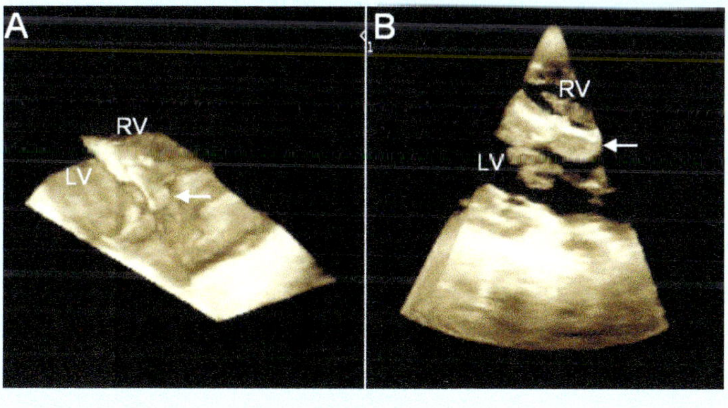

Figure 3-11

(A) Live real-time 3D TTE identification of the superior vena cava (SVC) behind the aorta (AO) imaged in parasternal long-axis view. A bounded echo-free space behind the aorta is imaged in a parasternal long-axis view. (B) Tilting of the full-volume 3D data set shows the bounded echo-free space (*arrowhead*) to be continuous with the right atrium. This is consistent with SVC. IVC, inferior vena cava; LA, left atrium; LV, left ventricle; RA, right atrium; RV, right ventricle; TV, tricuspid valve. (Reproduced with permission from Burri et al.[6] [Figs. 2A and 2C].)

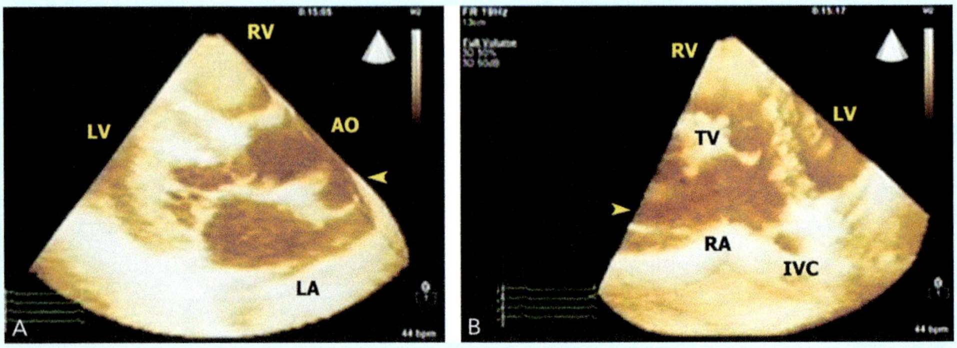

Figure 3-12

Live real-time 3D TTE. Apical examination. Reconstructed 3D volume of the left ventricle. (Reproduced with permission from Wang et al.[2] [Fig. 13D].)

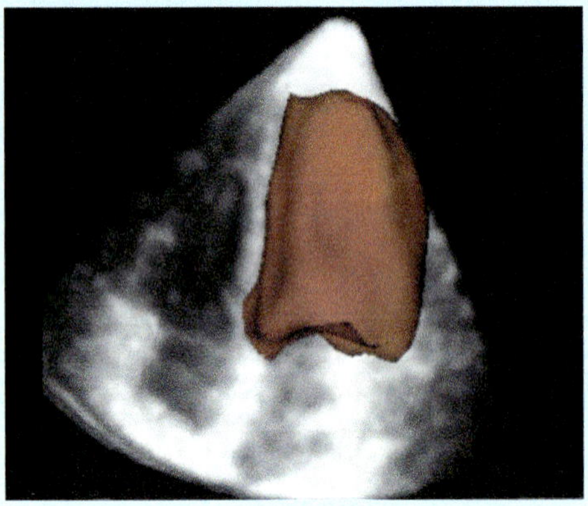

Figure 3-13

Live real-time 3DTTE. Apical examination. Cropping of the apical 3D dataset permits viewing of all four cardiac valves simultaneously. This is not possible using standard 2DE. AV, aortic valve; MV, mitral valve; PV, pulmonary valve; TV, tricuspid valve. (Reproduced with permission of Philips Medical Systems, Bothell, WA.)

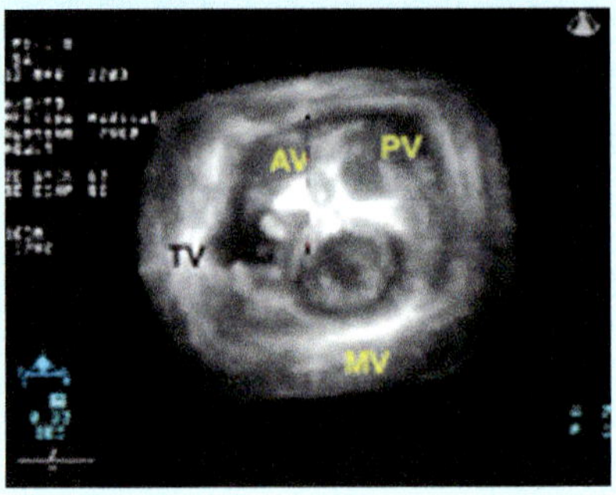

views can all be visualized from cropping the same 3D dataset. An especially interesting view that can facilitate appreciation of the anatomic relationship of the valves by visualizing all four cardiac valves simultaneously, in a manner not possible with 2DTTE, can also be obtained from the apical view (Fig. 3-13).[2]

Suprasternal view

The suprasternal view is the view that allows for visualization of the ascending aorta, aortic arch, and proximal descending aorta. From this view the vessels arising from the aortic arch, the pulmonary arteries, and the innominate veins can also be imaged (Fig. 3-14).[10]

Supraclavicular view

From the supraclavicular view, the entire length of the superior vena cava and the junction of the inferior vena cava with the right atrium can be well visualized. This view can also complement the suprasternal view in imaging the aortic arch and the major arteries and the adjacent veins (Fig. 3-15).[10]

Right parasternal view

The right parasternal window provides an essential view in the 3DTTE examination. This view can be very helpful especially in patients with right-sided heart enlargement, pericardial effusion, or ascending aortic dilatation, which push the right lung away from the sternum and provide an unobstructed view of cardiac structures.[10] In patients with atrial septal defect, for example, the entire septum can be visualized en face. This view is especially useful for the evaluation of the defect rim and the relation of the defect to the adjacent structures, which is crucial in deciding whether to use a percutaneous device to close the defect (Fig. 3-16).[11–13] Also from this view, the superior and inferior vena cavae and the connection of the coronary sinus to the right atrium as well as the pulmonary veins entering the left atrium can be well visualized. This view can also be used to visualize the right atrial appendage and the three leaflets of the tricuspid valve, which are difficult to see with 2DTTE. Other structures that can be seen from this view include the ascending aorta, the origin and proximal portion of the left main coronary artery, and the pulmonary valve and main pulmonary artery with its branches.

Figure 3-14

Live suprasternal 3DE examination demonstrating a long segment of the innominate artery (IA) branching from the aortic arch. AA, ascending aorta. (Reproduced with permission from Patel et al.[10] [Fig. 5A].)

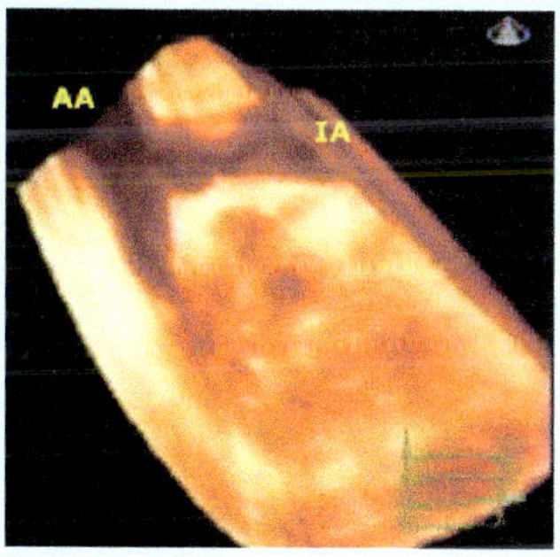

Figure 3-15

Live supraclavicular 3D TTE examination. Foreshortened image demonstrates both right and left innominate veins (RIV and LIV) joining to form the superior vena cava (SVC), which then enters into the right atrium (RA). A venous valve (V) is seen at the entrance of the SVC. Another venous valve (V1) is imaged at the junction of the azygos vein (AZ) and SVC. The inferior vena cava is also shown entering the RA inferiorly. AA, ascending aorta; CT (crista terminalis). (Reproduced with permission from Patel et al.[10] [Fig. 4A].)

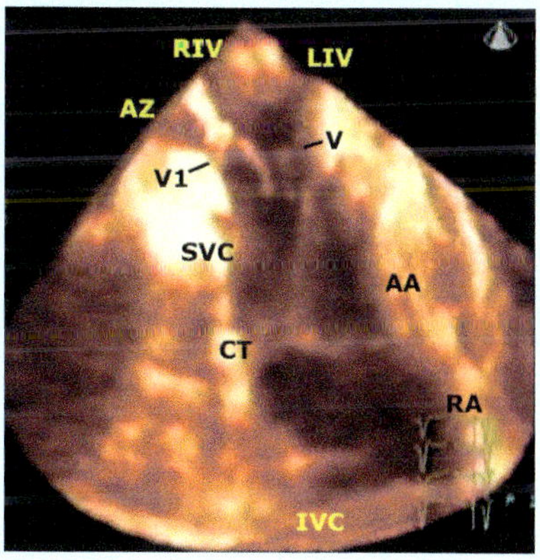

Figure 3-16

Live 3D right parasternal TTE examination of the atrial septum and superior and inferior vena cavae. *A*, The atrial septum (*), the entrance of the superior vena cava (SVC) into the right atrium, the base of the right atrial appendage (RAA), tricuspid valve (TV), and left atrium (LA) are shown. *B*, The previous image has been tilted to view the atrial septum (*) en face and to more clearly demonstrate the entrance of both the right upper and right lower pulmonary veins (RUPV and RLPV) into the LA. *C*, The entrance of the coronary sinus (CS) into the right atrium is shown. A longer segment of the SVC is demonstrated. RA, right atrium; RV, right ventricle. (Reproduced with permission from Patel et al.[10] [Figs. 1A-C].)

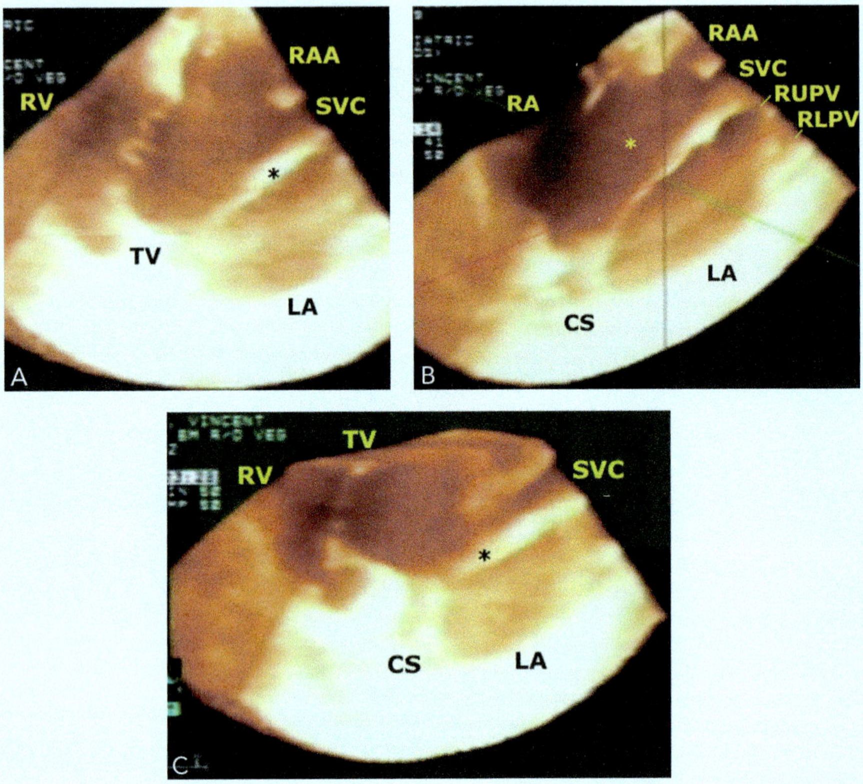

Subcostal view

The subcostal view can be extremely valuable for the visualization of any cardiac structure in patients with difficult acoustic windows from the traditional views in a manner very similar to the 2DTTE examination (Fig. 3-17).[14] In children, this view is particularly attractive for visualizing the left and right ventricles, the atria, all four cardiac valves, the pulmonary artery and its bifurcation, the inferior and superior vena cavae, and the interatrial septum. In the subcostal view, the interrogating ultrasound beam is perpendicular to the interatrial septum, which provides better assessment of this structure than do other views and allows for the visualization of atrial septal defects and other congenital defects, as will be described in other chapters.

Figure 3-17

Live real-time 3DTTE. Subcostal examination. Demonstrates several anatomic structures obtained from cropping of subcostally acquired 3D datasets. The *arrow* denotes the right ventricular apex. AS, interatrial septum; AV, aortic valve; LA, left atrium; LPA, left pulmonary artery; PV, pulmonary valve; RPA, right pulmonary artery. (Reproduced with permission from Nanda et al.[14] [Fig. 3-24G].)

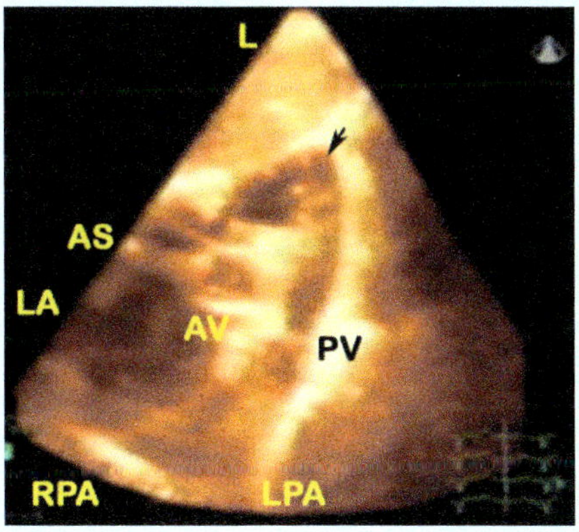

CONCLUSION

Thus far, 3DTTE has been used as a tool that complements rather than replaces the 2DTTE examination.[15] In practice, we use 3DTTE to provide incremental information that is not provided by the 2DTTE examination. Obviously, if the acoustic window is inadequate and the 2D images are suboptimal, then 3DTTE will not be able to improve the quality of the images. In such situations, 2DTEE may be more appropriate to provide the desired information. 3DTEE may be useful in combining the advantages of better image quality and the 3D perspective.[16] However, 3DTEE is not yet currently available for young infants and children.

REFERENCES

1. Hage FG, Nanda NC. Real-time three-dimensional echocardiography: a current view of what echocardiography can provide? *Indian Heart J.* 2009;61(2):146–155.
2. Wang XF, Deng YB, Nanda NC, et al. Live three-dimensional echocardiography: imaging principles and clinical application. *Echocardiography*. 2003;20(7):593–604.
3. Nanda NC, Kisslo J, Lang R, et al. Examination protocol for three-dimensional echocardiography. *Echocardiography*. 2004;21(8):763–768.
4. Singh V, Nanda NC, Agrawal G, et al. Live three-dimensional echocardiographic assessment of mitral stenosis. *Echocardiography*. 2003;20(8):743–750.
5. Mehmood F, Miller AP, Nanda NC, et al. Usefulness of live/real time three-dimensional transthoracic echocardiography in the characterization of ventricular septal defects in adults. *Echocardiography*. 2006;23(5): 421–427.
6. Burri MV, Mahan EF 3rd, Nanda NC, et al. Superior vena cava, right pulmonary artery or both: real time two- and three-dimensional transthoracic contrast echocardiographic identification of the echo-free space posterior to the ascending aorta. *Echocardiography*. 2007;24(8):875–882.
7. Qi X, Cogar B, Hsiung MC, et al. Live/real time three-dimensional transthoracic echocardiographic assessment of left ventricular volumes, ejection fraction, and mass compared with magnetic resonance imaging. *Echocardiography*. 2007;24(2):166–173.

8. Sugeng L, Mor-Avi V, Weinert L, et al. Quantitative assessment of left ventricular size and function: side-by-side comparison of real-time three-dimensional echocardiography and computed tomography with magnetic resonance reference. *Circulation.* 2006;114(7):654–661.
9. Mor-Avi V, Jenkins C, Kühl HP, et al. Real-time 3-dimensional echocardiographic quantification of left ventricular volumes: multicenter study for validation with magnetic resonance imaging and investigation of sources of error. *JACC Cardiovasc Imaging.* 2008;1(4):413–423.
10. Patel V, Nanda NC, Upendram S, et al. Live three-dimensional right parasternal and supraclavicular transthoracic echocardiographic examination. *Echocardiography.* 2005;22(4):349–360.
11. Mehmood F, Vengala S, Nanda NC, et al. Usefulness of live three-dimensional transthoracic echocardiography in the characterization of atrial septal defects in adults. *Echocardiography.* 2004;21(8):707–713.
12. Sinha A, Nanda NC, Misra V, et al. Live three-dimensional transthoracic echocardiographic assessment of transcatheter closure of atrial septal defect and patent foramen ovale. *Echocardiography.* 2004;21(8):749–753.
13. Singh A, Romp RL, Nanda NC, et al. Usefulness of live/real time three-dimensional transthoracic echocardiography in the assessment of atrioventricular septal defects. *Echocardiography.* 2006;23(7):598–608.
14. Nanda NC, Hsiung MC, Miller AP, et al. *Live/Real Time 3D Echocardiography.* Oxford, UK: Wiley-Blackwell; 2010.
15. Pothineni KR, Inamdar V, Miller AP, et al. Initial experience with live/real time three-dimensional transesophageal echocardiography. *Echocardiography.* 2007;24(10):1099–1104.
16. Ge S. How can we best image congenital heart defects? Are two-dimensional and three-dimensional echocardiography competitive or complementary? *J Am Soc Echocardiogr.* 2010 Jul;23(7):722–725.

CHAPTER

4

REAL-TIME THREE-DIMENSIONAL COLOR DOPPLER ECHOCARDIOGRAPHY

Shuping Ge, MD

ABSTRACT

Qualitative and quantitative real-time three-dimensional color Doppler echocardiography (RT3DCDE) has become an integral part of three-dimensional echocardiography (3DE) for the assessment of congenital and acquired heart disease. This chapter summarizes the available evidence on the use of qualitative and quantitative RT3DCDE methods for examining various flow abnormalities in congenital heart diseases (CHDs). Many of these methods can be incorporated into routine 3DE studies for diagnosis and assessment of CHD. Qualitative assessment and semiquantitative assessment of intra- and extracardiac flow and flow abnormalities as well as volumetric flow measurement by RT3DCDE and clinical applications for CHD are discussed.

INTRODUCTION

Conventional Doppler echocardiography, including pulsed-wave, continuous-wave, and color flow Doppler, is an integral modality for the diagnosis and assessment of congenital heart disease (CHD). In 1994, Belohlavek et al.[1] developed an algorithm to segment and reconstruct Doppler color flows in three dimensions in humans. This work first demonstrated the feasibility of three-dimensional (3D) reconstruction of selected color Doppler velocities on top of surrounding anatomy to allow appreciation of complex spatial velocity and flow patterns in cardiovascular diseases.[1] The early enthusiasm led to the development of commercially available systems that can be used to reconstruct laminar flow across the heart valve orifices[2,3] and to visualize turbulent flow in valve diseases.[4–6] At the same time, a quantitative 3D Doppler technique was developed and validated to reconstruct velocity signals to derive volumetric flow using in vitro and in vivo studies.[7,8]

The clinical use of 3D Doppler echocardiography became feasible after real-time 3D echocardiography (3DE) came to be available in the early 2000s.[9] This new technique was first used to assess valve disease qualitatively and quantitatively.[10–12] We developed a new technique to measure volumetric flow using real-time Doppler 3DE,[13] which stimulated the commercialization of this technique.[14] Other applications such as imaging of complex cardiac defects[15] and aortic and pulmonary arterial defects have also been demonstrated.[16]

Today, real-time 3D color Doppler echocardiography (RT3DCDE) has become an integral part of 3DE for assessing congenital and acquired heart disease.[17–19] This chapter summarizes the available evidence on the use of qualitative and quantitative RT3DCDE methods for examining various flow abnormalities in CHDs. Many of these methods can be incorporated into routine 3DE studies for diagnosis and assessment of CHD (Table 4-1). Qualitative assessment and semiquantitative assessment of intra- and extracardiac flow and flow abnormalities are discussed first, followed by volumetric flow measurement by RT3DCDE and clinical applications for CHD.

QUALITATIVE FLOW ASSESSMENT: INTRACARDIAC DEFECTS

One of the first applications of two-dimensional (2D) color Doppler flow is to demonstrate the property, direction, and magnitude of blood flow within the heart, such as color jets related to valve diseases, for diagnosis and semiquantitative assessment of flow abnormalities. The advent of RT3DCDE not only adds another dimension to imaging of these flow events but also permits understanding of the interaction of flow within cardiac chambers and vessels.

Valvular heart disease

Congenital pre- or postoperative valve diseases are common and can lead to significant valve stenosis and/or regurgitation. Many in vitro and in vivo studies have validated the utility of RT3DCDE for the diagnosis and assessment of valve diseases compared with the 2D color Doppler method (Tables 4-2 and 4-3).

To assess the severity of valve regurgitation, one can use 2D and Doppler echocardiography as recommended by the American Society of Echocardiography to measure (1) the size of the jet with or without normalization to the chamber size; (2) the proximal width of the jet or vena contracta; (3) the size of the proximal flow convergence region or proximal isovelocity surface area (PISA); (4) spectral Doppler features; (5) ventricular chamber size; and (6) quantitative regurgitant volume (RV), regurgitant fraction, and effective regurgitant orifice area (EROA).[20]

Studies have shown that RT3DCDE is more accurate and reproducible for measurement of the volumes of the regurgitant jet, area of the vena contracta, isovelocity surface area of the flow convergence region, and atrial or ventricular volumes. Therefore, it is superior and complementary to 2D echocardiography (2DE) and Doppler echocardiography for the qualitative and quantitative assessment of valve disease.

Table 4-1 Applications of RT3DCDE in CHD
Qualitative flow assessment
Intracardiac defects • Valve heart disease (e.g., mitral regurgitation) • Left-to-right shunt defects (e.g., ventricular septal defect)
Extracardiac defects • Aortic and pulmonary artery abnormalities (e.g., coarctation of aorta) • Pulmonary venous abnormalities
Flow measurements
SV and cardiac output Valve diseases Shunt defects

Table 4-2 Use of RT3DCDE to measure regurgitant jet volume from valve disease

Study					RT3DCDE vs. angiography grading		RT3DCDE vs. regurgitant volume		RT3DCDE vs. regurgitant fraction	
					2D jet area	3D jet volume	2D jet area	3D jet volume	2D jet area	2D jet volume
De Simone et al., 1999[6]	MR native	3DR	$n = 58$	3DR vs. angiography and 2D Doppler	$r = 0.73$	$r = 0.90$	$r = 0.66$	$r = 0.90$	$r = 0.68$	$r = 0.80$
De Simone et al., 1999[21]	MR repair	3DR	$n = 24$	3DR vs. 2D Doppler			$r = 0.40^a$	$r = 0.85$	$r = 0.45^a$	$r = 0.71$
De Simone et al., 1999[5]	MR native	3DR	$n = 63$	3DR vs. 2D Doppler				$r = 0.90$		$r = 0.76$
Lu et al., 2006[22]	AR native	RT	$n = 23$	RT3DCDE vs. 2DE				$r = 0.93$		$r = 0.88$
Sugeng et al., 2007[23]	MR/TR native	RT	$n = 56$	RT3DCDE vs. PISA				$r = 0.7–0.8$		

Abbreviations: 3DR, three-dimensional reconstructive; AR, aortic regurgitation; MR, mitral regurgitation; PISA, proximal isovelocity surface area; RT, real time; TR, tricuspid regurgitation.
$^aP > .05$.

Table 4-3 Vena contracta measurement using RT3DCDE

Study					3D VC vs. reference	2D VC vs. reference	3D VC × VTI vs. reference	2D VC × VTI vs. reference
Mori et al., 1999[24]	AR	3DR	$n = 6$	3DR vs. flow probe	$r = 0.99$		$r = 0.99$	
Ishii et al., 2001[25]	VSD	3DR	$n = 19$	3DR vs. catheterization			$r = 0.95$	
Khanna et al., 2004[11]	MR	RT	$n = 44$	RT3DCDE vs. angiography	$r = 0.88$	$r = 0.55$		
Fang et al., 2005[12]	AR	RT	$n = 56$	RT3DCDE vs. angiography/surgery	$r = 0.95$	$r = 0.92$		
Little et al., 2008[26a]	MR	RT	$n = 61$	RT3DCDE vs. Doppler EROA	$r = 0.87$	$r = 0.60$		
Pothineni et al., 2008[27]	PR	RT	$n = 82$	RT3DCDE vs. 2D color Doppler	$r = 0.76$		$r = 0.76$	
Marsan et al., 2009[28]	MR	RT	$n = 64$	RT3DCDE vs. CMR			$r = 0.94$; MD = −0.08 mL	MD = 2.9 mL
Shanks et al., 2010[29]	MR	RT	$n = 30$	RT3DCDE vs. CMR			MD = −2.32 mL	MD = −12.4 mL

Abbreviations: 3DR, three-dimensional reconstruction; AR, aortic regurgitation; EROA, effective regurgitant orifice area; MD, mean difference; MR, mitral regurgitation; PR, pulmonary regurgitation; RT, real time; VC, vena contracta; VSD, ventricular septal defect; VTI, velocity–time integral.

Jet volume by RT3DCDE

One of the first applications of RT3DCDE is to measure regurgitant jet volume from valve disease. Figure 4-1 demonstrates the methodology to measure jet volume by RT3DCDE. The validation studies are summarized in Table 4-2.[5,6,21–23] The available evidence has shown that RT3DCDE is superior to 2D color Doppler in delineating color jet size and geometry and qualifying jet volume, RV, and regurgitant fraction, especially for eccentric jets.[5,21] A major limitation is that most of these studies compared RT3DCDE with 2D and Doppler quantitative techniques or with angiography. Future study is warranted to validate these techniques using more accurate and independent references, such as cardiac magnetic resonance (CMR) imaging.

Vena contracta and RV

The geometry of the vena contracta or of the EROA varies among individual patients with valve disease. Many studies have confirmed that RT3DCDE is more accurate for the measurement of vena contracta (Fig. 4-2) and is independent of the geometric assumptions as related to 2D color Doppler flow. Table 4-3 summarizes the published studies validating the utility of vena contracta measurement using RT3DCDE.[11,12,24–30]

Figure 4-1

Jet volume measurement by 2DE and RT3DDE. *A*, Semiquantitative method for estimating jet severity as performed in two planes (two- and four-chamber views). Area of jet and left atrial area were traced. *B–I*, Methodology used to calculate jet volume to atrial ratio. Initially, the jet was aligned in two perpendicular views and regurgitant volume was calculated by tracing the largest area of jet in systole in eight slice planes, resulting in surface reconstruction to derive jet volume. In the same frame, atrial surface and volume (right) were reconstructed by tracing the atrium in eight equiangled planes. (With permission from Sugeng et al.[23])

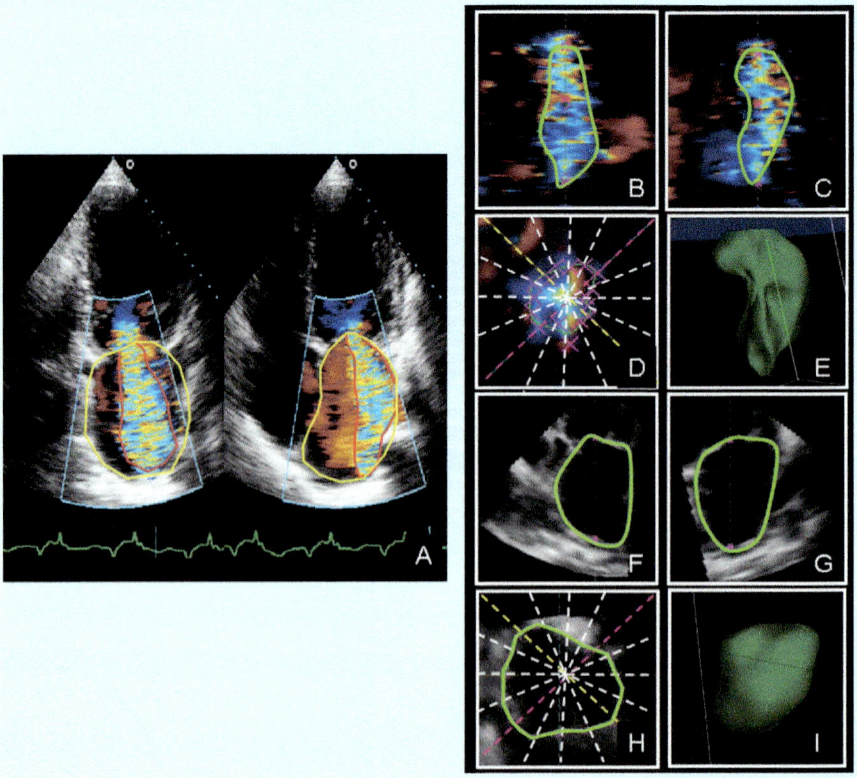

Figure 4-2

3D color Doppler assessment of the vena contracta or EROA. *A*, The 3D color Doppler data set is manually cropped using the plane perpendicular to the jet direction until the narrowest cross-sectional area of the jet is reached. *B*, In an en face view, the 3D EROA is measured by manual planimetry of the color Doppler signal. An example of an asymmetrical 3D EROA elongated along the leaflet coaptation line is provided, for which the hemispherical convergence method using geometric assumptions may not be applicable. (With permission from Shanks et al.[29])

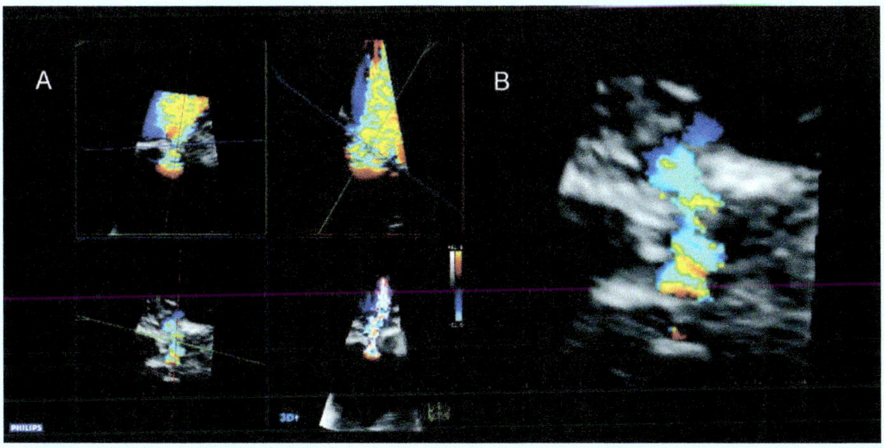

To measure the vena contracta using RT3DCDE, the color Doppler jet is obtained by RT3DCDE. The RT3DCDE system settings should be optimized first. The color box size is adjusted to include the entire jet. It is then crucial to obtain the highest temporal resolution, that is, frame rate, to avoid underestimation of the maximal jet volume and the vena contracta. Patient cooperation is important to avoid artifacts between subvolumes during image acquisition by electrocardiographic triggering. After the image is obtained, online or off-line analysis using multiplanar reconstruction mode is needed. The image is displayed in three orthogonal planes. Alignment of the cutting plane is needed to obtain a cross section that is smallest in area, that is, the vena contracta, for planimetry of the area by manual tracing of the color contours (Fig. 4-2).[29]

RV can be calculated as follows: RV = EROA × velocity–time integral (VTI). This method has been validated by comparing RV by 2D color Doppler, RT3DCDE, and CMR measurements.[28,29] Marsan et al.[28] performed a head-to-head comparison between RT3DCDE and velocity-encoded CMR for the assessment of functional mitral regurgitation. RV measured by RT3DCDE showed excellent correlation with RV measured by CMR (r = 0.94), and there was no significant difference between these techniques (mean difference = −0.08 mL/beat). Conversely, use of 2DE via the four-chamber view significantly underestimated RV (P = .006) compared with CMR (mean difference = 2.9 mL/beat). The 2D elliptical approach demonstrated a better agreement with CMR (mean difference = 1.6 mL/beat, P = .04). In another study, Shanks et al.[29] compared the accuracy of 2D and 3D transesophageal echocardiography (TEE) for quantification of mitral regurgitation, using MRI as the reference method. In this study, 2D TEE underestimated the RV by 21.6% when compared with 3D TEE and by 21.3% when compared with CMR. In contrast, 3D TEE underestimated the RV by only 1.2% when compared with CMR. Finally, one-third of the patients with grade 1 and 50% or more of the patients with grades 2 and 3 mitral regurgitation (MR), as assessed by 2D TEE, would have had their conditions upgraded to a more severe grade, based on the 3D TEE and MRI measurements. These studies suggest that transthoracic and transesophageal RT3DCDE may become a more accurate quantitative tool than 2DE, and a tool comparable to CMR, for assessing vena contracta, EROA, and RV for mitral regurgitation.

Table 4-4 PISA method for the measurement of valve regurgitation using RT3DCDE

Study		Reference	RT3DCDE vs. CWD	M mode	2D	3D
Li et al., 2000[36]	In vitro	Actual flow rate				$r = 0.97–0.99$
Coisne et al., 2002[35]	In vitro	Actual flow rate	−5.5%[a]	−32.1%[a]	−44.2%[*]	−2.6%[a]
Little et al., 2007[26b]	In vitro	Actual flow rate			$r = 0.69$[b]	$r = 0.96$[b]
Pirat et al., 2009[39]	In vitro	Actual flow rate			$r = 0.69$[c]	$r = 0.83$[c]

Abbreviation: CWD, continuous-wave Doppler.
[a]Percentage error.
[b]For mitral regurgitation.
[c]For aortic regurgitation.

Flow convergence region and PISA by RT3DCDE

Measurement of the proximal flow convergence region, or the PISA method, was initially employed to quantify the peak flow rate of regurgitant[31,32] or shunt flows[33] using 2D color Doppler flow mapping. In an ideal setting, the relationship can be simplified as follows: peak flow rate = $2 \times \pi \times R^2 \times$ aliasing velocity, where R is the radius of the hemispheric isovelocity shells. Studies have shown that other variables such as flow rate; orifice shape, size, and eccentricity; proximal flow constraint; and pulsatility all affect the accuracy of the flow rate computational algorithm.[34] In addition, the isovelocity shells in the proximal flow convergence region are not always hemispherical but are often ellipsoidal or skewed.

In vitro validation studies (Table 4-4)[25,35–37] suggest that RT3DCDE is a superior method for directly measuring the surface area of the isovelocity shells and can therefore improve the accuracy of this algorithm,[17,25,26,36–40] although other confounding factors such as Doppler angle alignment of the peripheral streamline flow and conversion from flow rate to flow volumes remain to be addressed. Further in vivo studies are needed to validate this promising technique.[26,35,36,39]

QUALITATIVE FLOW ASSESSMENT: EXTRACARDIAC DEFECTS

Congenital extracardiac arterial and venous abnormalities are commonly seen in isolation or in association with congenital intracardiac heart defects. This group of defects includes aortic arch, pulmonary artery, and systemic and pulmonary venous abnormalities. Unlike intracardiac structures and flows, which can usually be delineated well by 2D and color Doppler flow mapping, extracardiac arterial or venous abnormalities are often complex, tortuous, and difficult to comprehend using 2D and color Doppler standard views and sweeps. Other imaging modalities, such as computed tomography (CT), CMR, or angiography, may be needed to provide a definitive diagnosis and assessment of the 3D configuration of these abnormalities.

RT3DCDE has been applied to delineate these abnormalities.[15,16] After 3DE and 3D color Doppler echocardiography (3DCDE) images are obtained, one can choose color depression to remove grayscale images to stress flow and flow abnormalities in a fashion similar to "color Doppler angiography." Hlavacek et al.[16] demonstrated that it was feasible to show coarctation of the aorta, patent ductus arteriosus, hypoplastic aortic arch in hypoplastic left heart syndrome, and postoperative conditions in patients undergoing modified Blalock–Taussig shunt or arterial switch operation for complete transposition of the great arteries in 26 patients. We have also demonstrated the incremental value of RT3DCDE in complex CHD, such as aortopulmonary window. Furthermore, we studied 58 patients with vascular rings.[41] We showed that RT3DCDE provides a detailed 3D flow map, especially in patients with tortuous and complex 3D abnormalities, in a fashion similar to CT or CMR. These abnormalities include double aortic arch, right aortic arch, and pulmonary artery sling. Diagnostic accuracy was 100% in concordance with CT or CMR.

Limitations of current RT3DCDE include but are not limited to the following: (1) narrow 3D data set (it is sometimes difficult to include the entire heart in a single 3D data set for off-line analysis), (2) low frame rate, and (3) composite 3D image triggered by electrocardiography. Alignment artifact

Figure 4-3

(*A*), RT3DDE showing the 3D spatial relationship between the ascending aorta (Ao) and pulmonary artery (PA), i.e., aortopulmonary window (APW) and patent ductus arteriosus (PDA) from a suprasternal approach. (*B*), Cardiac catheterization and angiography of APW and associated lesions. (*C*), Intraoperative inspection of APW (red arrow) L, left; R, right. (With permission from Chen and Ge.[15])

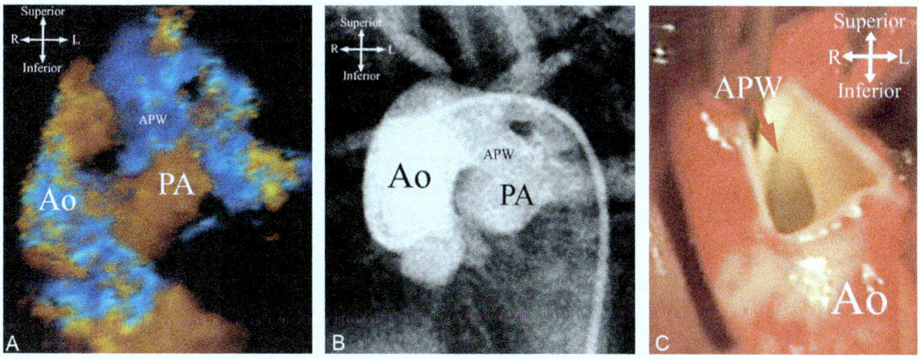

between subvolumes can occur. Technological advances are needed to make RT3DCDE a clinical tool for the evaluation of CHD.

QUANTITATIVE VOLUMETRIC FLOW MEASUREMENT

To quantify volumetric flow and assess cardiac output, valve disease, and shunt defect by conventional spectral Doppler echocardiography, one has to assume a flat and uniform velocity profile across the valve orifice and blood vessel. Therefore, the maximal velocity at the center of the flow profile represents the mean velocity across the cross-sectional area, an assumption that may lead to significant errors in volumetric flow calculation in humans by spectral Doppler techniques.[2,3,42] For example, Haugen et al.[2] showed that the ratio of maximum VTI to mean VTI was a mean of 1.3 (range: 1.1–1.6) across the mitral valve using a reconstructive 3D color Doppler technique. At the time of peak flow, the ratio of the maximum to the mean velocity was a mean of 1.5 (range: 1.2–2.6). By using a single sample volume in Doppler measurements of the maximum VTI, errors ranging from 10% to 60% may be introduced in calculations of stroke volumes (SVs) for the mitral valve,[2] and from 20% to 50% for the aortic valve.[3]

The RT3DCDE technique for quantifying volumetric flow is based on the Gaussian theorem: for any arbitrarily shaped control surface system, the flow rate passing through it equals the summation of all velocity components that are normal to the surface. The technique was first tested in 2D color Doppler flow mapping[43,44] and reconstructive 3DCDE.[7,45,46] We first became interested in volumetric flow measurement when RT3DCDE became available. We collaborated with Dr. Milan Sonka's laboratory in the Department of Electrical and Computer Engineering at the University of Iowa. We first demonstrated that volumetric flow across the mitral valve orifice by RT3DCDE correlated well with SV by phase velocity cine MRI at the ascending aorta (r = 0.92, mean difference = −5.2 ± 12.0 mL) and by left ventricular volumetric MRI measurement (r = 0.94, mean difference = −0.2 ± 10.3 mL).[13] In addition, compared with SV by real-time three-dimensional echocardiography (RT3DE), the correlation with volume flow was excellent for the mitral valve (r = 0.91), aortic valve (r = 0.89), and pulmonary valve (r = 0.89) but poor for the tricuspid valve (r = 0.20) by real-time three-dimensional Doppler echocardiography (RT3DDE). Agreement was good for

Figure 4-4

A volumetric flow measurement by RT3DDE. Top left and right, Two orthogonal sections of mitral valve (MV) flow. Hemispheric Gaussian control surface was placed at the level of the MV orifice. Bottom left, Region of interest was selected by tracing cross-sectional contours of color Doppler signals during diastolic phase. Bottom right, Flow rate curves and volumetric flow for MV were derived from the area under flow rate curve. (With permission from Lu.[14])

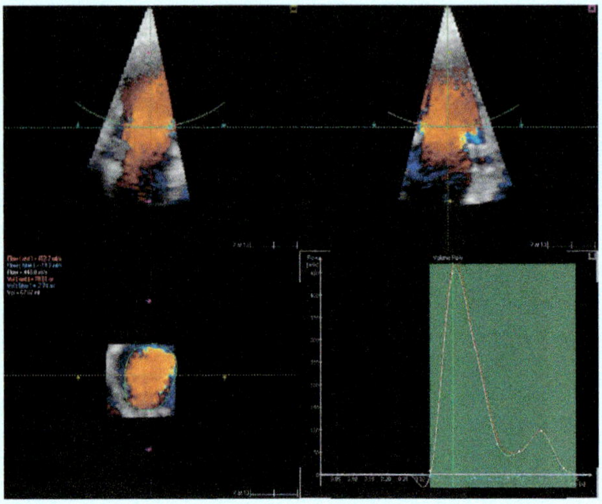

Figure 4-5

Flow rate curves and volumetric flow (VF) at aortic valve (AV) (*A*), mitral valve (MV) (*B*), pulmonary valve (PV) (*C*), and tricuspid valve (TV) (*D*) derived from measurements by RT3DDE. (Scales of VF are different.) (With permission from Lu.[14])

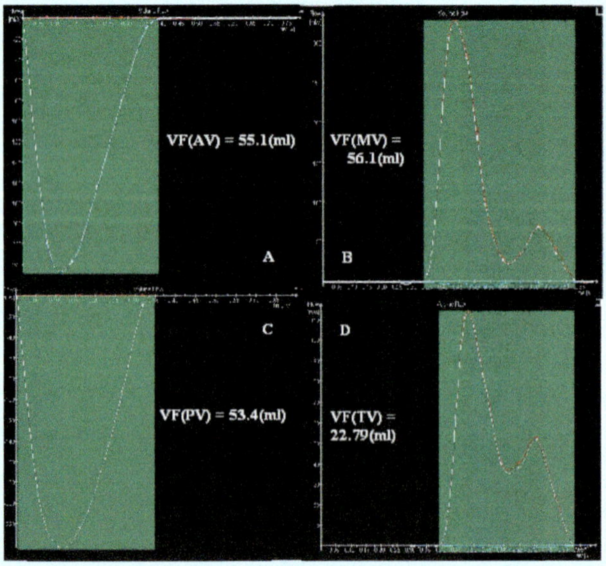

Table 4-5 Quantitative measurement of volumetric flow by RT3DCDE

Study		Reference	MV	AV	PV	TV
Ge et al., 2005[13]	Children (n = 13)	MRI	r = 0.92–0.94			
Li et al., 2005[47]	In vitro	Pulsatile pump		r = 0.98	0.99	
Pemberton et al., 2005[48a]	Animal (n = 16)	Flow probe		r = 0.96		
Pemberton et al., 2005[48a]	Children and adults (n = 55)	2DE		r = 0.95		
Lodato et al., 2007[49]	Adults (n = 47)	Thermodilution	r = 0.93; r = 0.75 (2D)	r = 0.94; r = 0.78 (2D)		
Lu et al., 2007[14]	Children (n = 19)	RT3DE	r = 0.91	r = 0.89	r = 0.89	r = 0.20

Abbreviations: 2DE, two-dimensional echocardiography; AV, aortic valve; MV, mitral valve; PV, pulmonary valve; TV, tricuspid valve.

the aortic valve (bias = 0.9 ± 5.0 mL), pulmonary valve (bias = −0.4 ± 5.7 mL), and mitral valve (bias = 4.1 ± 4.7 mL), and the tricuspid valve was markedly underestimated (bias = −24.4 ± 14.6 mL).[14] In vitro, in vivo, animal, and human validation studies are listed in Table 4-5.[13,14,47–49]

Another potentially important application of RT3DCDE is to assess aortic stenosis using the continuity equation: in aortic stenosis, aortic valve area = left ventricular outflow tract (LVOT) SV/LVOT VTI of continuous-wave Doppler, in which LVOT SV can be obtained by RT3DCDE.

Poh et al.[50] prospectively studied 68 patients with aortic stenosis (aged 74 ± 12 years). Correlation between aortic valve area using 2D and 3D derived SV was modest for the cohort overall (r = 0.71, P < .001) (mean difference was 0.11 ± 0.23 cm^2). Furthermore, validation of LVOT SV was performed by aortic flow probe in a sheep model with balloon inflation to mimic septal hypertrophy. In experimentally distorted LVOT geometry in sheep, RT3DE correlated better with flow probe assessment (r = 0.96, P < .001) than 2DE (r = 0.71, P = .006), suggesting possible skewing of velocity profiles in LVOT and its impact on flow quantification by 2D and 3D Doppler methods.

LIMITATIONS AND FUTURE DIRECTIONS

As the RT3DCDE technology evolves, we anticipate that the following advances will occur:

1. The RT3DCDE full and subvolume size will increase to include the entire heart.
2. It will become possible to acquire RT3DCDE in a single beat.
3. The temporal resolution (frame rate) will increase.
4. More versatile online and off-line tools will become available to visualize and measure flow and flow abnormalities.
5. More robust and semiautomated flow quantification tools will become available.[51,52]
6. RT3DCDE will become an integral method for the routine assessment of CHD.[33]

REFERENCES

1. Belohlavek M, Foley DA, Gerber TC, et al. Three-dimensional reconstruction of color Doppler jets in the human heart. *J Am Soc Echocardiogr*. 1994;7(6):553–560.
2. Haugen BO, Berg S, Brecke KM, et al. Velocity profiles in mitral blood flow based on three-dimensional freehand colour flow imaging acquired at high frame rate. *Eur J Echocardiogr*. 2000;1(4):252–256.

3. Haugen BO, Berg S, Brecke KM, et al. Blood flow velocity profiles in the aortic annulus: a 3-dimensional freehand color flow Doppler imaging study. *J Am Soc Echocardiogr.* April, 2002;15(4):328–333.
4. Shiota T, Jones M, Delabays A, et al. Direct measurement of three-dimensionally reconstructed flow convergence surface area and regurgitant flow in aortic regurgitation: in vitro and chronic animal model studies. *Circulation.* 1997;96(10):3687–3695.
5. De Simone R, Glombitza G, Vahl CF, et al. Three-dimensional color Doppler: a new approach for quantitative assessment of mitral regurgitant jets. *J Am Soc Echocardiogr.* 1999;12(3):173–185.
6. De Simone R, Glombitza G, Vahl CF, et al. Three-dimensional color Doppler: a clinical study in patients with mitral regurgitation. *J Am Coll Cardiol.* 1999;33(6):1646–1654.
7. Irvine T, Li XN, Mori Y, et al. A digital 3-dimensional method for computing great artery flows: in vitro validation studies. *J Am Soc Echocardiogr.* 2000;13(9):841–848.
8. Irvine T, Stetten GD, Sachdev V, et al. Quantification of aortic regurgitation by real-time 3-dimensional echocardiography in a chronic animal model: computation of aortic regurgitant volume as the difference between left and right ventricular stroke volumes. *J Am Soc Echocardiogr.* 2001;14(11):1112–1118.
9. Sugeng L, Spencer KT, Mor-Avi V, et al. Dynamic three-dimensional color flow Doppler: an improved technique for the assessment of mitral regurgitation. *Echocardiography.* 2003;20(3):265–273.
10. Shiota T, Jones M, Tsujino H, et al. Quantitative analysis of aortic regurgitation: real-time 3-dimensional and 2-dimensional color Doppler echocardiographic method: a clinical and a chronic animal study. *J Am Soc Echocardiogr.* 2002;15(9):966–971.
11. Khanna D, Vengala S, Miller AP, et al. Quantification of mitral regurgitation by live three-dimensional transthoracic echocardiographic measurements of vena contracta area. *Echocardiography.* 2004;21(8):737–743.
12. Fang L, Hsiung MC, Miller AP, et al. Assessment of aortic regurgitation by live three-dimensional transthoracic echocardiographic measurements of vena contracta area: usefulness and validation. *Echocardiography.* 2005;22(9):775–781.
13. Ge S, Bu L, Zhang H, et al. A real-time 3-dimensional digital Doppler method for measurement of flow rate and volume through mitral valve in children: a validation study compared with magnetic resonance imaging. *J Am Soc Echocardiogr.* 2005;18(1):1–7.
14. Lu X, Nadvoretskiy V, Klas B, et al. Measurement of volumetric flow by real-time 3-dimensional Doppler echocardiography in children. *J Am Soc Echocardiogr.* 2007;20(8):915–920.
15. Chen FL, Ge S. Aortopulmonary window demonstrated by real-time 3-dimensional echocardiography and color Doppler. *J Am Soc Echocardiogr.* 2007;20(11):1314.e7–1314.e8.
16. Hlavacek A, Lucas J, Baker H, et al. Feasibility and utility of three-dimensional color flow echocardiography of the aortic arch: the "echocardiographic angiogram." *Echocardiography.* 2006;23(10):860–864.
17. Matsumura Y, Fukuda S, Tran H, et al. Geometry of the proximal isovelocity surface area in mitral regurgitation by 3-dimensional color Doppler echocardiography: difference between functional mitral regurgitation and prolapse regurgitation. *Am Heart J.* 2008;155(2):231–238.
18. Hung J, Lang R, Flachskampf F, et al. 3D echocardiography: a review of the current status and future directions. *J Am Soc Echocardiogr.* 2007;20(3):213–233.
19. Ge S. How can we best image congenital heart defects? Are two-dimensional and three-dimensional echocardiography competitive or complementary? *J Am Soc Echocardiogr.* 2010;23(7):722–725.
20. Zoghbi WA, Enriquez-Sarano M, Foster E, et al. Recommendations for evaluation of the severity of native valvular regurgitation with two-dimensional and Doppler echocardiography. *J Am Soc Echocardiogr.* 2003;16(7):777–802.
21. De Simone R, Glombitza G, Vahl CF, et al. Three-dimensional color Doppler for assessing mitral regurgitation during valvuloplasty. *Eur J Cardiothorac Surg.* 1999;15(2):127–133.
22. Lu Q, Liu X, Xie M, et al. Real-time three-dimensional color Doppler flow imaging: an improved technique for quantitative analysis of aortic regurgitation. *J Huazhong Univ Sci Technolog Med Sci.* 2006;26(1):148–152.
23. Sugeng L, Weinert L, Lang RM. Real-time 3-dimensional color Doppler flow of mitral and tricuspid regurgitation: feasibility and initial quantitative comparison with 2-dimensional methods. *J Am Soc Echocardiogr.* 2007;20(9):1050–1057.
24. Mori Y, Shiota T, Jones M, et al. Three-dimensional reconstruction of the color Doppler-imaged vena contracta for quantifying aortic regurgitation: studies in a chronic animal model. *Circulation.* 1999;99(12):1611–1617.
25. Ishii M, Hashino K, Eto G, et al. Quantitative assessment of severity of ventricular septal defect by three-dimensional reconstruction of color Doppler-imaged vena contracta and flow convergence region. *Circulation.* 2001;103(5):664–669.

26a. Little SH, Pirat B, Kumar R, et al. Three-dimensional color Doppler echocardiography for direct measurement of vena contracta area in mitral regurgitation: in vitro validation and clinical experience. *JACC Cardiovasc Imaging.* November, 2008;1(6):695–704. [Epub November 18, 2008].
26b. Little SH, Igo SR, Pirat B, et al. In vitro validation of real-time three-dimensional color Doppler echocardiography for direct measurement of proximal isovelocity surface area in mitral regurgitation. *Am J Cardiol.* 2007;99(10):1440–1447.
27. Pothineni KR, Wells BJ, Hsiung MC, et al. Live/real time three-dimensional transthoracic echocardiographic assessment of pulmonary regurgitation. *Echocardiography.* 2008;25(8):911–917.
28. Marsan NA, Westenberg JJ, Ypenburg C, et al. Quantification of functional mitral regurgitation by real-time 3D echocardiography: comparison with 3D velocity-encoded cardiac magnetic resonance. *JACC Cardiovasc Imaging.* 2009;2(11):1245–1252.
29. Shanks M, Siebelink HM, Delgado V, et al. Quantitative assessment of mitral regurgitation: comparison between three-dimensional transesophageal echocardiography and magnetic resonance imaging. *Circ Cardiovasc Imaging.* 2010;3(6):694–700.
30. Velayudhan DE, Brown TM, Nanda NC, et al. Quantification of tricuspid regurgitation by live three-dimensional transthoracic echocardiographic measurements of vena contracta area. *Echocardiography.* 2006;23(9):793–800.
31. Recusani F, Bargiggia GS, Yoganathan AP, et al. A new method for quantification of regurgitant flow rate using color Doppler flow imaging of the flow convergence region proximal to a discrete orifice. An in vitro study. *Circulation.* 1991;83(2):594–604.
32. Bargiggia GS, Tronconi L, Sahn DJ, et al. A new method for quantitation of mitral regurgitation based on color flow Doppler imaging of flow convergence proximal to regurgitant orifice. *Circulation.* 1991;84(4):1481–1489.
33. Moises VA, Maciel BC, Hornberger LK, et al. A new method for noninvasive estimation of ventricular septal defect shunt flow by Doppler color flow mapping: imaging of the laminar flow convergence region on the left septal surface. *J Am Coll Cardiol.* 1991;18(3):824–832.
34. Shandas R, Gharib M, Sahn DJ. Nature of flow acceleration into a finite-sized orifice: steady and pulsatile flow studies on the flow convergence region using simultaneous ultrasound Doppler flow mapping and laser Doppler velocimetry. *J Am Coll Cardiol.* 1995;25(5):1199–1212.
35. Coisne D, Erwan D, Christiaens L, et al. Quantitative assessment of regurgitant flow with total digital three-dimensional reconstruction of color Doppler flow in the convergent region: in vitro validation. *J Am Soc Echocardiogr.* 2002;15(3):233–240.
36. Li XK, Irvine T, Wanitkun S, et al. Direct computation of multiple 3D flow convergence isovelocity surfaces from digital 3D reconstruction of colour Doppler data of the flow convergence region: an in vitro study with differently shaped orifices. *Eur J Echocardiogr.* 2000;1(4):244–251.
37. Matsumura Y, Saracino G, Sugioka K, et al. Determination of regurgitant orifice area with the use of a new three-dimensional flow convergence geometric assumption in functional mitral regurgitation. *J Am Soc Echocardiogr.* 2008;21(11):1251–1256.
38. Shiota T, Omoto R, Cobanoglu A, et al. Usefulness of transesophageal imaging of flow convergence region in the operating room for evaluating isolated patent ductus arteriosus. *Am J Cardiol.* 1997;80(8):1108–1112.
39. Pirat B, Little SH, Igo SR, et al. Direct measurement of proximal isovelocity surface area by real-time three-dimensional color Doppler for quantitation of aortic regurgitant volume: an in vitro validation. *J Am Soc Echocardiogr.* 2009;22(3):306–313.
40. Yosefy C, Levine RA, Solis J, et al. Proximal flow convergence region as assessed by real-time 3-dimensional echocardiography: challenging the hemispheric assumption. *J Am Soc Echocardiogr.* 2007;20(4):389–396.
41. Chen FL, Ge S. Utility of transthoracic three-dimensional color Doppler echocardiography for diagnosis of congenital aortic arch anomalies. *J Am Coll Cardiol.* 2007;49(9 suppl A):1005–1031.
42. Kvitting P, Hessevik I, Matre K, Segadal L. Three-dimensional cross-sectional velocity distribution in the ascending aorta in cardiac patients. *Clin Physiol.* 1996;16(3):239–258.
43. Sun Y, Ask P, Sjöberg BJ, et al. Estimation of volume flow rate by surface integration of velocity vectors from color Doppler images. *J Am Soc Echocardiogr.* 1995;8(6):904–914.
44. Kim WY, Poulsen JK, Terp K, Staalsen NH. A new Doppler method for quantification of volumetric flow: in vitro validation using color Doppler. *J Am Coll Cardiol.* 1996;27(1):182–192.
45. Kim WY, Poulsen JK, Terp K, et al. New semiautomated Doppler method for quantification of volumetric flow: intraoperative validation with multiplane transesophageal color Doppler imaging. *J Am Soc Echocardiogr.* 1997;10(4):330–336.
46. Mori Y, Rusk RA, Jones M, et al. A new dynamic three-dimensional digital color Doppler method for quantification of pulmonary regurgitation: validation study in an animal model. *J Am Coll Cardiol.* 2002;40(6):1179–1185.

47. Li X, Ashraf M, Thiele K, et al. A novel method for the assessment of the accuracy of computing laminar flow stroke volumes using a real-time 3D ultrasound system: in vitro studies. *Eur J Echocardiogr*. 2005;6(6):396–404. [Epub May 31, 2005].
48a. Pemberton J, Li X, Karamlou T, et al. The use of live three-dimensional Doppler echocardiography in the measurement of cardiac output: an in vivo animal study. *J Am Coll Cardiol*. 2005;45(3):433–438.
48b. Pemberton J, Li X, Kenny A, et al. Real-time 3-dimensional Doppler echocardiography for the assessment of stroke volume: an in vivo human study compared with standard 2-dimensional echocardiography. *J Am Soc Echocardiogr*. October, 2005;18(10):1030–1036.
49. Lodato JA, Weinert L, Baumann R, et al. Use of 3-dimensional color Doppler echocardiography to measure stroke volume in human beings: comparison with thermodilution. *J Am Soc Echocardiogr*. 2007;20(2):103–112.
50. Poh KK, Levine RA, Solis J, et al. Assessing aortic valve area in aortic stenosis by continuity equation: a novel approach using real-time three-dimensional echocardiography. *Eur Heart J*. 2008;29(20):2526–2535.
51. Thavendiranathan P, Liu S, Datta S, et al. Automated quantification of mitral inflow and aortic outflow stroke volumes by three-dimensional real-time volume color-flow Doppler transthoracic echocardiography: comparison with pulsed-wave Doppler and cardiac magnetic resonance imaging. *J Am Soc Echocardiogr*. January, 2012;25(1):56–65. [Epub November 21, 2011].
52. Thavendiranathan P, Liu S, Verhaert D, et al. Feasibility, accuracy, and reproducibility of real-time full-volume 3D transthoracic echocardiography to measure LV volumes and systolic function: a fully automated endocardial contouring algorithm in sinus rhythm and atrial fibrillation. *JACC Cardiovasc Imaging*. March, 2012;5(3):239–251.
53. Ge S. Automated measurement of stroke volumes by real-time three-dimensional Doppler echocardiography: coming of age? *J Am Soc Echocardiogr*. January, 2012;25(1):66–67.

CHAPTER

5

QUANTITATIVE MEASUREMENT OF VOLUMES, MASS, AND FUNCTION FOR THE LEFT, RIGHT, AND SINGLE VENTRICLES

Rula S. Balluz, MD, MPH; Shuping Ge, MD

ABSTRACT

Two methods of real-time three-dimensional echocardiography (RT3DE) for the measurement of left ventricular (LV) volume, mass, and ejection fraction (EF) are the manual method and the semiautomated method, the latter of which has advantages. 3DE compares favorably with other independent reference standards such as cardiac magnetic resonance (CMR) imaging in assessing LV volumes, mass, and EF in children. For the right ventricle (RV), although CMR is the clinical standard for quantitative analysis, the evidence of usefulness of quantitative RT3DE is increasing. Two RT3DE methods for measuring RV volumes and systolic function without geometric assumptions are the disc summation method and the Beutel semiautomated method. Limitations relate to image quality, border clarity, and the difficulty in imaging the entire RV. In single-ventricle defect, RT3DE requires no geometric assumptions and is potentially suited for quantification of volumes and EF. The capability of RT3DE to capture the entire LV in three dimensions also offers the opportunity to quantify regional wall motion, LV synchrony, strain and strain rate by RT3DE and 3D speckle tracking methodologies.

INTRODUCTION

Quantitative measurement of left ventricular (LV) volumes, mass, and function is one of the most common and important indications for echocardiography. These measurements are among the most powerful tools for diagnosis and prognosis of congenital and acquired heart diseases and for assessment of medical, percutaneous, and surgical interventions. Awareness is also growing of the importance of right ventricular (RV) volume, mass, and function in many cardiopulmonary diseases. Furthermore, there are challenges and opportunities to measure the volume, mass, and function of complex chambers such as the left atrium, right atrium, and the univentricular heart. As echocardiography continues to be the imaging modality of choice for these measurements, the strengths and limitations of M-mode, two-dimensional (2D), and recently three-dimensional (3D) echocardiographic (3DE) methodologies for accurate and reproducible measurement of these indices have been extensively investigated for congenital and acquired heart diseases.

Evidence suggests that 3DE provides improved accuracy and reproducibility over 2D methods for the measurement of LV volume and function calculation in adults[1,2] and children.[3–9] Data have accumulated on the utility of 3DE for measuring chamber volumes and function for the RV and for the single ventricle,[2,10–13] which may become more widely used in clinical and research arenas in the future. Finally, new advanced modes of analysis such as 3D strain and synchrony analysis by 3DE are promising methodologies that warrant further investigation.

LEFT VENTRICULAR VOLUMES, EJECTION FRACTION, AND MASS

Methods of analysis

Three-dimensional echocardiographic instrumentation and data acquisition for the LV are presented in earlier chapters in this volume. Two methods exist for the analysis of LV volume, mass, and ejection fraction (EF): the manual method and the semiautomated method using real-time 3DE (RT3DE).

The manual method. Quantitative RT3DE data acquisition and analysis of the LV are usually performed through an apical acoustic window using a matrix-array transducer. The images are first optimized using the biplane mode to visualize all LV epicardial and endocardial contours. Subsequently, a large conical 3D full-volume data set with a field of view to include the LV, preferably the entire heart, is acquired. The full-volume data set is usually compiled from one single volume or from four or more subvolumes with electrocardiographic (ECG) triggering. The subjects are asked to hold their breath during acquisition, if possible. RT3DE images can be processed offline using a dedicated software analysis package (Fig. 5-1).[3] The 3D data set is displayed in a four-tile image screen. A total of eight slices of the LV along its long axis are obtained from a short-axis reference image at 22.5° increments around a 180° plane. The endocardial and epicardial borders are traced manually at end-systole and end-diastole. The papillary muscles are included within the LV cavity. The LV volumes, stroke volumes (SV), and EF are calculated using the software to perform an interactive splice algorithm. The LV mass is calculated as follows: LV mass (in grams) = 1.04 × volume, where volume (in milliliters) = end-systolic volume (ESV) epicardial - ESV endocardial.

The semiautomated method. Semiautomated methods have many advantages over manual methods.[5] Figure 5-2 shows the analysis of RT3DE data sets using commercial software (3DQ-QLab, Philips Medical Systems, Eindhoven, The Netherlands) used in our laboratory. The 3D data are displayed in three different cross-sections that can be modified interactively using the following color-coding convention: apical four-chamber view displayed in a green box (Fig. 5-2, top left); apical two-chamber view displayed in a red box (Fig. 5-2, top right); and short-axis view displayed in a blue box (Fig. 5-2, bottom left). Using this convention, the two- and four-chamber views with the largest long-axis dimensions are selected in the first time frame of the data set, that is, in end-diastole. In these two planes, five points, including four points on the mitral annulus (two in each plane) and the apex in either plane, are manually initialized to define the endocardial surface. Then, the initial endocardial surface is manually adjusted in multiple apical planes, while including the papillary muscles in the LV cavity, and its position is corrected as necessary until the best match is verified. Then, the voxel count inside the endocardial surface is used to calculate the end-diastolic volume (EDV), without geometric modeling. This analysis is then repeated for the end-systolic frame, which is identified as the frame that showed the smallest LV cavity, resulting in a measurement of ESV. EF is calculated from the ESV and EDV using the standard formula.[14]

History, validation, and clinical application

The utilization of echocardiography to assess LV chamber size and function dates to the advent of this technology. Popp et al.[15] reported on the change of cardiac dimensions using M-mode echocardiography. Feigenbaum et al.[16] used these changes to assess LV function and correlated it to angiography. The correlation

Figure 5-1

Offline analysis of RT3DE data. *Top*, Two cross-sections (four- and two-chamber equivalent views) along the LV long axis from RT3DE data set. Epicardial and endocardial borders of a total of eight LV long-axis slices at 22.5° increments were manually traced to calculate LV indexes. *Bottom left*, Short-axis section of LV used as reference image to obtain eight LV long-axis slices. *Bottom right*, Cubical display of entire 3D endocardial (gray) and epicardial volumes (brown). (From Bu et al.[3])

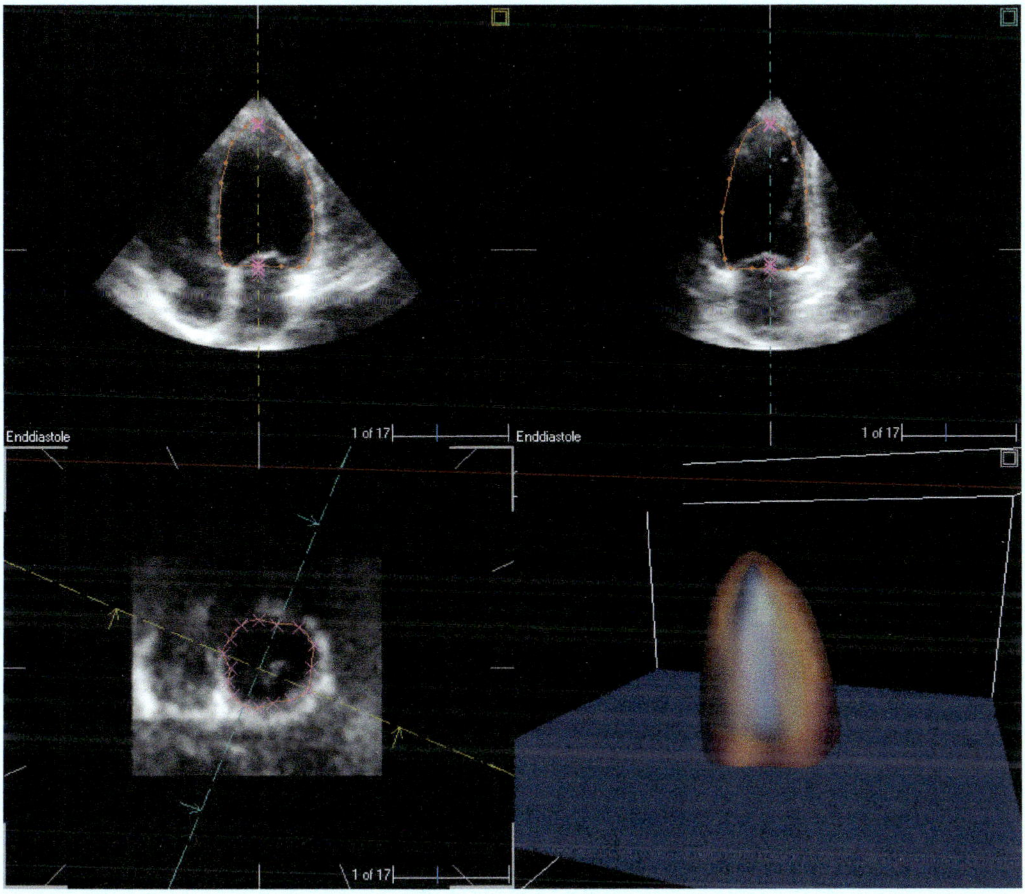

appeared good except in cases with dilatation and regional wall abnormalities. The development of 2DE allowed the utilization of LV area and the LV long axis to estimate volume. Wyatt et al.[17,18] showed that this technique was superior to M-mode, especially in asymmetrical hearts. This technique is limited by the fact that 3D measurements are extrapolated from 2D acquired data using geometrical assumptions. Also, on-axis cross-sectional images may not be accurate because the whole surface of the heart is not visualized. Finally, there may be problems with foreshortening the long axis of the ventricle. The logical next step is the development of 3D constructions of the LV to assess volumes and function.

Dekker et al.[19] first attempted to create 3D images with a mechanical arm, which resulted in creating a 3D model of the LV. Many investigators also published measurements of LV volumes using similar techniques with in vivo validation using animal and human models.[20–22] Sapin et al.[23] assessed LV volume using a 2D apical biplane method and 3D acoustic locator technique in 39 patients 1–4 hours before the patients underwent cineventriculography. These investigators concluded that the correlation between cineventriculography and 3DE was excellent, and the observed error was almost half the error obtained using

Figure 5-2

Semiautomated 3DE algorithm for measurement of LVEDV, LVESV, and LVEF. Apical four-chamber view is displayed in the green box (*top left*); apical two-chamber view displayed in the red box (*top right*); and the short-axis view is displayed in a blue box (*bottom left*). (From Lu et al.[5])

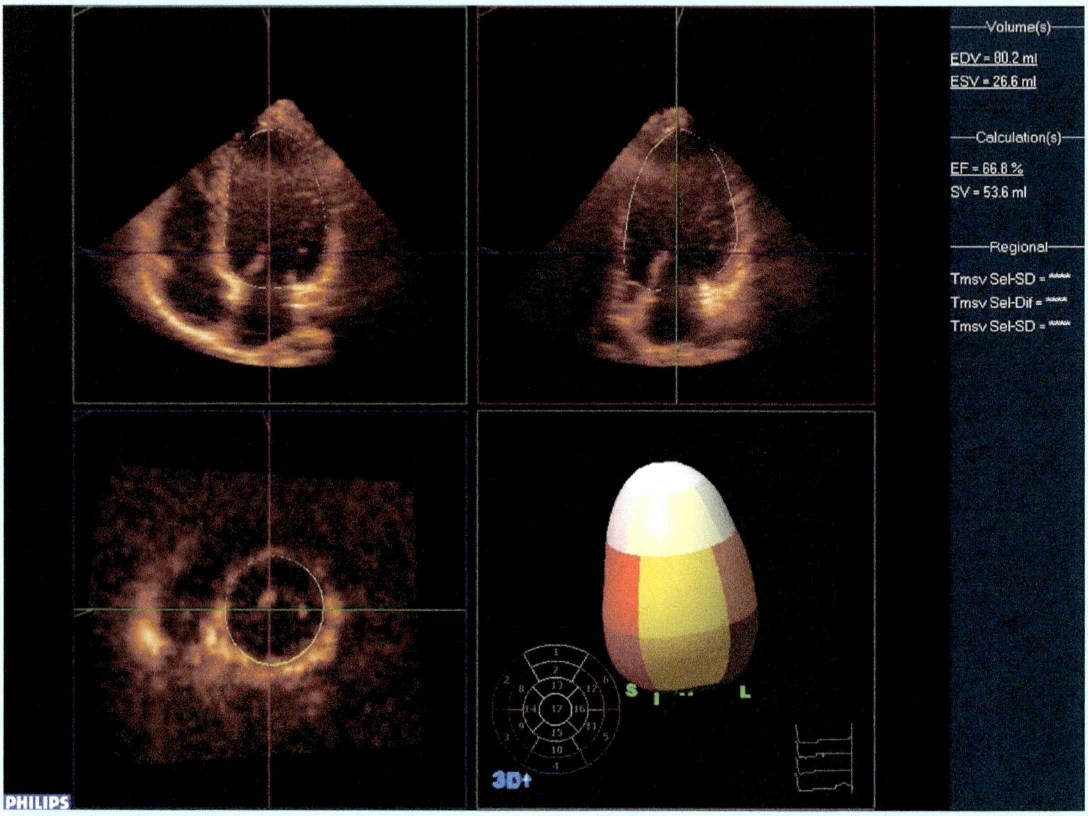

2D measurement. Keller[24] also used the 3D technique to assess LV volume and mass in comparison with both 2DE and cardiac magnetic resonance (CMR) imaging. This group also showed better correlation between 3D and CMR and small interobserver variability. Gopal et al.[25] used the free-hand scanning technique to compare 3D imaging with both 2D imaging and CMR in patients with abnormal ventricles. They studied 34 patients with abnormal ventricles and showed that the free-hand 3DE technique was superior to both M-mode and 2D measurement of LV function in this population compared to CMR. The ability of 3D technology to overcome geometric assumptions, avoid image positioning errors, and provide a surface reconstruction algorithm was the basis for this improvement, as confirmed by many subsequent studies.[26–29]

The advent of RT3DE generated a renewed enthusiasm for potential clinical use in the adult population. RT3DE has been shown to have excellent correlations with CMR for assessing chamber volumes and EF in adults, but it underestimates LV volumes with insignificant difference for the EF between the two modalities. Most studies found the differences in volume calculations to be more significant with dilated and abnormal ventricles.[30] Some experts propose including the endocardial surface with the trabeculations to improve the correlation with CMR.[31–33] Others suggest increasing the number of planes to better delineate the endocardial surface in an attempt to eliminate geometric assumptions, especially in abnormal ventricles.[34,35] Others have had more success using direct volumetric measurement through the use of semiautomated border detection. Table 5-1[29,32,34,36–44] summarizes large adult cohorts in the literature for validations of LV volumes by RT3DE in comparison with CMR, computed tomography (CT), angiography, and radionuclide scanning.

Table 5-1 Major studies comparing RT3DE with CMR for LV volume, mass, and EF

Study	Patients (*n*)	Imaging modality	Correlation coefficient (EDV/ESV/EF)
Caiani et al. (2005)[36]	46	CMR vs RT3DE	0.97/0.97/0.93
Jacobs et al. (2006)[37]	50	CMR vs RT3DE	0.89/0.92/0.86
Jenkins et al. (2006)[38]	110	CMR vs RT3DE	0.86/0.91/0.81
Nikitin et al. (2006)[39]	64	CMR vs RT3DE	0.97/0.98/0.94
Krenning et al. (2007)[40]	39	CMR vs RT3DE CMR vs RT3DE (contrast-enhanced borders)	0.86/0.94/0.81 0.97/0.96/0.94
Pouleur et al. (2008)[42]	83	CMR vs RT3DE	0.97/0.98/0.94
Qi et al. (2007)[41]	58	CMR vs RT3DE	0.94/0.92/0.91
Soliman et al. (2007)[34]	53	CMR vs RT3DE full-volume reconstruction CMR vs RT3DE multiplane interpolation	0.99/0.99/0.98 0.97/0.98/0.94
Chukwu et al. (2008)[29]	69	CMR vs RT3DE improved estimation with increased plane	0.93/0.87/0.66 biplane 0.97/0.89/0.61 4 plane 0.98/089/0.60 6 plane 0.99/0.95/0.95 8 plane 0.99/0.95/0.8 4 voxel-based
Mor-Avi et al. (2008)[32]	92	CMR vs RT3DE Multicenter study	0.91/0.93/0.81
Macron et al. (2010)[43]	66	CMR vs RT3DE single vs multibeat acquisition	0.92/0.93/0.85 single beat (not good resolution) 0.94/0.94/0.92 2 beats 0.93/0.94/0.88 4 beats Fewer beats → better estimation
Chang et al. (2011)[44]	109	CMR vs RT3DE single beat	0.94/0.91/0.91

Abbreviations: CMR, cardiac magnetic resonance; EF, ejection fraction; EDV, end-diastolic volume; ESV, end-systolic volume; RT3DE, real-time three-dimensional echocardiography.

Real-time 3DE has also been applied in adults with congenital heart disease for the measurement of LV volumes. van den Bosch et al.[45] studied 32 patients ranging from 19 to 51 years with complex congenital heart disease, including tetralogy of Fallot, RV obstructive lesions, and transposition of the great vessels after atrial switch surgery. Compared with CMR, RT3DE underestimated LV volume, but the difference was not statistically significant. These investigators found good correlations in LVEDV, LVESV, and LVEF between RT3DE by manual border detection and CMR, with correlation coefficients (r) = 0.98, 0.97, and 0.94, respectively. Correlations in LVEDV, LVESV, and EF were modest between CMR and RT3DE using automatic border detection in this study of ventricles with altered geometries (r = 0.79, 0.83, and 0.54, respectively).

Left ventricular mass

Real-time 3DE has also been utilized for the assessment of LV mass. The technique requires identification of both endocardial and epicardial borders. This has made estimation of LV mass more challenging in adult studies. A major challenge is the difficulty in visualizing the apex for mass calculation. However, validation studies showed better correlation between RT3DE and CMR compared with estimating LV mass estimation using M-mode or 2D methods, which have been reproduced in many adult studies.[5,38,42]

Meta-analysis. Shimada and Shiota[46] conducted a meta-analysis to assess the sources of errors in the evaluation of LV by 3DE. Their analysis included 3055 subjects in 95 studies. The study showed significant underestimation bias of both LVEDV and LVESV by RT3DE compared with CMR. The bias for the estimation of LVEF was not statistically significant. Sources of error included female sex, and in recent publications, presence of congenital heart disease and studies with larger patient numbers, which were associated with more underestimation in the analysis. Semiautomatic border detection and the use of matrix-array transducer were associated with less underestimation. Despite the differences between RT3DE volumetric estimation of the LV and CMR, the literature supports the role of RT3DE as both accurate and reproducible in assessing LV volume and LVEF, although it is not interchangeable with other radiologic modalities.

Shimada and Shiota[47] published another meta-analysis evaluating the use of RT3DE to assess LV mass. This analysis assessed 25 studies including 671 comparisons. Studies published in 2004 or earlier showed high heterogeneity (I(2) = 69%) and significant underestimation of LV mass by 3DE (–5.7 g, 95% confidence interval –11.3 to –0.2, P = 0.04). Studies published between 2005 and 2007 were still heterogeneous (I(2) = 60%) but showed less systematic bias (–0.5 g, 95% confidence interval –2.5 to 1.5, P = 0.63). In contrast, studies published in 2008 or later were highly homogeneous (I(2) = 3%) and showed excellent accuracy (–0.1 g, 95% confidence interval –2.2 to 1.9, P = 0.90). Investigation of factors affecting the bias revealed that evaluation of cardiac patients compared with healthy volunteers led to greater bias (P<0.05). In conclusion, this meta-analysis elucidates the underestimation of LV mass by 3DE, improvement of the technique over the past decade, and factors affecting the degree of bias. These data provide a detailed basis for improving the accuracy of 3DE, an indispensable step toward further clinical application.

Currently, for transthoracic and transesophageal assessment of LV volumes and EF, 3DE is recommended over the use of 2DE, as 3DE has been clearly demonstrated to provide more accurate and reproducible measurements.[2]

Left ventricle analysis in children

Although M-mode and 2DE recordings are widely used to assess LV size, mass, and global systolic function in children with congenital and acquired heart disease, in many defects LV or ventricular septal geometric or functional alterations diminish the accuracy and reproducibility of these measurements. Many validation studies have demonstrated that 3DE compares favorably with other independent reference standards such as CMR and is superior for assessing LV volumes, mass, and EF in children as well as adults (Table 5-2).[3–9]

Table 5-2 RT3DE for LV volumes, mass, and function in children

Study	Patients (*n*)	RT3DE compared with other methods	Methods	LV indices	Correlation
Bu et al. (2005)[3]	19	CMR	Long-axis, 8 planes	LVEDV, LVESV, LV mass, LVEF, SV	$r = 0.86–0.97$
Iino et al. (2007)[4]	25	LV angiography	Semiautomated	LVEDV and LVEF	$r = 0.979–0.996$
Lu et al. (2008)[5]	20	CMR	4-plane, 8-plane semiautomated	LVEDV, LVESV, LV mass, LVEF, SV	$r = 0.85–0.9$
Riehle et al. (2008)[6]	12	CMR	Semiautomated	LVEDV, LVESV, LV mass, LVEF, SV	$r = 0.93–0.99$, 0.69 for EF
Friedberg et al. (2010)[7]	35	CMR	Disc summation	LVEDV, LVESV, LVEF	$r = 0.90–0.96$
Hascoet et al. (2010)[8]	50	RT3DE	Semiautomated (Qlab vs TomTec)	LVEDV, LVESV, LV mass, LVEF, SV	$r > 0.97$ but 0.79 for EF
Laser et al. (2010)[9]	49	CMR	2 Ultrasound systems/ semiautomated	LVEDV and LVESV	$r = 0.91–0.95$

Abbreviations: CMR, cardiac magnetic resonance; EF, ejection fraction; EDV, end-diastolic volume; ESV, end-systolic volume; LV, left ventricular; RT3DE, real-time three-dimensional echocardiography.

Since our first validation of RT3DE by CMR,[3] seven RT3DE studies have been published comparing measurements of LV volumes, mass, and EF with CMR measurements.[3–9] These reports showed excellent correlation, agreement, and reproducibility for volumes and mass between the two modalities but only modest advantages in the measurement of EF. We have also found that RT3DE using a semiautomated method is more accurate and reproducible than M-mode or Simpson's 2D biplane method and is as efficient as 2DE in children.[5] These findings suggest that the American Society of Echocardiography's recommendation that in adults LV should be quantified using RT3DE may also be applied to children.[1,2]

Studies of LV mass assessment in children are very limited. However, the available studies report excellent correlations between RT3DE and CMR, although RT3DE overestimated LV mass in comparison with CMR in most of these studies. Inter- and intraobserver variability in this assessment are excellent.[3,5–7] These data suggest that RT3DE quantification of LV mass is feasible for clinical applications, although the normal ranges of LV volumes, mass, and EF in various age groups must still be defined.

RIGHT VENTRICULAR VOLUMES, EJECTION FRACTION, AND MASS

Because of the complex geometry of the right ventricle (RV), clinical assessment of its size, mass, and EF has largely been qualitative. However, the importance of RV chamber size and systolic function has increasingly been recognized in both pediatric and adult heart disease. Many volume and pressure overloading conditions can cause remodeling and dysfunction of the RV. Studies in children who have undergone repair of tetralogy of Fallot have shown that longitudinal follow-up of RV and LV remodeling and dysfunction is crucial to guide timely intervention to replace the pulmonary valve to avoid failure of the RV, arrhythmia, and sudden cardiac death. Although CMR has been established as a clinical standard for quantitative analysis of the RV, quantitative RT3DE may be useful in many instances, for example, as a potential screening tool and in those in whom CMR is contraindicated or not available. Because of the cost, portability, and availability of RT3DE and the growing evidence of the utility of RV3DE, the application of RV3DE for quantitative analysis of the RV may increase in the future.

Methods of analysis

Two RT3DE methods are available for measuring RV volumes and systolic function without geometric assumptions: the disc summation method[10] (Fig. 5-3) and the Beutel semiautomated method[11] (Fig. 5-4).

Data acquisition. Real-time 3DE is performed using an apical window and views and a matrix-array transducer. The images are first optimized using biplane mode, a simultaneous display of modified four- and two-chamber views, to visualize the RV inflow and outflow tracts. Subsequently, a full-volume 3D data set with optimized angle to include the entire RV, line density, and frame rate is acquired. The full-volume data set is compiled from a single full-volume set or from ECG-triggered acquisition of subvolumes. The subjects are asked to hold their breath during acquisition.

The disc summation method. All RT3DE images are processed offline using a dedicated analysis software package.[10] The 3D data set is displayed in a four-tile image screen (Fig. 5-3A). By using the navigation tools and manipulation of the *x*, *y*, and *z* planes of the data set, the RV images are displayed in short-axis views

Figure 5-3

The disc summation method for the measurement of RV volumes and EF in children. Manual tracing of the RV endocardial contours was performed on a stack of short-axis images. The four-chamber views and coronal views are used as reference images. Simpson's principle is used to derive RVEDV, RVESV, and RVEF. (From Lu et al.[10])

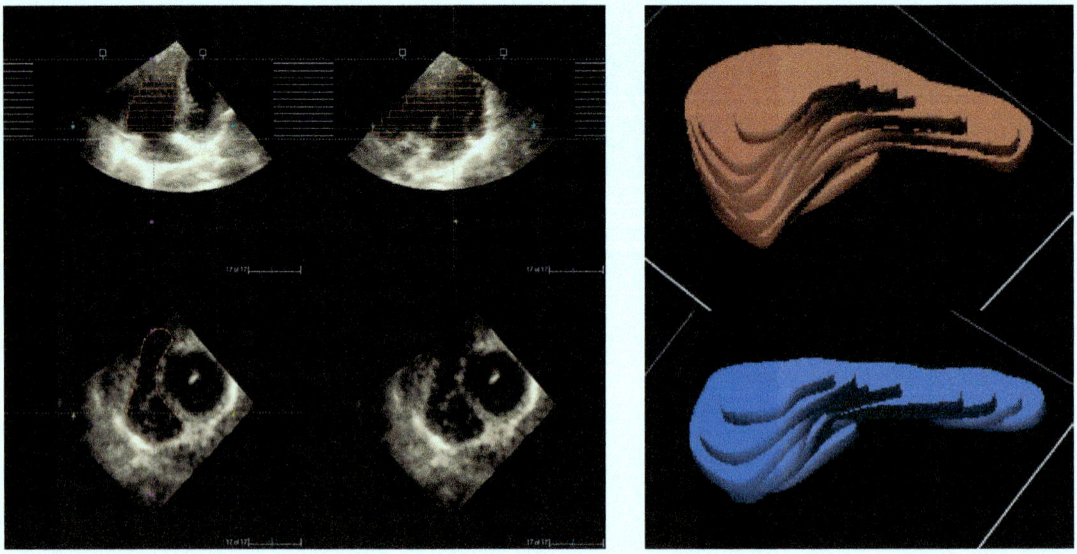

Figure 5-4

The semiautomated method for the measurement of the RV indices.

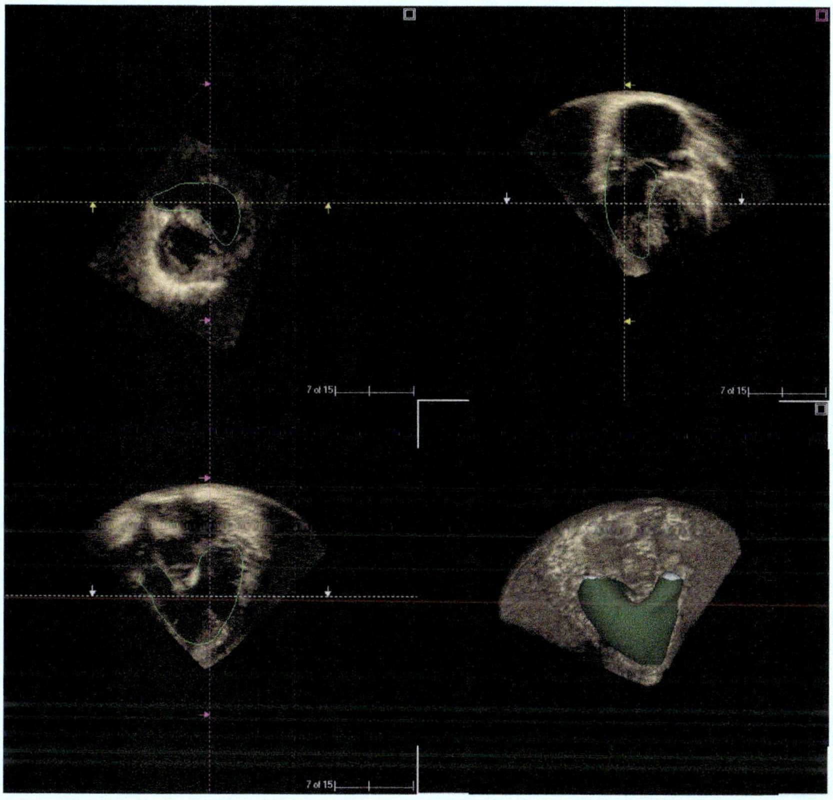

from the apex to the base for measurement of RV volumes. Three reference views—modified four-chamber, two-chamber, and dynamic short-axis views (Fig. 5-3)—are used to assist in the identification of the RV inflow, trabecular, and outflow portions for endocardial border tracing. RV volume measurement starts from the tricuspid annulus by a set of short-axis disks parallel to the tricuspid annulus and ends at the RV apex. The RV end-systolic and end-diastolic endocardial borders are traced manually in contiguous 5-mm slices. Large trabeculations and papillary muscles are not included in chamber volumes. These volumetric slices (planimetered area × slice thickness) are summated based on Simpson's principle to provide the RV volumes in end-systole and end-diastole (Fig. 5-3). The RVEF is calculated as: RVEF (%) = (EDV – ESV)/EDV × 100%.

The Beutel semiautomated method. Analysis through the Beutel semiautomated method is performed with dedicated software (Fig. 5-4).[11] All RT3DE data are imported and analyzed in three sets of views: a sagittal view (to profile the tricuspid valve and RV inflow), a four-chamber view (to profile the apex), and a coronal view (to profile the RV inflow and the outflow), to obtain all the major landmarks of the RV. Manual tracings of these landmarks are adjusted before the algorithm fills in the rest of the endocardial borders to calculate the RV volumes by summing the areas for each slice through the complete volume data set. Contrast, zoom, shading, and color are used to improve delineation of the endocardium. The software analysis uses a semiautomated border detection algorithm with manual correction options based on normal as well as pathologic RV modeling. Global and tripartite (inflow, trabecular, and outlet portion of the RV) ESV, EDV, SV, and EF are computed.

Validation and clinical studies

Unlike the LV, there is no established geometric model that can be used for quantitative analysis of RV volumes, mass, and function. Clinical evaluation of RV size and function is largely qualitative for both adults and children. Quantitative analysis of the RV becomes a major potential application for 3DE, especially since RT3DE hardware and software have become available. Initial validation studies of RV volumes and EF quantification by 3DE were based on in vitro and in vivo models.[48–54] Multiple clinical studies in adults followed, comparing RT3DE volumes with CMR (Table 5-3).[55–60]

RV analysis in children and in patients with congenital heart disease. Our group[10] used a disc-summation method and studied 20 normal children between the ages of 6 and 18 years comparing RV volumes and function obtained with RT3DE versus CMR. We found excellent correlation between RT3DE and CMR, with correlation coefficients of 0.96, 0.98, and 0.89 for RVESV, RVEDV, and RVEF, respectively.

Table 5-3 3DE studies for assessing right ventricular volumes and ejection fraction in comparison with CMR

Study	Age (y)	Patients (*n*)	Patient characteristics	Imaging modality	Correlation coefficients	Results
Kjaergaard et al. (2006)[55]	59–78	30	Normal subjects and CVD	CMR vs TTE	EDV/ESV 0.56/0.62	Volume overestimation NS; EF underestimation
Nesser et al. (2006)[56]	23–74	20	Normal subjects and CVD	CMR vs TTE/ TEE	TEE EDV/ESV/EF 0.97/0.92/0.84 TTE EDV/ESV/EF 0.95/0.94/0.85	ESV overestimation by both TEE, TTE, NS; EDV underestimation by both TEE, TTE, NS EF underestimation
Gopal et al. (2007)[57]	42–70	17	Healthy volunteers	CMR vs TEE	RT3DE disc summation RVEDV/ESV/EF 0.9/0.8/0.8 Apical rotation RVEDS/ESV/EF 0.8/0.8/0.7	RV volume underestimation both 2D and 3D with superior correlation between RT3DE and CMR
Jenkins et al. (2007)[58]	51–73	50	CVD	CMR vs TTE	EDC/ESV/EF 0.6/0.55/0.72	Better correlation between RT3DE and CMR compared to 2D and CMR
Sugeng et al. (2010)[59]	35–71	28	Congenital heart disease and other CVD	CMR vs TTE, CT	TTE EDV/ESV/EF 0.87/0.89/0.877	Volume underestimation of by RT3DE; wider range of error, overestimation of volumes by CT
Leibundgut et al. (2010)	33–62	80	CVD	CMR vs TTE	RVEDV/ESV/EF 0.84/0.83/0.72	Volume underestimation by RT3DE, EF, NS

Abbreviations: CMR, cardiac magnetic resonance; CVD, cardiovascular disease; EF, ejection fraction; ESV, end-systolic volume; NS, no significance; RT3DE, real-time three-dimensional echocardiography; TEE, transesophageal echocardiography; TTE, transthoracic echocardiography.

We also found good inter- and intraobserver variability. There was small but significant underestimation of RV volume, especially RVEDV, by RT3DE compared with CMR. The differences were not statistically significant for RVESV and RVEF. Niemann et al.[11] used a Beutel semiautomated method to study 17 adults and 16 children with congenital heart disease, including tetralogy of Fallot, transposition of the great arteries, truncus arteriosus, atrial septal defect, ventricular septal defect (VSD), coarctation of the aorta, and atrioventricular septal defect. They used a semiautomated border detection method in comparison with CMR. Excellent correlation was obtained, with correlation coefficients of 0.99 for RVESV, 0.95 for RVEDV, and 0.97 for EF.

As seen in adults with cardiovascular disease,[61–67] including congenital heart disease,[62–67] quantitative analysis of RV volumes and EF using RT3DE is also feasible in children. The limitations of RT3DE for quantitative analysis of the RV are related to image quality, border clarity, and the difficulty imaging the entire RV, especially in patients with an enlarged RV, such as those who have undergone repair of tetralogy of Fallot.

Meta-analysis. Shimada et al.[68] performed a meta-analysis of published studies comparing assessment of RV volumes and EF by RT3DE versus CMR. The analysis included 23 studies and 807 adults and children. They concluded that compared with CMR, 3DE significantly underestimated RVESV, RVEDV, and EF, particularly in patients with larger volumes (>200 mL) and in younger patients (≤18 years). There was no improvement for the analysis with time. The use of matrix-array transducer did not improve the correlation, either. There was no statistical difference with the use of automated compared with manual border detection. Although RT3DE is highly promising for the evaluation of RV indices, further investigation is warranted to address the limited feasibility and accuracy for clinical use.[2]

SINGLE VENTRICULAR VOLUMES, EJECTION FRACTION, AND MASS

One of the most complex types of congenital heart disease in children is the functional single ventricle. These patients often require two to three stages of palliation, ultimately resulting in a Fontan type of palliation, and they often have long-term structural and functional complications, arrhythmias, exercise intolerance, and limited neurodevelopmental outcomes. RT3DE requires no geometric assumptions and is ideally suited for quantification of volumes and EF for this type of congenital heart disease.

Altman et al.[69] first used acoustic spatial locator 3D reconstructive technology to assess the volume and EF of single ventricles with LV morphology, comparing 3DE with 2DE and CMR. They studied 12 patients and showed superior agreement with less data scatter in ESV, EDV, mass, and EF between 3DE (bias 3.4 ± 5.5 mL, 14.2 ± 8.3 mL, 5.8 ± 8.4 g, and 4.4% ± 5.3%, respectively) and CMR than between 3DE and 2DE (-2.9 ± 8.1 mL, 2.9 ± 10.4 mL, -8.3 ± 12.0 g, and 8.5% ± 10.3%, respectively). The inter- and intraobserver variabilities were more favorable for 3DE (5.7%–7.1%) compared with CMR than for 3DE compared with 2DE (10%–24%). Altman et al. concluded that 3DE provides estimates of ventricular volumes, EF, and mass that are comparable to CMR in this select group of patients with single ventricles of LV morphology.

Soriano et al.[70] applied RT3DE for the estimation of volumes, mass, and EF in patients with single ventricles using a disc-summation technique. RT3DE was feasible in 27 of 29 patients (93%). The RT3DE EDV correlated well but was smaller than with CMR, and 3DE EF was smaller than with CMR. There was no significant difference in the measurements of ESV or mass. The 3DE interobserver differences for mass and volumes were not significant except for the measurement of EF. Intraobserver differences were not significant. Soriano et al. speculated that the modest correlation in EF between RT3DE and CMR was related in part to the small range of EFs in this single-ventricle population. This study suggested that RT3DE quantification of EDV, ESV, mass, and EF in patients with single ventricles is feasible, reproducible, and reasonably accurate, except in the measurement of EF and warrants further validation.

We[71] showed that a long-axis, eight-plane Simpson's technique is also feasible to assess volumes and EF for the functional single ventricle. Furthermore, our study showed that EF values are an independent predictor of transplant-free survival for this group. EF less than 40% is associated with significantly lower rates of transplant-free survival in this group of patients.

3D ANALYSIS OF REGIONAL WALL MOTION, SYNCHRONY, AND STRAIN

Regional wall motion and synchrony

The capability of RT3DE to capture the entire LV in three dimensions offers the opportunity not only to assess global LV function more accurately and reproducibly but also to quantify the regional function of the 16 LV segments and to assess LV interventricular synchrony. To analyze LV regional function and synchrony, the cyclic changes of the volumes of each of the 16 LV segments are plotted against time over the course of the cardiac cycle (Fig. 5-2). The volume curves and plots allow measurement of volume changes of each segment (i.e., segmental motion) and temporal differences of each segment to minimum volume (i.e., synchrony). Regional minimal volume (i.e., maximal contraction) normally occurs at the same time in ventricular systole for all segments. The systolic dyssynchrony index (SDI) is calculated as the standard deviation of time to regional minimal volume of the segments.

Studies in the pediatric literature have validated the use of this new technology to assess LV synchrony in volume and pressure loading conditions, the effect of ventricular septal patch repair to LV synchrony, and outcome of resynchronization therapy in patients with a single ventricle with LV morphology. Kobayashi et al.[72] prospectively studied 27 children with end-stage renal disease (13 on peritoneal dialysis and 14 on hemodialysis) and 29 normal controls. SDI was normalized to cardiac cycle duration (SDIp). SDIp (16 segments) and LV mass were significantly greater in the hemodialysis group. SDI and SDIp (16 segments) improved after a hemodialysis session ($P < 0.05$); LV mass and LV mass index remained unchanged. LV dyssynchrony was significantly greater in patients with LV hypertrophy compared with those without. Their study demonstrated an association between LV volume load and LV hypertrophy with significant LV dyssynchrony in end-stage renal disease. SDI may provide a sensitive marker for mechanistic and early detection of LV dysfunction.

Veeram et al.[73] studied patients with large VSDs who underwent surgical patch closure during infancy. They investigated the long-term effects of the presence of akinetic patch in the ventricular septum and postoperative right bundle branch block (RBBB) on LV mechanical synchrony and global systolic function. Their study showed that pediatric patients 5–10 years after VSD patch closure have normal LV function. The presence of the RBBB was associated with mechanical dyssynchrony and tendency toward LV dilatation in this group of patients. Veeram et al. demonstrated that RT3DE is a sensitive technique for assessing LV synchrony in postoperative VSD patients, especially those with RBBB, who require long-term follow-up for potential complications.

Finally, Bacha et al.[74] performed multisite pacing studies in 26 patients undergoing stepwise single-ventricle palliation. RT3DE was used in 10 subjects. They observed significant response to multisite pacing, including (1) improvement in QRS duration in 24 of 26 patients (93.9 ± 17.5 ms vs 71.7 ± 10.8 ms; $P < 0.001$); (2) increase in systolic blood pressure in 25 of 26 patients (86.3 ± 20.0 mm Hg vs 93.8 ± 20.2 mm Hg; $P < 0.001$); (3) increase in cardiac index in 21 of 22 patients (3.2 ± 0.8 vs 3.7 ± 1.0 L × min^{-1} × m^{-2}; $P < 0.001$); and (4) improvement in index of asynchrony in eight of 10 patients (10.3 ± 4.8 vs 6.0 ± 1.4; $P < 0.04$). The study suggests that RT3DE is potentially useful in assessing cardiac resynchronization therapy even in cases with complex geometries.

Strain analysis by RT3DE

Conventional indices of regional and global ventricular function, defined by endocardial excursion, such as fractional shortening and EF, are considered to be load-dependent.[75,76] Myocardial velocities by tissue Doppler imaging (TDI) do not rely on geometric assumptions but are inherently unidimensional, angle-dependent, variable with aging, and influenced by anthropometrics and heart rate.[77,78] Myocardial strain has been shown to be more robust for assessment of regional ventricular myocardial function using both echocardiography and CMR.[79–83] TDI-based strain analysis has been extensively validated and has been shown to be limited as a one-dimensional and angle-dependent method.[79] Recently, 2D speckle tracking echocardiography (2DSTE) has been introduced as a new method to quantify myocardial strain. This technique measures myocardial deformation by means of frame-by-frame tracking and motion analysis of speckles within B-mode images.

Validation studies with tagged CMR and sonomicrometry in adults[79,80] and children[84,85] have provided evidence that 2DSTE is a reliable method for determining ventricular myocardial function. 2DSTE has many limitations, however. First, myocardial deformation measurement by 2DSTE is affected by loss of speckles due to motion outside the imaging plane.[86] Second, 2DSTE has limited reproducibility, likely owing to the variabilities in the choice of image planes and lack of standardization in image analysis.[87] Finally, the analysis is cumbersome and six planes are needed for complete analysis, which is a major limitation for automation and potential clinical use.

Recently, the advent of three-dimensional speckle tracking echocardiography (3DSTE) has shown the potential to overcome the limitations of 2DSTE imaging for the assessment of LV global and regional systolic function. This method tracks the motion of speckles within the scan volume, allowing more complete and accurate assessment of myocardial deformation in 3D space[88–91] by avoiding the loss of speckles due to out-of-plane motion. 3DSTE has been validated for the quantification of LV volumes[91] and LV wall motion in ischemic heart disease[92] in adults. Nonetheless, data are scarce and incomplete for children with or without congenital heart disease.[84,85,93] Thus, feasibility, reproducibility, maturational changes, and normal values in this population must be shown before these indices can be used for assessing LV function for diagnosis, prognosis, and risk stratification of various congenital and acquired heart diseases in the young before and after medical, percutaneous, and surgical intervention.

We used RT3DE to study 256 consecutive healthy subjects using full-volume 3D data acquisition with a 3D matrix-array transducer.[94] Study subjects were divided into five age groups: group 1 (birth to age 1 year); group 2 (1–5 years); group 3 (6–9 years); group 4 (10–13 years); and group 5 (14–18 years). The 3D LV global strain (GS), global longitudinal peak systolic strain (GLS), global radial peak systolic strain (GRS), and global circumferential peak systolic strain (GCS) values were determined using modality-independent software (Fig. 5-5). A total of 228 cases (89%) were adequate for analysis and 28 cases (11%) were excluded, including

Figure 5-5

Three-dimensional speckle tracking echocardiography (3DSTE) offline analysis. *A*, Position the landmarks. First, select one of the long-axis views, place mitral valve (MV) landmark at the annulus level in the middle of the MV, and place apex landmark at the apex. Then, select short-axis view. Place aortic valve (AV) landmark at valve level in the middle of the AV. *B*, Semiautomated endocardial border identification and tracking. *C*, Manual tracking revision, if needed. *D*, LV systolic strain parameters can be calculated and displayed.

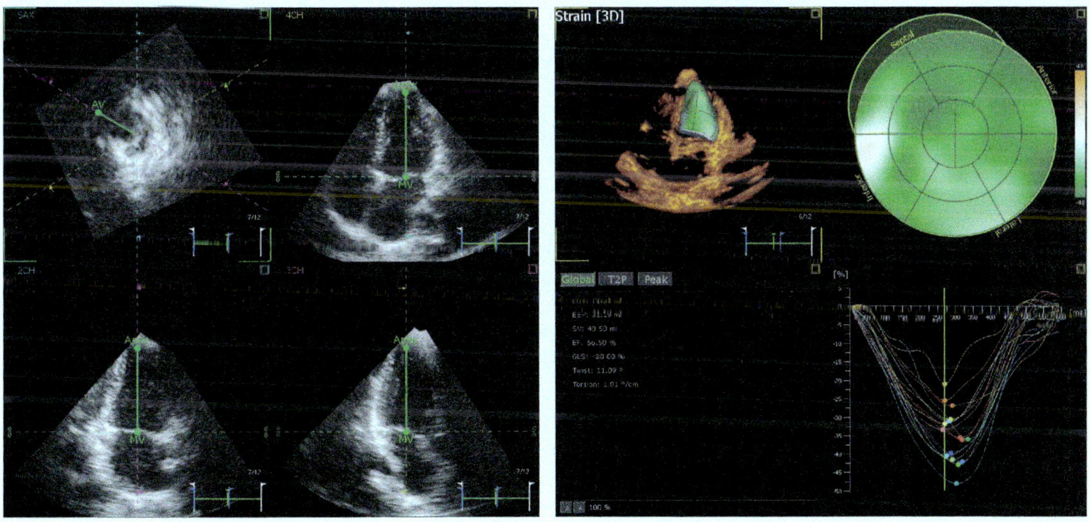

10 cases excluded owing to the low frame rates as determined by the system and 18 cases excluded owing to poor 3D images. We found statistically significant differences among the five age groups for GLS and GCS, but no statistical difference between the age groups for GRS and GS values. Multiple linear regression analyses showed that LV and RV dimension, mass, volume, and EF were significantly associated with GLS, GAS, GRS, and GCS. The interobserver variability of 3D systolic strain parameters ranged from 1.2% to 9.5%, and intraobserver variability ranged from 0.5% to 3.8%. Our study concluded that global 3D systolic strain measurement using the new 3D RT STE is feasible and reproducible in children. GLS and GCS are higher in early puberty and lower in late puberty compared with infancy and early childhood. GRS and GS have no maturational changes. Future work will define the Z-scores for these measurements and in various congenital and acquired heart diseases for potential clinical application and research.

To use this new methodology to evaluate LV strain and function, Saltijeral et al.[95] evaluated 30 consecutive, nonselected obese children and 42 healthy volunteer children using a similar RT3DE wall motion tracking method. They found statistically significant differences in interventricular septum thickness, LV posterior wall thickness, LV EDV, LV ESV, left atrium volume, LV mass, and lateral annulus peak velocity between the groups as well as in all the 3D wall motion tracking variables. By multivariate logistic regression analysis, the strongest relationship with obesity was found for LV average circumferential strain (β coefficient = 0.74; $r^2 = 0.55$; $P = 0.003$). Their data suggested that obesity-related cardiomyopathy is associated not only with structural cardiac changes but also with myocardial deformation changes occurring in childhood. Assessment of LV circumferential strain using 3D wall motion tracking is a marker with promising sensitivity for identifying obesity-related cardiomyopathy.

FUTURE PERSPECTIVES

Much evidence suggests that in the presence of adequate image quality, LV volumes, mass, and EF measurements by 3DE agree more closely with CMR measurements and have better reproducibility than does 2DE, making 3DE the modality of choice for the everyday clinical evaluation of LV volumes and EF. Quantitative analysis of volumes, mass, and EF for the RV and for single ventricles holds great promise and warrants future investigation. New modes of regional wall motion, strain, and LV dyssynchrony assessment using RT3DE are in the forefront of active research. Future advancements in hardware are expected to allow acquisition of wide-angle 3D data from the entire heart in a single cardiac cycle, with higher spatial and temporal resolution. We anticipate that further development in automatic quantitative analysis algorithms and software will make RT3DE an integral clinical methodology for diagnosis, prognosis, and assessment of medical, percutaneous, and surgical intervention for congenital heart disease.[96]

REFERENCES

1. Hung J, Lang R, Flachskampf F, et al. American Society of Echocardiography. 3D echocardiography: a review of the current status and future directions. *J Am Soc Echocardiogr*. 2007;20(3):213–233.
2. Lang RM, Badano LP, Tsang W, et al. EAE/ASE recommendations for image acquisition and display using three-dimensional echocardiography. *J Am Soc Echocardiogr*. 2012;25(1):3–46.
3. Bu L, Munns S, Zhang H, et al. Rapid full volume data acquisition by real-time 3-dimensional echocardiography for assessment of left ventricular indexes in children: a validation study compared with magnetic resonance imaging. *J Am Soc Echocardiogr*. 2005;18:299–305.
4. Iino M, Shiraishi H, Ichihashi K, et al. Volume measurement of the left ventricle in children using real-time three-dimensional echocardiography: comparison with ventriculography. *J Cardiol*. 2007;49:221–229.
5. Lu X, Xie M, Tomberlin D, et al. How accurately, reproducibly, and efficiently can we measure left ventricular indices using M-mode, 2-dimensional, and 3-dimensional echocardiography in children? *Am Heart J*. 2008;155:946–953.
6. Riehle TJ, Mahle WT, Parks WJ, et al. Real-time three-dimensional echocardiographic acquisition and quantification of left ventricular indices in children and young adults with congenital heart disease: comparison with magnetic resonance imaging. *J Am Soc Echocardiogr*. 2008;21:78–83.

7. Friedberg MK, Su X, Tworetzky W, et al. Validation of 3D echocardiographic assessment of left ventricular volumes, mass, and ejection fraction in neonates and infants with congenital heart disease: a comparison study with cardiac MRI. *Circ Cardiovasc Imaging*. 2010;3:735–742.
8. Hascoet S, Brierre G, Caudron G, et al. Assessment of left ventricular volumes and function by real time three-dimensional echocardiography in a pediatric population: a TomTec versus QLAB comparison. *Echocardiography*. 2010;27:1263–1273.
9. Laser KT, Bunge M, Hauffe P, et al. Left ventricular volumetry in healthy children and adolescents: comparison of two different real-time three-dimensional matrix transducers with cardiovascular magnetic resonance. *Eur J Echocardiogr*. 2010;11:138–148.
10. Lu X, Nadvoretskiy V, Bu L, et al. Accuracy and reproducibility of real-time three-dimensional echocardiography for assessment of right ventricular volumes and ejection fraction in children. *J Am Soc Echocardiogr*. 2008;21:84–89.
11. Niemann PS, Pinho L, Balbach T, et al. Anatomically oriented right ventricular volume measurements with dynamic three-dimensional echocardiography validated by 3-Tesla magnetic resonance imaging. *J Am Coll Cardiol*. 2007;50:1668–1676.
12. Soriano BD, Hoch M, Ithuralde A, et al. Matrix-array 3-dimensional echocardiographic assessment of volumes, mass, and ejection fraction in young pediatric patients with a functional single ventricle: a comparison study with cardiac magnetic resonance. *Circulation*. 2008;117:1842–1848.
13. Fu M, Choi G, Xie MX, et al. Quantitative real-time 3D echocardiography predicts adverse outcomes in functional single ventricle patients. *J Am Soc Echocardiogr*. 2010;23:B54.
14. Mor-Avi V, Jenkins C, Kuhl HP, et al. Real-time 3-dimensional echocardiographic quantification of left ventricular volumes: multicenter study for validation with magnetic resonance imaging and investigation of sources of error. *JACC Cardiovasc Imaging*. 2008;1(4):413–423.
15. Popp RL, Wolfe SB, Hirata T, Feigenbaum H. Estimation of right and left ventricular size by ultrasound: a study of the echoes from the interventricular septum. *Am J Cardiol*. 1969;24:523–530.
16. Feigenbaum H, Popp RL, Wolfe SB, et al. Ultrasound measurements of the left ventricle: a correlative study with angiocardiography. *Arch Intern Med*. 1972;129:461–467.
17. Wyatt HL, Heng MK, Meerbaum S, et al. Cross-sectional echocardiography. II. Analysis of mathematic models for quantifying volume of the formalin-fixed left ventricle. *Circulation*. 1980;61:1119–1125.
18. Wyatt HL, Meerbaum S, Heng MK, et al. Cross-sectional echocardiography. III. Analysis of mathematic models for quantifying volume of symmetric and asymmetric left ventricles. *Am Heart J*. 1980;100:821–828.
19. Dekker D, Piziali RL, Dong E. A system for ultrasonically imaging the human heart in three dimensions. *Comput Biomed Res*. 1974;7:544–553.
20. Matsumoto M, Inoue M, Tamura S, et al. Three-dimensional echocardiography for spatial visualization and volume calculation of cardiac structures. *J Clin Ultrasound*. 1981;9:157–165.
21. Ariet M, Geiser EA, Lupkiewicz SM, et al. Evaluation of a three-dimensional reconstruction to compute left ventricular volume and mass. *Am J Cardiol*. 1984;54:415–420.
22. Moritz WE, Pearlman AS, McCabe DH, et al. An ultrasonic technique for imaging the ventricle in three dimensions and calculating its volume. *IEEE Trans Biomed Eng*. 1983;30:482–491.
23. Sapin PM, Schroder KM, Gopal AS, et al. Comparison of two- and three-dimensional echocardiography with cineventriculography for measurement of left ventricular volume in patients. *J Am Coll Cardiol*. 1994;24:1054–1063.
24. Keller AM. Positional localization: three-dimensional transthoracic echocardiographic techniques for the measurement of cardiac mass, volume, and function. *Echocardiography*. 2000,17:745–748.
25. Gopal AS, Schnellbaecher MJ, Shen Z, et al. Freehand three-dimensional echocardiography for determination of left ventricular volume and mass in patients with abnormal ventricles: comparison with magnetic resonance imaging. *J Am Soc Echocardiogr*. 1997;10(8):853–861.
26. Siu SC, Rivera JM, Guerrero JL, et al. Three-dimensional echocardiography. In vivo validation for left ventricular volume and function. *Circulation*. 1993, 88:1715–1723.
27. Kupferwasser I, Mohr-Kahaly S, Stähr P, et al. Transthoracic three-dimensional echocardiographic volumetry of distorted left ventricles using rotational scanning. *J Am Soc Echocardiogr*. 1997;10(8):840–852.
28. Nosir YF, Salustri A, Kasprzak JD, et al. Left ventricular ejection fraction in patients with normal and distorted left ventricular shape by three-dimensional echocardiographic methods: a comparison with radionuclide angiography. *J Am Soc Echocardiogr*. 1998;11(6):620–630.
29. Chukwu EO, Barasch E, Mihalatos DG, et al. Relative importance of errors in left ventricular quantitation by two-dimensional echocardiography: insights from three-dimensional echocardiography and cardiac magnetic resonance imaging. *J Am Soc Echocardiogr*. 2008;21(9):990–997.

30. Gutiérrez-Chico JL, Zamorano JL, Pérez de Isla L, et al. Comparison of left ventricular volumes and ejection fractions measured by three-dimensional echocardiography versus by two-dimensional echocardiography and cardiac magnetic resonance in patients with various cardiomyopathies. *Am J Cardiol.* 2005;95(6):809–813.
31. Corsi C, Lamberti C, Catalano O, et al. Improved quantification of left ventricular volumes and mass based on endocardial and epicardial surface detection from cardiac MR images using level set models. *J Cardiovasc Magn Reson.* 2005;7:595–602.
32. Mor-Avi V, Jenkins C, Kuhl HP, et al. Real-time 3D echocardiographic quantification of left ventricular volumes: multicenter study for validation with magnetic resonance imaging and investigation of sources of error. *J Am Coll Cardiol Imaging.* 2008;1:413–423.
33. Mor-Avi V, Sugeng L, Weinert L, et al. Fast measurement of left ventricular mass with real-time three-dimensional echocardiography: comparison with magnetic resonance imaging. *Circulation.* 2004;110: 1814–1818.
34. Soliman OI, Krenning BJ, Geleijnse ML, et al. Quantification of left ventricular volumes and function in patients with cardiomyopathies by real-time three-dimensional echocardiography: a head-to-head comparison between two different semiautomated endocardial border detection algorithms. *J Am Soc Echocardiogr.* 2007;20:1042–1049.
35. Yao GH, Li F, Zhang C, et al. How many planes are required to get an accurate and timesaving measurement of left ventricular volume and function by real-time three-dimensional echocardiography in acute myocardial infarction? *Ultrasound Med Biol.* 2007;33:1572–1578.
36. Caiani EG, Corsi C, Zamorano J, et al. Improved semiautomated quantification of left ventricular volumes and ejection fraction using 3-dimensional echocardiography with a full matrix-array transducer: comparison with magnetic resonance imaging. *J Am Soc Echocardiogr.* 2005;18(8):779–788.
37. Jacobs LD, Salgo IS, Goonewardena S, et al. Rapid online quantification of left ventricular volume from real-time three-dimensional echocardiographic data. *Eur Heart J.* 2006;27:460–468.
38. Jenkins C, Chan J, Hanekom L, et al. Accuracy and feasibility of online three-dimensional echocardiography for measurement of left ventricular parameters. *J Am Soc Echocardiogr.* 2006;19:1119–1128.
39. Nikitin NP, Constantin C, Loh PH, et al. New generation 3-dimensional echocardiography for left ventricular volumetric and functional measurements: comparison with cardiac magnetic resonance. *Eur J Echocardiogr.* 2006;7:365–372.
40. Krenning BJ, Kirschbaum SW, Soliman OI, et al. Comparison of contrast agent-enhanced versus non-contrast agent-enhanced real-time three-dimensional echocardiography for analysis of left ventricular systolic function. *Am J Cardiol.* 2007;100(9):1485–1489.
41. Qi X, Cogar B, Hsiung MC, et al. Live/real time three-dimensional transthoracic echocardiographic assessment of left ventricular volumes, ejection fraction, and mass compared with magnetic resonance imaging. *Echocardiography.* 2007;24(2):166–173.
42. Pouleur AC, le Polain de Waroux JB, Pasquet A, et al. Assessment of left ventricular mass and volumes by three-dimensional echocardiography in patients with or without wall motion abnormalities: comparison against cine magnetic resonance imaging. *Heart.* 2008;94(8):1050–1057.
43. Macron L, Lim P, Bensaid A, et al. Single-beat versus multibeat real-time 3D echocardiography for assessing left ventricular volumes and ejection fraction: a comparison study with cardiac magnetic resonance. *Circ Cardiovasc Imaging.* 2010;3(4):450–455.
44. Chang SA, Lee SC, Kim EY, et al. Feasibility of single-beat full-volume capture real-time three-dimensional echocardiography and auto-contouring algorithm for quantification of left ventricular volume: validation with cardiac magnetic resonance imaging. *J Am Soc Echocardiogr.* 2011;24(8):853–859.
45. van den Bosch AE, Robbers-Visser D, Krenning BJ, et al. Real-time transthoracic three-dimensional echocardiographic assessment of left ventricular volume and ejection fraction in congenital heart disease. *J Am Soc Echocardiogr.* 2006;19:1–6.
46. Shimada YJ, Shiota T. A meta-analysis and investigation for the source of bias of left ventricular volumes and function by three-dimensional echocardiography in comparison with magnetic. *Am J Cardiol.* 2011;107(1):126–138.
47. Shimada YJ, Shiota T. Meta-analysis of accuracy of left ventricular mass measurement by three-dimensional echocardiography. *Am J Cardiol.* April 26, 2012. [Epub ahead of print]
48. Jiang L, Handschumacher MD, Hibberd MG, et al. Three-dimensional echocardiographic reconstruction of right ventricular volume: in vitro comparison with two-dimensional methods. *J Am Soc Echocardiogr.* 1994;7(2):150–158.
49. Jiang L, Siu SC, Handschumacher MD, et al. Three-dimensional echocardiography. In vivo validation for right ventricular volume and function. *Circulation.* 1994;89(5):2342–2350.
50. Shiota T, Jones M, Chikada M, et al. Real-time three-dimensional echocardiography for determining right ventricular stroke volume in an animal model of chronic right ventricular volume overload. *Circulation.* 1998;97(19):1897–1900.

51. Ota T, Fleishman CE, Strub M, et al. Real-time, three-dimensional echocardiography: feasibility of dynamic right ventricular volume measurement with saline contrast. *Am Heart J.* 1999;137(5):958–966.
52. Chen G, Sun K, Huang G. In vitro validation of right ventricular volume and mass measurement by real-time three-dimensional echocardiography. *Echocardiography.* 2006;23:395–399.
53. Hoch M, Vasilyev NV, Soriano B, et al. Variables influencing the accuracy of right ventricular volume assessment by real-time 3-dimensional echocardiography: an in vitro validation study. *J Am Soc Echocardiogr.* 2007;20:456–461.
54. Liu YN, Deng YB, Liu BB, Zhang QY. Rapid and accurate quantification of right ventricular volume and stroke volume by real-time 3-dimensional triplane echocardiography. *Clin Cardiol.* 2008;31(8):378–382.
55. Kjaergaard J, Petersen CL, Kjaer A, Schaadt BK, et al. Evaluation of right ventricular volume and function by 2D and 3D echocardiography compared to MRI. *Eur J Echocardiogr.* 2006;7:430–438.
56. Nesser HJ, Tkalec W, Patel AR, et al. Quantitation of right ventricular volumes and ejection fraction by three dimensional echocardiography in patients: comparison with magnetic resonance imaging and radionuclide ventriculography. *Echocardiography.* 2006;23:666–680.
57. Gopal AS, Chukwu EO, Iwuchukwu CJ, et al. Normal values of right ventricular size and function by real-time 3-dimensional echocardiography: comparison with cardiac magnetic resonance imaging. *J Am Soc Echocardiogr.* 2007;20:445–455.
58. Jenkins C, Chan J, Bricknell K, StrudwickM, Marwick TH. Reproducibility of right ventricular volumes and ejection fraction using real-time three-dimensional echocardiography: comparison with cardiac MRI. *Chest.* 2007;131:1844–1851.
59. Sugeng L, Mor Avi V, Weinert L, et al. Multimodality comparison of quantitative volumetric analysis of the right ventricle. *JACC Cardiovasc Imaging.* 2010;3:10–18.
60. Leibundgut G, Rohner A, Grize L, et al. Dynamic assessment of right ventricular volumes and function by real-time three-dimensional echocardiography: a comparison study with magnetic resonance imaging in 100 adult patients. *J Am Soc Echocardiogr.* 2010;23:116–126.
61. Iriart X, Montaudon M, Lafitte S, et al. Right ventricle three-dimensional echography in corrected tetralogy of Fallot: accuracy and variability. *Eur J Echocardiogr.* 2009;10(6):784–792.
62. Grewal J, Majdalany D, Syed I, et al. Three-dimensional echocardiographic assessment of right ventricular volume and function in adult patients with congenital heart disease: comparison with magnetic resonance imaging. *J Am Soc Echocardiogr.* 2010;23(2):127–133.
63. Grapsa J, O'Regan DP, Pavlopoulos H, et al. Right ventricular remodelling in pulmonary arterial hypertension with three-dimensional echocardiography: comparison with cardiac magnetic resonance imaging. *Eur J Echocardiogr.* 2010;11(1):64–73.
64. Grison A, Maschietto N, Reffo E, et al. Three-dimensional echocardiographic evaluation of right ventricular volume and function in pediatric patients: validation of the technique. *J Am Soc Echocardiogr.* 2007;20:921–929.
65. Khoo NS, Young A, Occleshaw C, Cowan B, Zeng IS, Gentles TL. Assessments of right ventricular volume and function using three-dimensional echocardiography in older children and adults with congenital heart disease: comparison with cardiac magnetic resonance imaging. *J Am Soc Echocardiogr.* 2009;22(11): 1279–1288.
66. van der Hulst AE, Roest AA, Holman ER, et al. Real-time three-dimensional echocardiography: segmental analysis of the right ventricle in patients with repaired tetralogy of fallot. *J Am Soc Echocardiogr.* 2011;24(11):1183–1190.
67. van der Zwaan HB, Geleijnse ML, McGhie JS, et al. Right ventricular quantification in clinical practice: two-dimensional vs. three-dimensional echocardiography compared with cardiac magnetic resonance imaging. *Eur J Echocardiogr.* 2011;12(9):656–664.
68. Shimada YJ, Shiota M, Siegel RJ, Shiota T. Accuracy of right ventricular volumes and function determined by three-dimensional echocardiography in comparison with magnetic resonance imaging: a meta-analysis study. *J Am Soc Echocardiogr.* 2010;23(9):943–953.
69. Altmann K, Shen Z, Boxt LM, et al. Comparison of three-dimensional echocardiographic assessment of volume, mass, and function in children with functionally single left ventricles with two-dimensional echocardiography and magnetic resonance imaging. *Am J Cardiol.* 1997;80(8):1060–1065.
70. Soriano BD, Hoch M, Ithuralde A, et al. Matrix-array 3-dimensional echocardiographic assessment of volumes, mass, and ejection fraction in young pediatric patients with a functional single ventricle: a comparison study with cardiac magnetic resonance. *Circulation.* 2008;117:1842–1848.
71. Fu M, Choi G, Xie MX, et al. Quantitative real-time 3D echocardiography predicts adverse outcomes in functional single ventricle patients. *J Am Soc Echocardiogr.* 2010;23:B54.
72. Kobayashi D, Patel SR, Mattoo TK, et al. The impact of change in volume and left-ventricular hypertrophy on left-ventricular mechanical dyssynchrony in children with end-stage renal disease. *Pediatr Cardiol.* March 23, 2012. [Epub ahead of print]

73. Veeram Reddy SR, Du W, Zilberman MV. Left ventricular mechanical synchrony and global systolic function in pediatric patients late after ventricular septal defect patch closure: a three-dimensional echocardiographic study. *Congenit Heart Dis.* 2009;4(6):454–458.
74. Bacha EA, Zimmerman FJ, Mor-Avi V, et al. Ventricular resynchronization by multisite pacing improves myocardial performance in the postoperative single-ventricle patient. *Ann Thorac Surg.* 2004;78(5):1678–1683.
75. Dragulescu A, Mertens LL. Developments in echocardiographic techniques for the evaluation of ventricular function in children. *Arch Cardiovasc Dis.* 2010;103:603–614.
76. Pacileo G, Di Salvo G, Limongelli G, et al. Echocardiography in congenital heart disease: usefulness, limits and new techniques. *J Cardiovasc Med.* 2007;8:17–22.
77. Gorscan J III, Strum DP, Mandarino WA, Gulati VK, Pinsky MR. Quantitative assessment of alterations in regional left ventricular contractility with color-coded tissue Doppler echocardiography. *Circulation.* 1997;95:2423–2433.
78. Eidem BW, McMahon CJ, Cohen RR, et al. Impact of cardiac growth on Doppler tissue imaging velocities: a study in healthy children. *J Am Soc Echocardiogr.* 2004;17:212–221.
79. Korinek J, Wang J, Sengupta PP, et al. Two-dimensional strain—a Doppler-independent ultrasound method for quantitation of regional deformation: validation in vitro and in vivo. *J Am Soc Echocardiogr.* 2005;18:1247–1253.
80. Admunsen BH, Helle-Valle T, Edvardsen T, et al. Noninvasive myocardial strain measurement by speckle tracking echocardiography: validation against sonomicrometry and tagged magnetic resonance imaging. *J Am Coll Cardiol.* 2006;47:789–793.
81. Young AA, Axel L, Dougherty L, Bogen DK, Parenteau CS. Validation of tagging with MR imaging to estimate material deformation. *Radiology.* 1993;188:101–108.
82. Amundsen BH, Helle-Valle T, Edvardsen T, et al. Noninvasive myocardial strain measurement by speckle tracking echocardiography: validation against sonomicrometry and tagged magnetic resonance imaging. *J Am Coll Cardiol.* 2006;47:789–793.
83. Moore CC, Lugo-Olivieri CH, McVeigh ER, Zerhouni EA. Three-dimensional systolic strain patterns in the normal human left ventricle: characterization with tagged MR imaging. *Radiology.* 2000;214:453–466.
84. Marcus KA, Mavinkurve-Groothuis AM, Barends M, et al. Reference values for myocardial two-dimensional strain echocardiography in a healthy pediatric and young adult cohort . *J Am Soc Echocardiogr.* 2011;24:625–636.
85. Lorch SM, Ludomirsky A, Singh GK. Maturational and growth-related changes in left ventricular longitudinal strain and strain rate measured by two-dimensional speckle tracking echocardiography in healthy pediatric population. *J Am Soc Echocardiogr.* 2008;21:1207–1215.
86. Geyer H, Caracciolo G, Abe H, et al. Assessment of myocardial mechanics using speckle tracking echocardiography: fundamentals and clinical applications. *J Am Soc Echocardiogr.* 2010;23:351–69.
87. Bansal M, Cho GY, Chan J, et al. Feasibility and accuracy of different techniques of two-dimensional speckle based strain and validation with harmonic phase magnetic resonance imaging. *J Am Soc Echocardiogr.* 2008;21:1318–1325.
88. D'Hooge J, Konofagou E, Jamal F, et al. Two-dimensional ultrasonic strain rate measurement of the human heart in vivo. *IEEE Trans Ultrason Ferroelectr Freq Control.* 2002;49:281–286.
89. Perez de Isla L, Balcones DV, Fernandez-Golfin C, et al. Three-dimensional-wall motion tracking: a new and faster tool for myocardial strain assessment: comparison with two dimensional wall motion tracking. *J Am Soc Echocardiogr.* 2009;22:325–330.
90. Gayat E, Ahmad H, Weinert L, et al. Reproducibility and inter-vendor variability of left ventricular deformation measurements by three-dimensional speckle-tracking echocardiography. *J Am Soc Echocardiogr.* 2011;24:878–885.
91. Nesser HJ, Mor-Avi V, Gorissen W, et al. Quantification of left ventricular volumes using three dimensional echocardiographic speckle tracking: comparison with MRI. *Eur Heart J.* 2009;30:1565–1573.
92. Maffessanti F, Nesser HJ, Weinert L, et al. Quantitative evaluation of regional left ventricular function using three-dimensional speckle tracking echocardiography in patients with and without heart disease. *Am J Cardiol.* 2009;104:1755–1762.
93. Bussadori C, Moreo A, Di Donato M, et al. A new 2D-based method for myocardial velocity strain and strain rate quantification in a normal adult and pediatric population: assessment of reference values. *Cardiovasc Ultrasound.* 2009;13:7–8.
94. Zhang L, Gao J, Xie M, Yin P, Liu W, Li Y, Klas B, Sun J, Balluz R, Ge S. Left ventricular three-dimensional global systolic strain by real-time three-dimensional speckle-tracking in children: feasibility, reproducibility, maturational changes, and normal ranges. *J Am Soc Echocardiogr.* 2013 Aug;26(8):853–859.
95. Saltijeral A, Isla LP, Pérez-Rodríguez O, et al. Early myocardial deformation changes associated to isolated obesity: a study based on 3D-wall motion tracking analysis. *Obesity.* 201;19(11):2268–2273.
96. Zhang L, Xie MX, Balluz R, Ge S. Real-time 3-dimensional echocardiography for evaluation of congenital heart defects: state of the art. *Echocardiography.* 2012;29(2):232–241.

CHAPTER

6

THREE-DIMENSIONAL ECHOCARDIOGRAPHY OF ATRIAL SEPTAL DEFECT

David A. Roberson, MD; Vivian Wei Cui, MD

ABSTRACT

Atrial septal defects (ASDs) of secundum, primum, sinus venosus, and coronary sinus types are demonstrated in great detail with three-dimensional echocardiography (3DE). Although three-dimensional (3D) transthoracic echocardiography is helpful, 3D transesophageal echocardiography (TEE) is most useful to demonstrate all relevant anatomic details, guide interventional catheter therapy to close an ASD, assist in intraoperative surgical treatment, and analyze ASDs that are created or enlarged for palliation of complex congenital heart disease. The five currently available modalities of 3DE are X plane, live 3D, 3D zoom, full-volume 3DE, and 3D color mode. Each has its strengths, limitations, and specific usefulness. This chapter reviews the anatomy of the various types of ASD and presents images from the available 3D imaging modalities, focusing primarily on 3D TEE imaging of ASD.

INTRODUCTION

Atrial septal defect (ASD) has an incidence of approximately one per 1000 live births,[1] making it the fourth most common congenital cardiac anomaly. The four types of ASD in decreasing order of incidence are secundum ASD, primum ASD, sinus venosus ASD, and coronary sinus ASD.[2] Within our practice, the relative incidence of each type of ASD is secundum 87%, primum 11%, sinus venosus 2%, and coronary sinus defect 0.4%. The left-to-right shunt caused by a moderate-sized or large ASD results in chronic right-sided heart volume overload; pulmonary overcirculation; and, if is left untreated, potential pulmonary hypertension. Therefore, an ASD of significant size requires closure by device or surgery.[3] Most secundum ASDs are amenable to transcatheter device closure[4]; however, approximately 15% of secundum ASDs and all of the other three types of ASD require surgical treatment. Additionally, a modified type of ASD that is intentionally created or enlarged by surgery or interventional catheter procedure is becoming increasingly common in this era of successful single-ventricle palliation.

This chapter focuses on transesophageal echocardiography (TEE) imaging of ASDs, a relatively new and very important application. It will become clear that the capability of three-dimensional echocardiography (3DE) to demonstrate surfaces, volumes, and spatial relationships of anatomic structures has advanced considerably and that the method provides unique views and insights into the dynamic anatomy of the atrial septum and defects therein. I present a historical perspective on 3DE, followed by a discussion on ASD types, 3DE modalities, three-dimensional (3D) TEE protocol, best views, and the role of 3D TEE in ASD.

HISTORICAL PERSPECTIVE

Early 3DE technology was dependent on 3D images reconstructed from two-dimensional (2D) transthoracic echocardiograms. Marx et al.[5] first reported some of the unique and useful 3D images of secundum ASD that were successfully reconstructed from transthoracic 2D images. This endeavor was labor intensive and resulted in images of limited resolution. Acar et al.[6] subsequently reported that the 3D en face images of secundum ASD reconstructed from 2D images were useful and accurately demonstrated the shape, size, and rim features. In the same year, Cao et al.[7] reported that visualization of the number of orifices, ASD shape, and surrounding structures was enhanced using reconstructed 3D images derived from 2D TEE images. The development of a real-time matrix array 3D transthoracic transducer initiated the era of real-time, rather than reconstructed, 3D image acquisition and viewing of ASD. Van den Bosch et al.[8] reported that 3DE provided important information and enhanced understanding of secundum ASD anatomy, physiology, and treatment with better accuracy, improved image quality, and very short processing time compared with prior technology. Initial reports of the use of 3D TEE appeared in 2009. Taniguchi et al.[9] demonstrated the feasibility, utility, speed, and accuracy of real-time 3D TEE used during secundum ASD device closure. In 2010, Faletra et al.[10] described in great detail the anatomy of the right atrium and atrial septum as it applies to electrophysiologic issues and Pushparajah et al.[11] presented a collection of images from various types of ASDs.

The progress of 3D transthoracic echocardiography (TTE) and TEE technology to demonstrate secundum ASD is beautifully demonstrated in these reports. The 3DE of non-secundum-type ASDs has been reported in only a few case reports. This chapter includes examples of secundum ASDs as well as the other three types of nonsecundum ASDs.

TYPES OF ASDS

The secundum ASD (**Figs. 6-1–6-8**) is located within the oval fossa, and its size and shape are quite variable. The size of the defect is a function of the size of the limbic margins or rims, which are located on the right atrial side of the septum, and the size and number of holes within the septum primum, which is located on the left atrial side of the atrial septum. Important features to define are defect size, shunt size and direction, location, rim sizes, number of orifices, balloon size during interventional closure procedures, device position, device configuration, and the features of any residual shunt after device placement. Very large defects or those with deficiency of the superior, inferior, or posterior rims may not be amenable to device closure because the rim tissue is insufficient to securely place the ASD closure device. Although aortic rim deficiency is the most common, it usually does not preclude device placement as the device can be wrapped around the aorta provided it does not significantly indent or distort the aortic sinus of Valsalva. Secundum ASD size varies considerably over the cardiac cycle, with an area change ranging from 25% to 75%. 3DE is ideal for demonstrating the relationship of the ASD and the closure device to surrounding structures. The amount of right atrial and right ventricular enlargement generally reflects the size of the left-to-right shunt, although one must also consider the contribution of tricuspid valve insufficiency and pulmonary hypertension to chamber enlargement in the right side of the heart. The quantitation of volumetric flow through an ASD is also possible, as discussed in Chapter 4.

The primum ASD (**Figs. 6-9** and **6-10**) is located adjacent to the atrioventricular valves, and its long axis parallels the atrioventricular valve annulus, generally along an anterior/superior to posterior/inferior axis. The apical margin of the defect is comprised of the atrioventricular valves, which are coplanar in this defect owing to deficiency of the atrioventricular septum. Primum ASDs vary in size but are usually at least medium sized, and the shape is oval to almost rectangular in some cases. A cleft mitral valve or an accessory commissure of the mitral valve is typically present, along with varying degrees of mitral insufficiency and tricuspid insufficiency. Key anatomic features to define are the size of the defect and shunt, abnormalities of the atrioventricular valves (especially the mitral valve cleft), chordal attachments of the mitral valve, and the presence and severity of subaortic stenosis.

Figure 6-1

Right atrial and left atrial en face views of secundum ASD acquired in 3D zoom mode, demonstrating the major anatomic landmarks including the superior vena cava (SVC), inferior vena cava (IVC), aorta (Ao), left and right pulmonary veins (LPV and RPV), and septum primum (SP). A, anterior; L, left; P, posterior; R, right; S, superior.

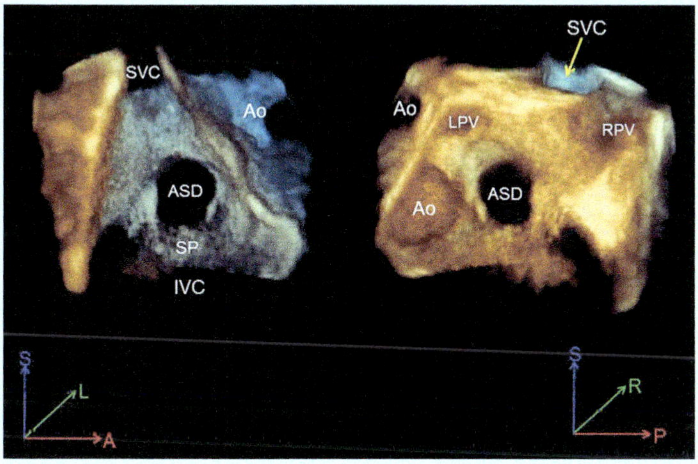

Figure 6-2

En face view of a centrally located secundum ASD with well-developed rims. This image was acquired in 3D zoom mode and viewed from the right side. The ASD rims are 1, superior vena cava (SVC); 2, aortic (Ao); 3, atrioventricular; 4, inferior vena cava (IVC); 5, right pulmonary vein. A, anterior; L, left; S, superior.

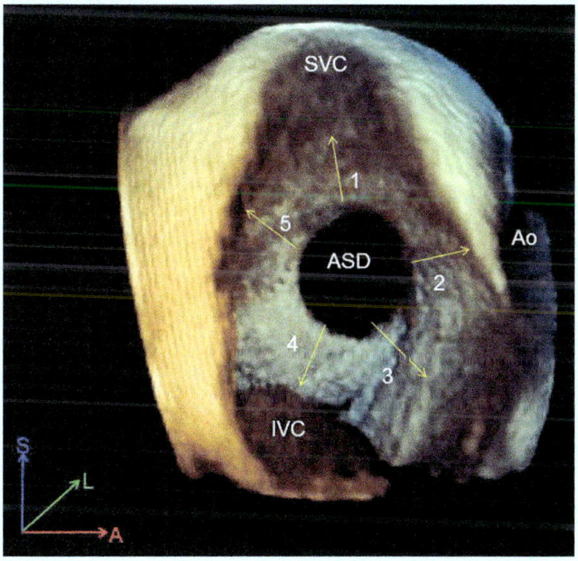

Figure 6-3

Views of secundum ASDs with deficient rims: an ASD is present (asterisk) with deficient superior vena cava (SVC) rim (upper left) obtained with transgastric sagittal live 3D mode, deficient aortic rim (center) seen from a right atrial (RA) en face view obtained with 3D zoom mode, and a deficient inferior vena cava (IVC) rim (lower right) seen from an RA en face view obtained with 3D zoom mode. Arrows point to the respective rim deficiency. Ao, aorta; LA, left atrium; RPA, right pulmonary artery.

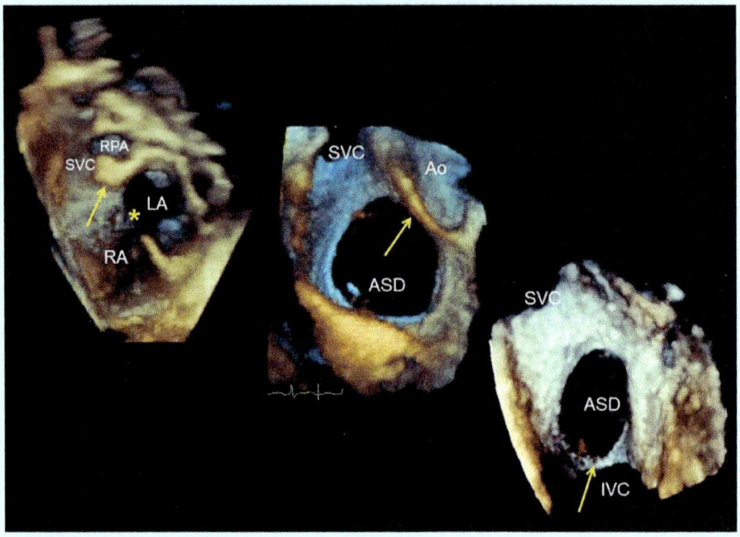

Figure 6-4

Sagittal (left) and posterior (right) deep transgastric views of a secundum ASD (asterisk) acquired in live 3D mode. Note the views of the right atrial appendage (RAA), right pulmonary vein (RPV), tricuspid valve (TV), superior rim (S), and inferior rim (I). These views are particularly useful for measuring superior and inferior rims and septal length during device closure. The left panel demonstrates superior rim deficiency. LA, left atrium; RPA, right pulmonary artery; A, anterior; P, posterior; R, right; SVC, superior vena cava.

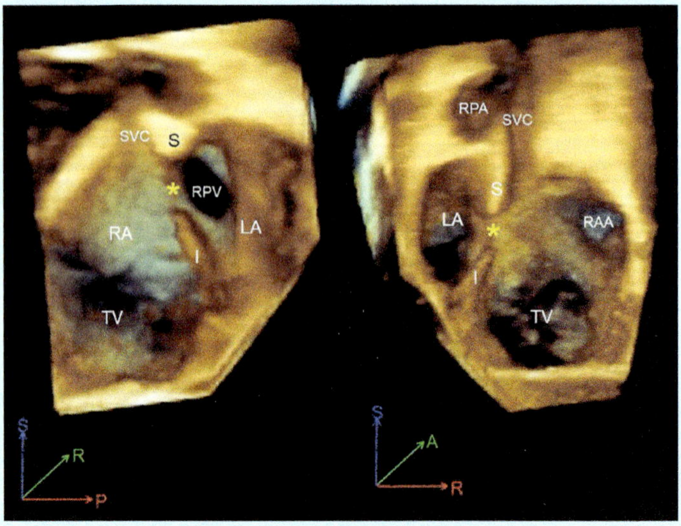

Figure 6-5

Right atrial (RA) (left panel) and left atrial (LA) (right panel) en face views acquired in 3D zoom mode of a multiple-orifice secundum ASD in which a band of septum primum divides the secundum ASD into smaller posterior and larger anterior portions. A, anterior; IVC, inferior vena cava; L, left; P, posterior; R, right; RPV, right pulmonary vein; SVC, superior vena cava.

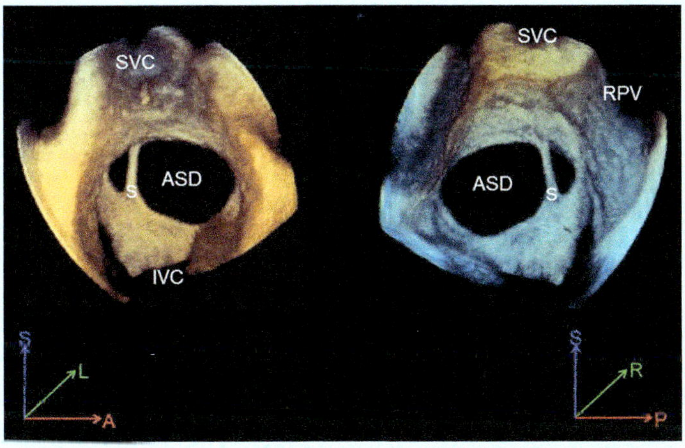

Figure 6-6

Right atrial (RA) (left panel) and left atrial (LA) (right panel) en face views acquired in 3D zoom mode of a multiple-orifice secundum ASD in which there are two fenestrations (1 and 2) in the septum primum. Ao, aorta; SVC, superior vena cava.

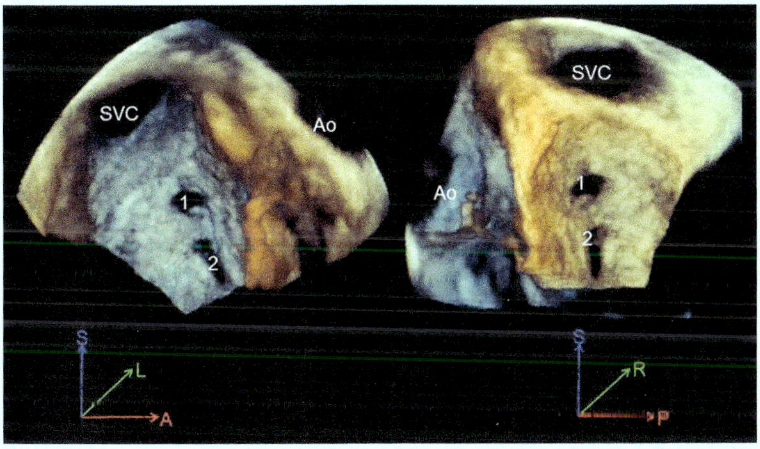

Sinus venosus ASDs (Figs. 6-11 and 6-12) are located at the junction of either caval vein to the atrium and are associated with superior vena cava override of the defect in the superior type and inferior vena cava override in the inferior type. Anomalous pulmonary venous drainage of some or all of the right pulmonary veins is usually present. The superior type is much more frequent (83% superior type vs. 17% inferior type in our series) and is more often associated with anomalous right pulmonary vein connections than the inferior type. Key features to define are ASD size and location, vena caval override, and pulmonary vein connections.

Figure 6-7

Right atrial (RA) en face images acquired in 3D zoom mode of secundum ASDs (asterisks) with atypical septum primum. On the left is a triangle-shaped ASD and on the right is an atrial septal aneurysm (arrow). A, anterior; Ao, aorta; IVC, inferior vena cava; L, left; S, superior; SVC, superior vena cava; TV, tricuspid valve.

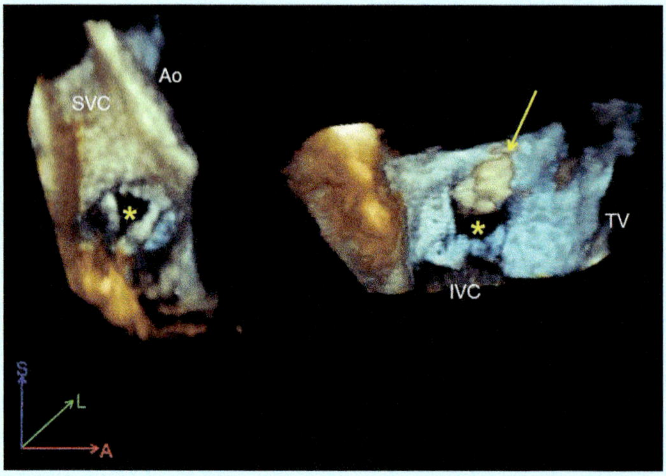

Figure 6-8

A view of malalignment of the septum secundum and septum primum components of the atrial septum obtained by cropping and viewing a 3D zoom acquisition of the atrial septum from the posterior. The ASD is located at the asterisk. A, anterior; R, right; RA, right atrium; S, superior; SVC, superior vena cava; S1, septum primum; S2, septum secundum.

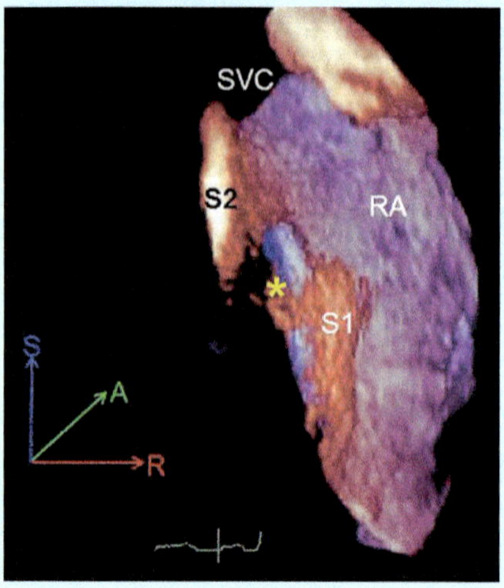

Coronary sinus ASD (Fig. 6-13) is a very rare anomaly, representing less than 1% of all ASDs. In our practice, we have encountered only three such ASDs in 23 years. The defect is associated with complete or partial unroofing of the coronary sinus into the left atrium and usually presents with a persistent left superior vena cava to coronary sinus connection. There is a left-to-right shunt from the left atrium through the coronary sinus orifice into the right atrium. The coronary sinus orifice is often enlarged and retains its usual position adjacent to the tricuspid valve annulus. Unlike the primum ASD, in the coronary sinus ASD there is no deficiency of the atrioventricular septum; therefore, the atrioventricular valves maintain their normal offset position, with the tricuspid valve septal leaflet attachments being a few millimeters more apical than the mitral valve as seen in the four-chamber view.

The term *modified ASD* (Figs. 6-14–6-16) refers to ASDs that are created or enlarged by interventional catheterization technique or surgery. One type is performed in order to provide unobstructed blood flow between the atria. This type is located within the confines of the oval fossa, unless it is inadvertently

Figure 6-9

3D full-volume views of a primum ASD as seen from the right side (left panel) and the left side (right panel) (yellow arrows). A, anterior; Ao, aorta; L, left; LA, left atrium; LV, left ventricle; MV, mitral valve; PA, pulmonary artery; RA, right atrium; RV, right ventricle; S, superior; TV, tricuspid valve.

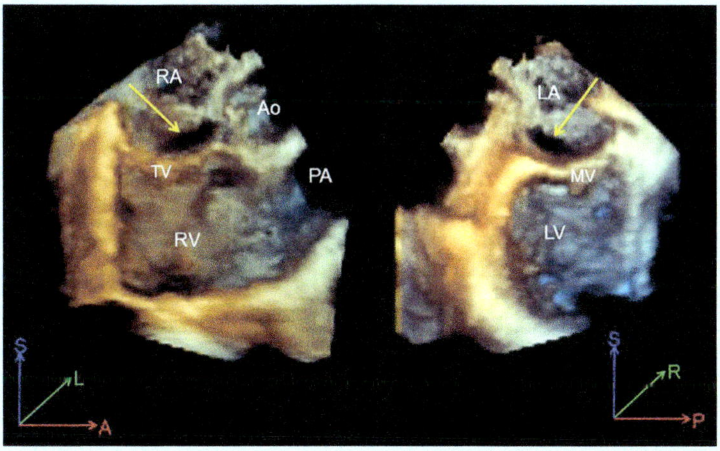

Figure 6-10

A 3D full-volume four-chamber view of primum ASD (asterisk) in the left panel and 3D zoom view of cleft mitral valve (red arrow) as seen from the left atrium in the right panel. A, anterior; AL, anterior leaflet; Ao, aorta; AS, atrial septum; I, inferior; L, left; LA, left atrium; LAA, left atrial appendage; LV, left ventricle; ML, mural leaflet; MV, mitral valve; P, posterior; PA, pulmonary artery; PL, posterior leaflet; RA, right atrium; RV, right ventricle; S, superior; TV, tricuspid valve; VS, ventricular septum.

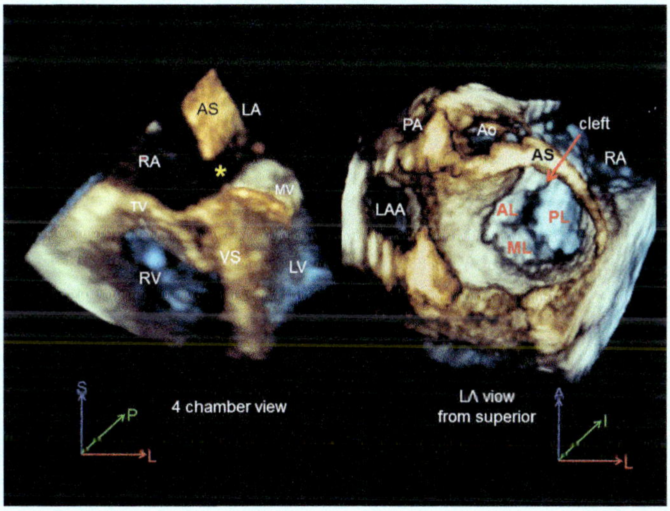

enlarged beyond its rims. An example of this type of defect is found in Norwood palliation of hypoplastic left heart. Another type of modified ASD is a Fontan fenestration, which is located between the side of the circulation, which receives the systemic venous return and connects to the pulmonary arteries, and the functional left-sided atrium, which receives the pulmonary venous return. This atrial-level communication

Figure 6-11

3D full-volume views (left and right) and 3D color Doppler flow map (bottom) of superior-type sinus venosus ASD (asterisks). The view at upper left is a long-axis view; note the anomalous right pulmonary vein (RPV) to the superior vena cava (SVC). The upper right is a posterior aspect view; note the SVC override. The 3D color Doppler flow map shows the abnormal RPV to SVC flow. A, anterior; AS, atrial septum; I, inferior; L, left; LA, left atrium; P, posterior; R, right; RA, right atrium; RAA, right atrial appendage; RPA, right pulmonary artery; S, superior; TV, tricuspid valve.

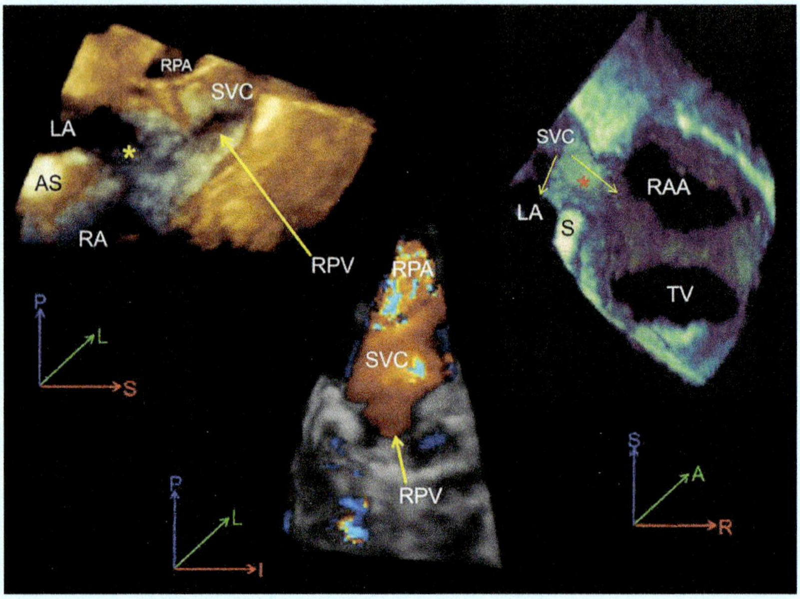

Figure 6-12

3D zoom acquisition right atrial (RA) en face and long-axis views of inferior sinus venosus ASD. A, anterior; CS, coronary sinus; EV, eustachian valve; IVC, inferior vena cava; L, left; LA, left atrium; P, posterior; S, superior; SVC, superior vena cava; TV, tricuspid valve.

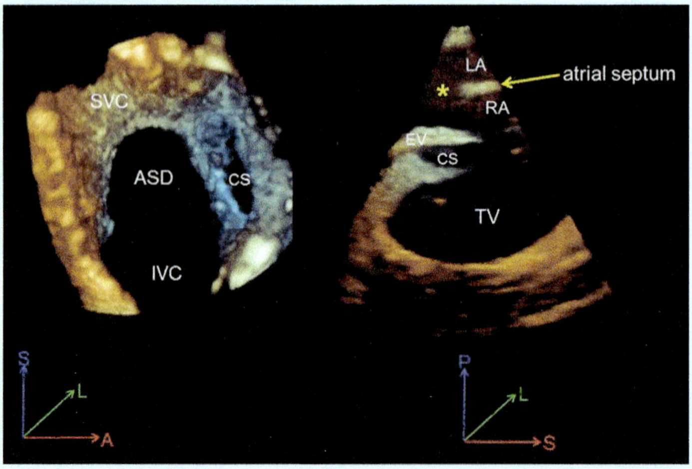

Figure 6-13

3D full-volume four-chamber images of coronary sinus ASD (arrows). On the left is a four-chamber view and on the right a left atrial (LA) oblique en face view. L, left; LV, left ventricle; MV, mitral valve; P, posterior; RA, right atrium; RV, right ventricle; S, superior.

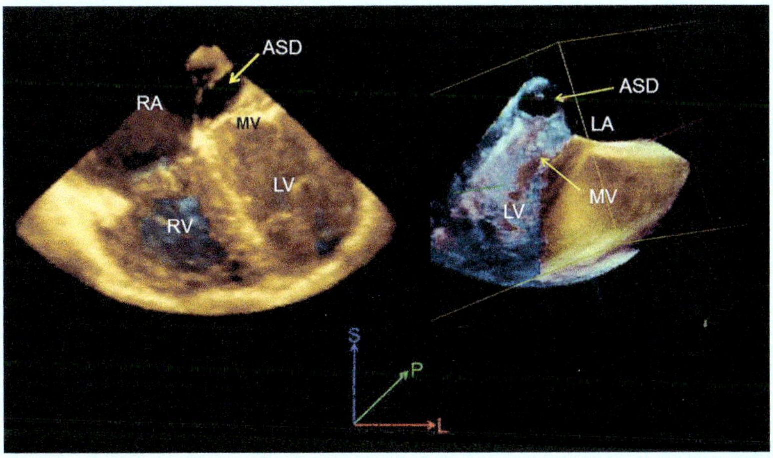

Figure 6-14

3D full-volume views from the left side of a restrictive ASD in tricuspid atresia (left). After balloon atrial septostomy, the ASD is larger (right). LV, left ventricle; P, posterior; R, right; S, superior; S1, septum primum.

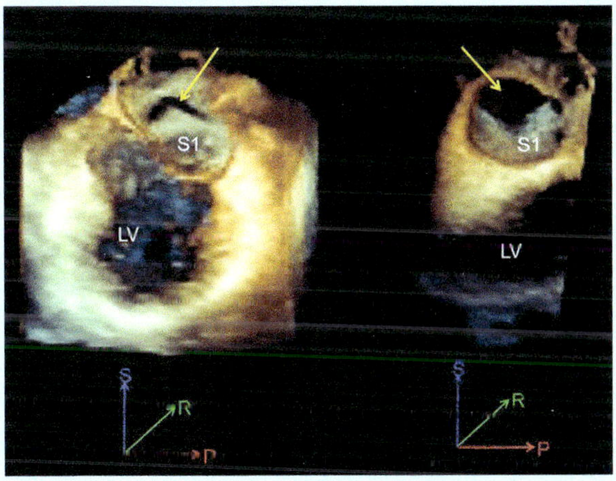

allows a route for right-to-left shunting, thereby providing decompression of high Fontan circuit pressures and maintenance of systemic cardiac output. Fenestrations are variably positioned according to the preference of the surgeon, although a rightward posterolateral location not far from the pulmonary veins is a fairly common location.

Figure 6-15

3D full-volume view from the right side of a nonrestrictive ASD in hypoplastic left heart after Norwood procedure. A, anterior; Ao, aorta; L, left; NeoAo, neoaorta; RV, right ventricle; S, superior; TV, tricuspid valve.

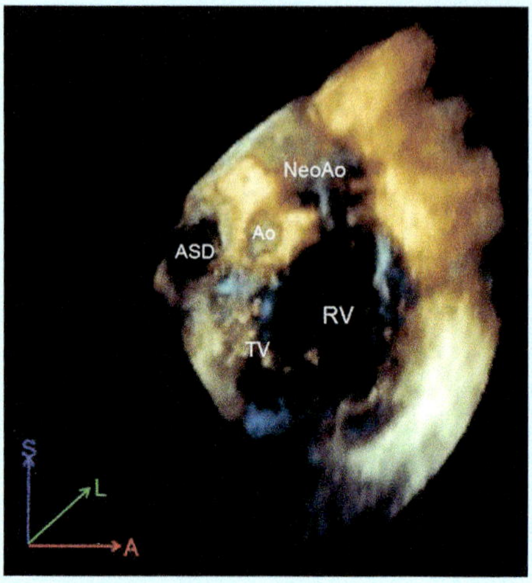

Probably the most important current application of echocardiography in the treatment of ASD is to guide interventional device closure. Important views related to sizing balloon and devices are presented in Figures 6-17–6-20.

3DE IMAGING MODALITIES

The five currently available 3DE modes on the equipment that we currently use include X-plane, live 3D, 3D zoom, full-volume 3DE, and 3D color Doppler flow analysis. Each has its own strengths, limitations, and utility for 3DE evaluation of ASDs.

X-plane mode

X-plane 3D imaging uses a 3D transducer to display simultaneous orthogonal 2D images. The plane of dissection of the reference image and the angle between the two simultaneous biplane images are adjustable and are defined

Figure 6-16

3D color Doppler flow map of a right-to-left shunt through a Fontan fenestration (F) (left). A live 3D mode demonstration Amplatzer patent foramen ovale device (AGA Medical Corp., Plymouth, Minnesota) was placed, closing the fenestration (right). L, left; LA, left atrium; P, posterior; S, superior.

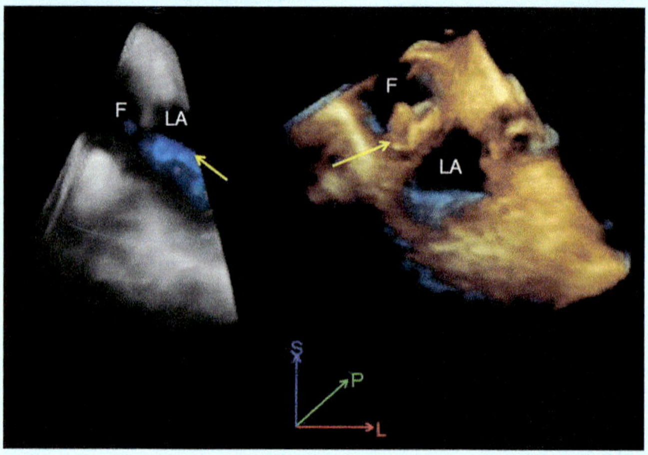

Figure 6-17

X-plane simultaneous biplane views (long axis, left) (short axis, right) of the sizing balloon waist diameter. LA, left atrium; RA, right atrium.

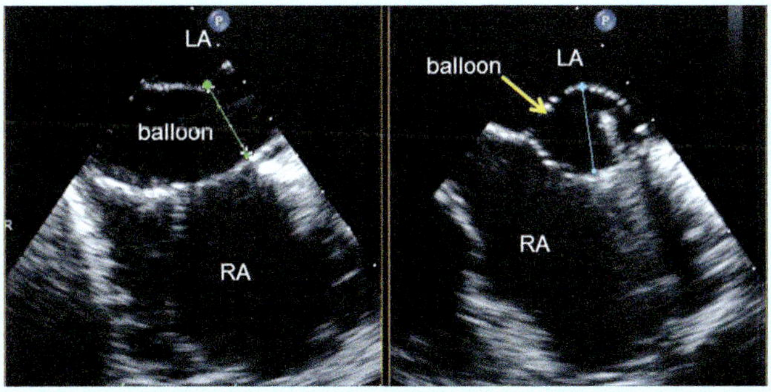

Figure 6-18

Multiple views of the Amplatzer ASD closure device (D). CS, coronary sinus; LA, left atrium; RA, right atrium; SVC, superior vena cava.

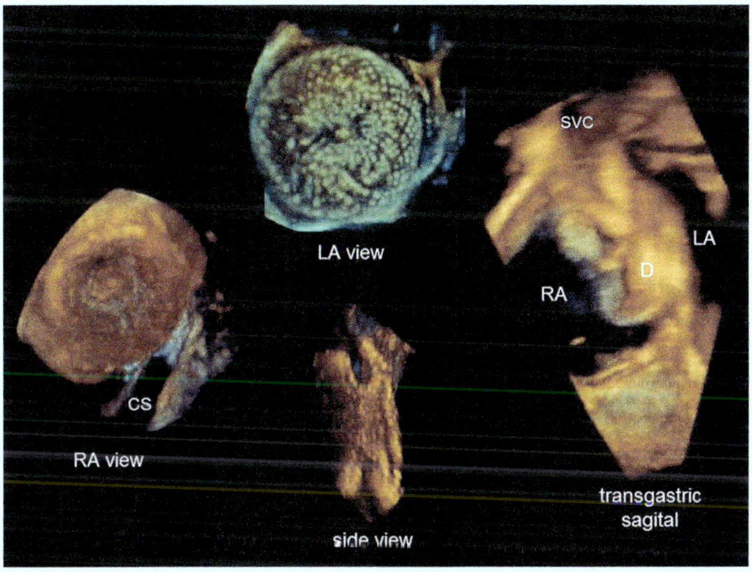

by the sonographer. It is the echocardiographic analog of biplane angiographic imaging. Color Doppler flow mapping is also available in X-plane imaging. X-plane imaging is useful to define spatial relationships and to ensure that characteristics such as ASD length and width and color Doppler flow mapping of jet widths are being measured in the correct plane.

Figure 6-19

Live 3D views of the aorta being deformed by an Amplatzer device (left disk, LD; and right disk, RD). On the left, the device is indenting the aorta. On the right, the aorta is being compressed between the left and right atrial disks. Ao, aorta; I, inferior; L, left; LA, left atrium; P, posterior; RA, right atrium; RV, right ventricle.

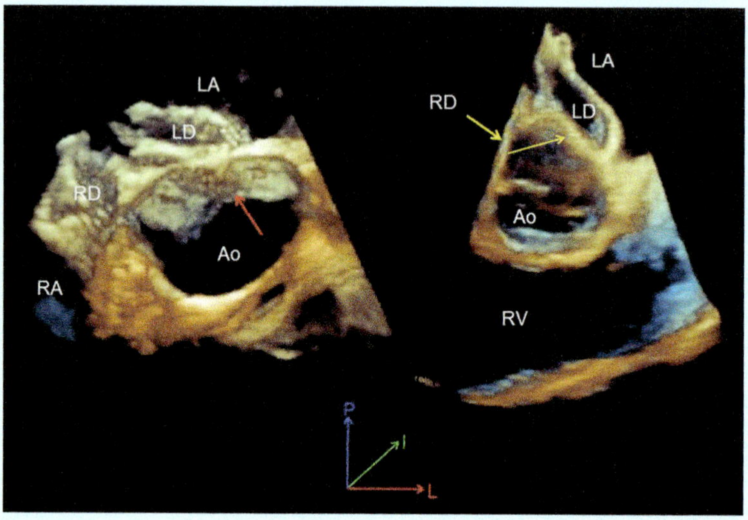

Figure 6-20

3D zoom short-axis view of the three spirals (1, 2, 3) of a Helex device (Gore, Newark, Delaware). L, left; LA, left atrium; P, posterior; RA, right atrium; S, superior.

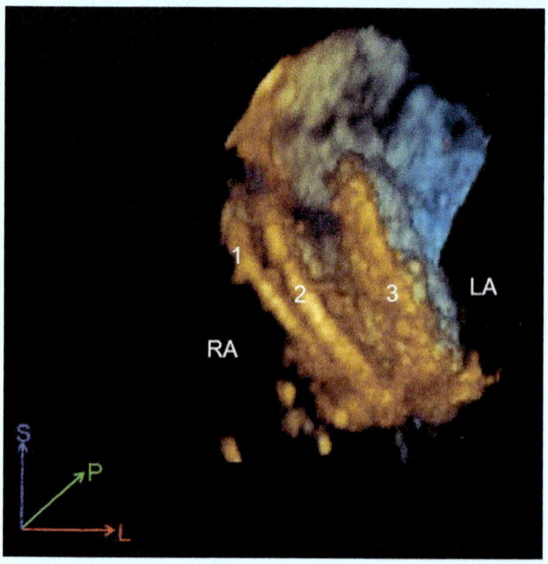

Live 3D mode

The live 3D mode consists of a 15°–25° wide wedge of live 3DE. It has high frame rates of 23–60 per second with high resolution. Two settings are available for live 3D. The first, medium-resolution live 3D, has a slightly larger sample volume and slightly lower resolution. The second setting is high-resolution live 3D, which has a slightly smaller sample volume and higher resolution. There is only a minimal difference between these two settings in clinical practice. The anterior to posterior position of the sector can be adjusted without moving the transducer by using the elevation setting. A lateral steering adjustment to shift the sector rightward or leftward is also available. The live 3D mode is much less affected by heart rate and respiration and is devoid of stitch artifact, thereby making it very useful during ASD device deployment. Provided that the entire structure of interest can be included within the small image sector volumetric wedge, this is our preferred 3D TEE imaging mode. In order to demonstrate the entirety of the anatomy of interest in 3D, it is often necessary to position the structure of interest in the far field of the live 3D echo sector because this is the region where the sector is thickest. The live 3D acquisitions are quite useful when obtained from the deep transgastric sagittal bicaval view, which places the ASD in the far field where the 3D echo sector is largest. This is particularly useful when the ASD extends far posteriorly and is therefore positioned close to the esophagus. In these cases, the narrow apex of the midesophagus to the upper esophagus image sector views may prevent imaging of the entire ASD from the standard TEE transducer positions.

3D zoom mode

3D zoom has live real-time imaging with a user-defined trapezoid-shaped 3D sample volume having adjustable height, width, and imaging depth. 3D zoom is the most reliable modality to provide the most useful en face views of the right and left sides of the atrial septum. In these views, the type, size, location, and rims of the ASD typically are seen very well. These views are also used for quantitative dynamic analysis and determination of final closure device configuration. They can also be used to monitor device deployment. The main limitation of this modality at this time is that 3D zoom frame rates are quite slow at 6–16 per second. Hopefully, further revisions will alleviate this problem in the near future.

Full-volume 3D mode

Full volume 3D mode has a large pyramid-shaped sample volume 80°–90° wide that is formed by rapid reconstruction from four to seven contiguous live 3D wedges stitched together over four to seven heartbeats. A wide field of view demonstrates defects and their surrounding structures well. The frame rate and resolution are high, similar to live 3D imaging. Use of this modality is necessary to acquire images in order to perform right- and left-ventricle 3D volume measurements. It is limited, however, by stitch artifact, which can be severe at faster heart rates. Breath holding is also very important in order to minimize the stitch artifact. Full-volume 3D mode also requires postacquisition cropping, which results in a usually short delay between image acquisition and useful display of the 3D image. Although echocardiographers can tolerate this slight delay, in my experience surgeons and interventional cardiologists may not be so patient.

3D color Doppler flow mode

3D color Doppler flow analysis is a rapid reconstruction modality acquired over four to seven heart beats in a fashion similar to full-volume 3DE. It has a sample volume approximately half the size of the standard 3D volume but with color Doppler flow analysis superimposed over the anatomic structures. Frame rates range from approximately 20 to 45 per second.

All five modalities have multiple adjustable parameters including gain, contrast, smoothing, image algorithms, color adjustments, color depth shading adjustments, and so forth. The four formats other than X-plane imaging can be cropped in three orthogonal planes or using a single adjustable plane after acquisition. All images can be rotated through 180° in orthogonal planes. Images are acquired and stored digitally in the usual fashion. Image manipulation, cropping, and quantification can be performed on the ultrasound platform or on a digital review station. All five of the 3DE modalities and all of the cropping and quantitative techniques are available for transthoracic transducers, which come in pediatric and adult sizes, and in a transesophageal transducer that can be used in patients weighing more than 20 kg.

3D TRANSTHORACIC PROTOCOL

Following a defined protocol is important in performing TTE to assess congenital heart diseases, as recommended by the American Society of Echocardiography.[12] During the course of this protocol, specific 3D data sets may be acquired. In infants and children, 3D full-volume, 3D color Doppler, live 3D, and X-plane imaging from subcostal coronal and sagittal views and from the apical view are most useful. 3D zoom has frame rates that are too low for smaller children, and we do not use it routinely. In adults, the subcostal images are often of limited quality, especially for sinus venosus ASD. Therefore, in adults we suggest obtaining images from the parasternal short-axis view, including 3D acquisitions using the 3D zoom mode. In larger patients in whom ASD is suspected but not clearly defined, we recommend 3D TEE.

3D TRANSESOPHAGEAL PROTOCOL

We recommend acquiring 3D images of ASD from the upper esophagus, midesophagus, shallow transgastric, and deep transgastric positions. At the upper esophagus position, obtain a basal transverse view at 0° to 15° array orientation and also obtain a basal short-axis view at 30° to 60°. 3D zoom mode is quite useful in this position as it provides right- and left-sided en face views of the atrial septum. Live 3D or 3D zoom can be used to assess device deployment in real time from whichever of these positions best demonstrates the ASD in a given patient. Note that the acoustic power output of the 3D TEE transducer is quite high so that adjustment of gain, compression, and brightness settings down to the lower ranges is required to demonstrate fine anatomic details.

At the midesophagus level, obtain a four-chamber view at 0°–20° transducer array orientation in order to obtain a full-volume acquisition for quantitation of 3D ventricular volumes. The coronary sinus is usually seen best at this position by using slight transducer retroflexion. Also, in this position a bicaval view can be obtained by spinning the transducer array to 90°–120° and twisting the transducer shaft clockwise. This view is used to obtain additional right- and left-sided en face views of the atrial septum in 3D zoom mode. It is also used to assess the cavoatrial junction to determine whether a sinus venosus ASD is present, analyze the superior and inferior rims of the atrial septum, detect vena cava override, and view anomalous right pulmonary venous return. By orienting the 3D image to view it from a posterior aspect and cropping the image from the posterior to the anterior direction, a view can be obtained that demonstrates the dynamic change in alignment between the primum and the secundum septum.

Further insertion to the shallow transgastric position reveals short- and long-axis views of the ventricles and ventricular septum in order to assess ventricular size, septal contour, and ventricular function. Next, deep transgastric views are accomplished in four steps: from a standard midesophagus four-chamber view, advance the transducer 5–15 cm depending on patient size, anteflex 90°, twist the transducer shaft clockwise approximately one-quarter to one-half turn, and slowly withdraw until a deep transgastric view appears (usually, the view of the left ventricular outflow tract is the first apparent view). Once the left ventricular outflow tract view is obtained, spin the transducer array to 120° and twist the transducer shaft clockwise to demonstrate a sagittal bicaval view of the atrial septum. This view is used to demonstrate inferior rim size, vertical dimension of the ASD, superior rim size, and the total length of the atrial septum. Spinning the transducer array back to 0°–20° and slightly deeper insertion will result in a four-chamber view. Additional or modified images may be needed in some cases in order to provide optimal delineation of the ASD and surrounding structures.

If time allows, we use all four different anatomic 3DE modes, including live 3D, 3D zoom, full-volume 3D, and X-plane imaging. We apply 3D color flow analysis in whichever view provides the best color Doppler flow mapping apparent on color Doppler 2DE. If time is limited, we concentrate on the three real-time, live modalities using 3D zoom modality to acquire en face views of the atrial septum from either basal short-axis or bicaval view and to monitor device deployment from the deep transgastric bicaval view, basal short-axis view, or midesophageal bicaval view. 3D full-volume views from the apical and deep transgastric views are obtained in each case if time allows.

BEST 3D TEE VIEWS OF ASD

The important anatomic features of ASD are best demonstrated using the following views. The right atrium en face view provides clear anatomic visualization of the type of ASD present; its shape, size, location, number of orifices; size of the ASD rims; and the size of the coronary sinus. The left atrium en face view demonstrates the type of ASD present, the right pulmonary vein posterior rim, and phasic changes in ASD size and shape.

A transgastric sagittal view is very useful as it best demonstrates the inferior and superior rims, caval veins, septal length, and device configuration and orientation during deployment. This view is ideal to demonstrate the inferior rim, which can be difficult to see clearly from esophageal position views. The posterior view best demonstrates the alignment between septum primum and septum secundum in secundum ASD and caval vein override of the ASD in sinus venosus ASD. The posterior aspect views also show the changing alignment of the septum primum and septum secundum over the cardiac cycle and the curvilinear anatomy of the atrial septum.

STATUS AND ROLE OF 3DE IN ATRIAL SEPTAL DEFECTS

The development of matrix array real-time live 3D TTE and TEE and related software has made the 3D imaging of ASD rapid and accurate. Qualitative and quantitative analyses are feasible and rapid. It is now possible to perform actual real-time 3D TTE and TEE imaging using live 3D and 3D zoom modes or very rapid reconstruction with 3D full-volume and color Doppler 3DE modes. Image quality, resolution, frame rate, ease of use, and quantitative capabilities have clearly improved markedly over prior technologies. 3D visualization of surfaces, volumes, dynamic changes, surrounding anatomy, unique views, and advanced quantitation can now be performed rapidly and accurately. These developments overcome many of the barriers that have limited the clinical application and advancement from 2D to 3D TEE imaging. However, technical limitations persist; further experience must be gained and protocols and training must be developed before a paradigm shift from 2DE to 3DE as the main clinical imaging modality can be contemplated at most centers. For now, 3D TEE has an expanding and complementary role to 2D TEE. Currently, 3D TEE is limited to patients weighing 20 kg or more; however, 3D TTE can be performed even in preterm infants, although rapid heart rates and respirations limit the use of full-volume 3D and 3D zoom modes in this population.

3D TTE and TEE are feasible with high diagnostic accuracy and provide additional detailed anatomic data. Speed, resolution, ease of application, and quantitative capabilities continue to improve. Limitations persist despite extensive technical improvements. Ideal 3DE image acquisition features should include live 3D cropping, faster frame rates, penetration to greater depths, and single-frame full-volume acquisition.

REFERENCES

1. Hoffman JI, Kaplan S. The incidence of congenital heart disease. *J Am Coll Cardiol*. 2002;39(12):1890–1900.
2. Bharati, S and Lev, M. Atrial septal defect, secundum. In: Bharati S, Lev M, eds. *The Pathology of Congenital Heart Disease: A Personal Experience with More than 6,300 Congenitally Malformed Hearts*. Armonk, NY: Futura Publishing; 1996:451–490.
3. Porter CJ, Feldt RH, Edwards WD, Seward JB, Schaff HV. In: Moss AJ, Adams FH, Emmanouilides GC, eds. *Moss and Adams' Heart Disease in Infants, Children and Adolescents: Including the Fetus and Young Adult*. Vol 1 (Atrial septal defects). 7th ed. Baltimore, MD: Williams & Wilkins; 1995:687–703.
4. Butera G, Romagnoli E, Carminati M, et al. Treatment of isolated secundum atrial septal defects: impact of age and defect morphology in 1,013 consecutive patients. *Am Heart J*. 2008;156(4):706–712.
5. Marx GR, Fulton DR, Pandian NG, et al. Delineation of site, relative size and dynamic geometry of atrial septal defects by real time three-dimensional echocardiography. *J Am Coll Cardiol*. 1995;25(2):482–490.
6. Acar P, Saliba Z, Bonhoeffer P, et al. Influence of atrial septal defect anatomy in patient selection and assessment of closure with the Cardioseal device; a three-dimensional transoesophageal echocardiographic reconstruction. *Eur Heart J*. 2000;21(7):573–581.
7. Cao QL, Radtke W, Berger F, et al. Transcatheter closure of multiple atrial septal defects. Initial results and value of two- and three-dimensional transoesophageal echocardiography. *Eur Heart J*. 2000;21(11):941–947.
8. van den Bosch AE, Ten Harkel DJ, McGhie JS, et al. Characterization of atrial septal defect assessed by real-time 3-dimensional echocardiography. *J Am Soc Echocardiogr*. 2006;19(6):815–821.
9. Taniguchi M, Akagi T, Watanabe N, et al. Application of real-time three-dimensional transesophageal echocardiography using a matrix array probe for transcatheter closure of atrial septal defect. *J Am Soc Echocardiogr*. 2009;22(10):1114–1120.

10. Faletra FF, Ho SY, Auricchio A. Anatomy of right atrial structures by real-time 3D transesophageal echocardiography. *JACC Cardiovasc Imaging*. 2010;3(9):966–975.
11. Pushparajah K, Miller OI, Simpson JM. 3D echocardiography of the atrial septum: anatomical features and landmarks for the echocardiographer. *JACC Cardiovasc Imaging*. 2010;3(9):981–984.
12. Lai WW, Geva T, Shirali GS, et al. Guidelines and standards for performance of a pediatric echocardiogram: a report from the Task Force of the Pediatric Council of the American Society of Echocardiography. *J Am Soc Echocardiogr*. 2006;19(12):1413–1430.

CHAPTER 7

THREE-DIMENSIONAL ECHOCARDIOGRAPHIC ASSESSMENT OF VENTRICULAR SEPTAL DEFECT

Sinai C. Zyblewski; Anthony M. Hlavacek, MD; Robert H. Anderson, BSc, MD

ABSTRACT

Three-dimensional (3D) reconstruction has revolutionized our appreciation of the location and phenotypic features of holes between the ventricles. The approach we use to categorize holes between the ventricles can be used not only for isolated defects seen in patients with concordant atrioventricular and ventriculoarterial connections but also for defects seen in patients with more complex malformations of the heart. All ventricular septal defects, when viewed from the right ventricle, can be placed in one of three groups: defects with exclusively muscular borders, those with fibrous continuity in their posteroinferior rim between the leaflets of an arterial and an atrioventricular valve, and those with fibrous continuity between the leaflets of the two arterial valves. Attention must also be directed to the way the hole opens into the right ventricle (to the right ventricular inlet, the apical component of the right ventricle, or the ventricular outlet) and to the malalignment between the outlet septum and the remainder of the muscular septum. The 3D analysis of these features is outlined.

INTRODUCTION

Holes between the ventricles are the most frequently encountered congenital cardiac malformations. Although several issues relating to their categorization and description remain contentious, these can largely be resolved when using three-dimensional echocardiography (3DE). Surprisingly, although multiple articles have been written comparing the value of the three-dimensional (3D) approach with more conventional echocardiographic techniques,[1–3] to the best of our knowledge, apart from our own previous review, none have sought to use the 3D approach to assess the anatomic categorization of the various defects. Characterization of the defects is usually based on the anatomy of the normal ventricular septum. The knowledge of normal anatomy now provided by appropriate 3DE interrogation shows that some of the holes, notably those opening directly beneath both arterial valvar leaflets, cannot exist in an otherwise normally constructed heart, since the essence of these defects is absence of the freestanding muscular subpulmonary infundibulum. These, and other, subtle anatomic features do not seem to be generally appreciated. They are now demonstrated with exquisite accuracy using 3D interrogation. Such analysis also shows that fundamental differences exist between the defects often described as being of the "atrioventricular canal" type. In this chapter, therefore, we concentrate on showing how the use of 3D reconstruction can revolutionize the appreciation of the location and phenotypic features of holes between ventricles. We further show that the system we recommend for description can be used not only for the so-called isolated defects, these being the ones seen in patients with concordant atrioventricular and ventriculoarterial connections, but also for the defects seen in patients with more complex malformations of the heart.[4]

CATEGORIZATION OF VENTRICULAR SEPTAL DEFECTS

Several disparate approaches are currently used for categorizing holes between the ventricles. If we had our druthers, we would prefer to describe "holes between the ventricles," since there is no uniform agreement on the plane of space to be described as a "ventricular septal defect." It is this lack of a uniform definition that underscores some of the differences between the systems used previously to distinguish different anatomic defects. One time-honored system placed the holes in one of four types identified numerically.[5] The definining feature chosen for each of the groups in this system, however, is far from being uniform. Defects placed in the first category are those that occupy the area that, in the normal heart, is usually closed by the membranous part of the interventricular septum. These defects, therefore, are defined by their phenotypic morphology, specifically the presence in the posteroinferior margin of fibrous continuity between the leaflets of the aortic and tricuspid valves (Fig. 7-1). The second group is also defined on the basis of phenotypic morphology, the paradigm for this group being that the holes have exclusively muscular borders (Fig. 7-2). But these holes can occupy markedly different parts of the muscular ventricular septum (compare Fig. 7-2A and B). This fact illustrates the need, when describing the defects, to account not only for their phenotypic morphology but also for the way they open into the right ventricle.

Figure 7-1

Phenotypic features of the so-called type 1 ventricular septal defect. There is fibrous continuity in the posteroinferior margin of the defect between the leaflets of the aortic and tricuspid valves. Based on this feature, we describe such defects as being perimembranous, irrespective of how they open into the right ventricle.

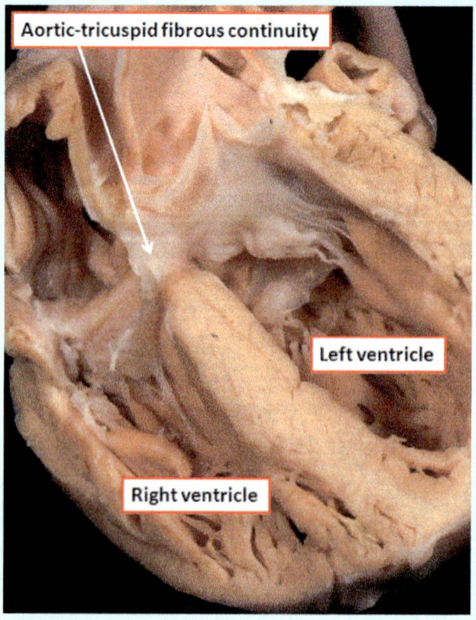

Figure 7-2A and B

Two defects that would be categorized as type 2. Both have exclusively muscular borders; but the hole shown in panel *A* opens into the inlet of the right ventricle (RV), whereas that shown in panel *B* opens into the right ventricular outlet.

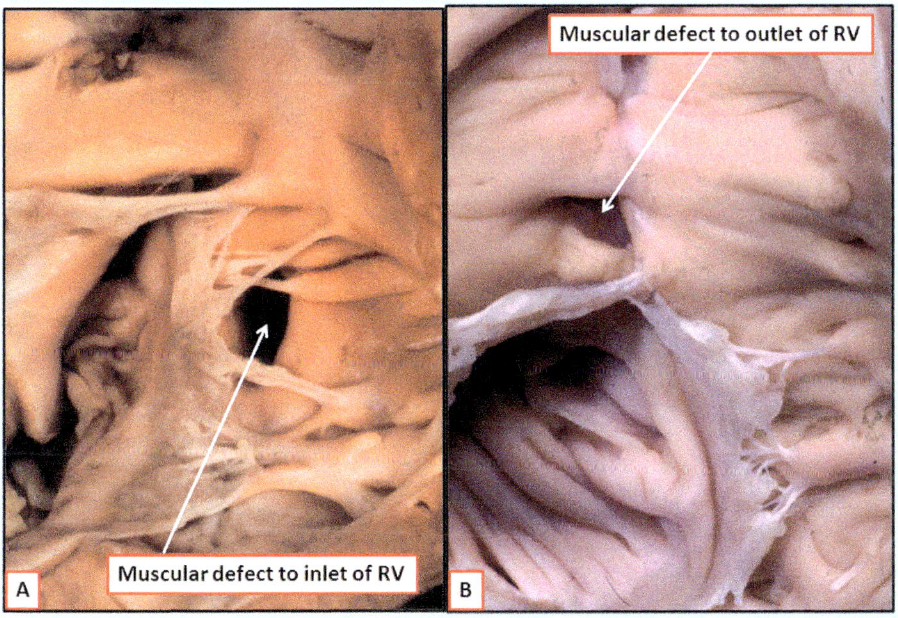

The patients making up the third group are unified because the holes open directly beneath the leaflets of both arterial valves. These holes can also differ in their phenotyic morphology, depending on whether their posteroinferior margins are muscular (Fig. 7-3A) or fibrous (Fig. 7-3B).

If there is fibrous continuity posteroinferiorly, then patients with such defects are also rightly considered as belonging in the first group. It is the patients who are allegedly to be placed in the fourth group that give the greatest problems, since according to the initial classification these patients are supposed to have atrioventricular canal defects. It is now well established that the essential phenotypic feature of the atrioventricular canal defect is the commonality of the atrioventricular junction.[6] It is then a fact that patients with this phenotypic feature can, indeed, possess defects that confine shunting at the ventricular level (Fig. 7-4A). Previous investigators, nonetheless, have also described patients with straddling and overriding of the tricuspid valve as having atrioventricular canal defects,[7] seemingly ignoring the fact that such patients have separate right and left atrioventricular junctions (Fig. 7-4B).

Some also consider that patients with large holes adjacent to the site of the membranous septum should be cataegorized as having atrioventricular canal defects.[8] When it is recognized that the defining feature of these holes is the presence of fibrous continuity posteroinferiorly between the leaflets of the aortic and tricuspid valves, then these patients are obviously also placed appropriately in the first group, providing that it is recognized that the holes predominantly open into the inlet of the right ventricle. The problems that potentially exist with the time-honored approach to categorization, therefore, can be resolved simply by separating the defects initially on the basis of their phenotypic morphology and then describing the way they open into the right ventricle.

In a second popular categorization,[8] those holes that open directly beneath both arterial valvar leaflets are recognized as a discrete group, but described on the basis of conal hypoplasia. A further feature of this system of categorization is to emphasize the malalignment that frequently exists between the conal septum and the remainder of the muscular ventricular septum, as exemplified by the morphologic features of tetralogy of Fallot (Fig. 7-5). We also recognize the need to take note of this feature, but we know that septal malalignment is not confined to patients with tetralogy of Fallot. Even those with unequivocal tetralogy, furthermore, can show

Figure 7-3A and B

Two defects that would be classified as type 3 in the time-honored system. They differ in that the hole shown in panel *A* has a muscular posteroinferior rim, which protects the atrioventricular conduction axis, whereas the hole shown in panel *B* exhibits aortic–tricuspid continuity, which means that the hole is also perimembranous. We describe these defects as being doubly committed and juxta arterial.

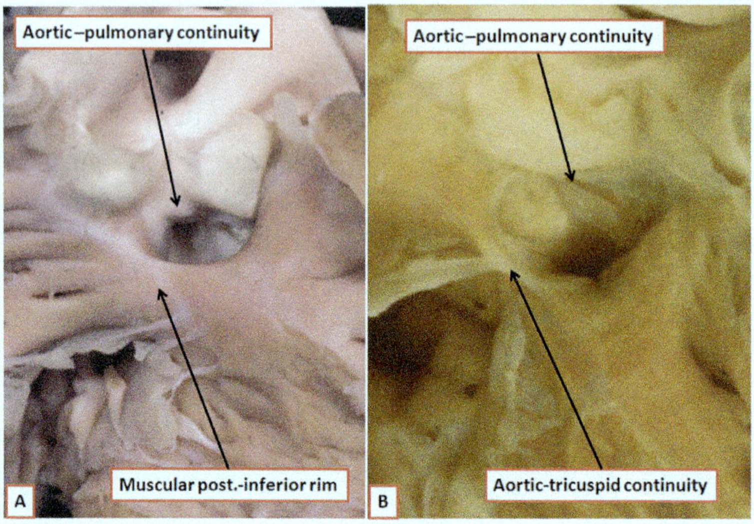

Figure 7-4A and B

Two holes opening into the inlet of the right ventricle. In the hole shown in panel *A* (star), the valvar leaflets bridge through the defect and are tethered in both right and left ventricles. This is because the heart has a common atrioventricular junction. The bridging leaflets are tethered to the underside of the atrial septum so that shunting through an atrioventricular septal defect is confined at the ventricular level. The hole shown in panel *B* is also associated with a valve tethered in both ventricles, but in this instance the valve is tricuspid rather than common. This heart does not have an atrioventricular canal. Double-headed arrows show the separate right and left atrioventricular junctions. The phenotypic feature is malalignment of the atrial and ventricular septal structures (stars).

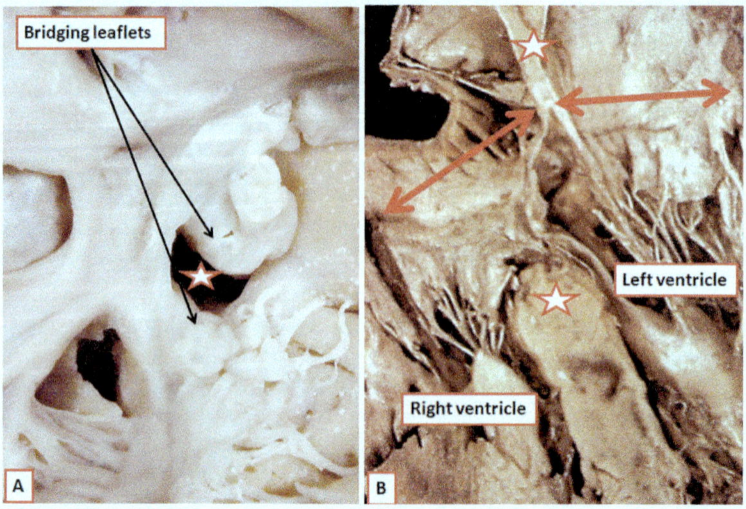

Figure 7-5A, B, and C

Hearts with malalignment between the outlet septum (muscular in panels *A* and *B*, and fibrous in panel *C*) and the remainder of the muscular ventricular septum. All, therefore, show conoventricular malalignment. The defects differ markedly, nonetheless, in terms of their phenotype. The heart shown in panel *A* has a perimembranous defect, whereas that shown in panel *B* is muscular and the one seen in panel *C* is doubly committed and juxta arterial.

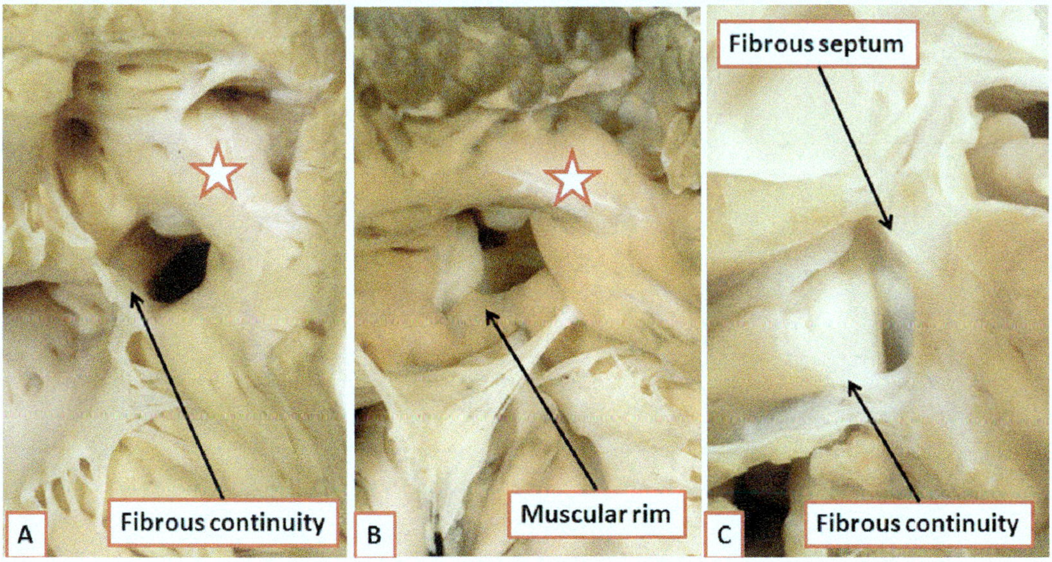

marked phenotypic variability when grouped together because of so-called conoventricular malalignment (Fig. 7-5B and C).

The system we advocate for differentiating the various defects has evolved from the categorization that was initially popularized in Europe.[9] This approach was based on the concept that all ventricular septal defects, when viewed from the right ventricle, could be placed in one of three groups. These groups are made up of defects with exclusively muscular borders (Fig. 7-2); those with fibrous continuity in their posteroinferior rim between the leaflets of an arterial and an atrioventricular valve (Fig. 7-1); and those with fibrous continuity between the leaflets of the two arterial valves, the patients falling in this latter group also, in some circumstances, satisfying the criteria for placement in the second group (Fig. 7-3). In addition to the phenotypic features, this system mandates that attention be directed to at least two other features. The first is the way in which the hole opens into the right ventricle. This can be to the right ventricular inlet, apical component of the right ventricle, or ventricular outlet, with large defects often opening in a confluent fashion to all parts of the right ventricle. The second feature requiring diagnosis and description is malalalignment between the septal components. Most commonly, this involves malalignment between the outlet septum, which can be muscular or fibrous, and the remainder of the muscular septum. The malalignment can be toward the right ventricle, as in tetralogy of Fallot (Fig. 7-5), or toward the left ventricle, a feature typically associated with coarctation or interruption of the aortic arch when the ventriculoarterial connections are concordant (Fig. 7-6A) but with subpulmonary stenosis in the setting of discordant ventriculoarterial connections (Fig. 7-6B). As we will show, all these features lend themselves to 3D analysis.

3D analysis also reveals the size of the defects, and whether or not they show features of spontaneous reduction in size, or even spontaneous closure. When properly employed, therefore, the 3D technique provides all the necessary clinical information for the diagnosis and treatment of patients with ventricular septal defects.

Figure 7-6A and B

Hearts with malalignment of the muscular outlet septum (star), but toward the left ventricle rather than the right ventricle as shown in Figure 7-5. The malalignment produces subaortic obstruction in the heart shown in panel *A*, which has concordant ventriculoarterial connections, but subpulmonary obstruction in the heart shown in panel *B*, which has concordant atrioventricular and discordant ventriculoarterial connections, or transposition.

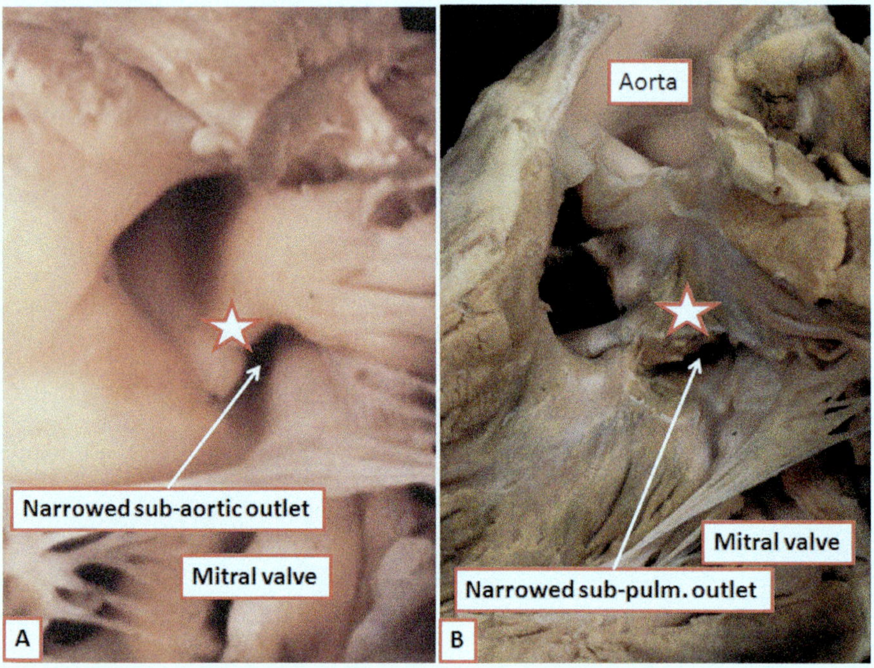

NORMAL VENTRICULAR SEPTUM

The normal ventricular septum has extensive muscular components and a very small fibrous component. The fibrous part is usually known as the membranous septum. The extensive muscular septum is not related, as might be expected, to the components of the ventricles themselves. It was Goor and Lillehei[10] who first pointed to the advantages gained from describing the ventricles in terms of their inlet, outlet, and apical trabecular components, rather than "sinus" and "conus." The tripartite approach to description, however, is less well suited to the ventricular septum. In hearts with separate right and left atrioventricular junctions, very little of the normal muscular ventricular septum interposes between the ventricular inlets. This is because, in the normal situation, the subaortic outflow tract interposes between the orifice of the mitral valve and the ventricular septum (Fig. 7-7). Because of this wedging of the subaortic area, the membranous septum interposes between the left ventricular outlet component and both the right-sided chambers, the attachment of the hinge of the septal leaflet of the tricuspid valve dividing the fibrous septum into atrioventricular and interventricular components (Fig. 7-8). The larger part of the extensive muscular septum interposes between the apical ventricular components. There is virtually no muscular septum interposed between the ventricular outlets, the leaflets of the pulmonary valve being lifted away from the base of the ventricular mass by the freestanding infundibular sleeve (Fig. 7-9).

The roof of the normal right ventricle is the so-called crista supraventricularis, or the supraventricular crest. 3D interrogation is able to show that the greater part of the crest, which separates the leaflets of the tricuspid and pulmonary valves, is formed by the parietal wall of the right ventricle, or the ventriculoinfundibular fold

Figure 7-7A and B

3DE images showing how, in the normal heart, the subaortic outflow tract interposes between the mitral valve and the septum (star in panel *B*). Panel *A* is reconstructed to show the four-chamber projection, whereas panel *B* shows the arrangement as seen in short axis. As seen in panel *B*, the muscular septum adjacent to the subaortic area (double-headed arrow) is an inlet–outlet septum. This explains why ventricular septal defects opening in the perimembranous position are directly subaortic.

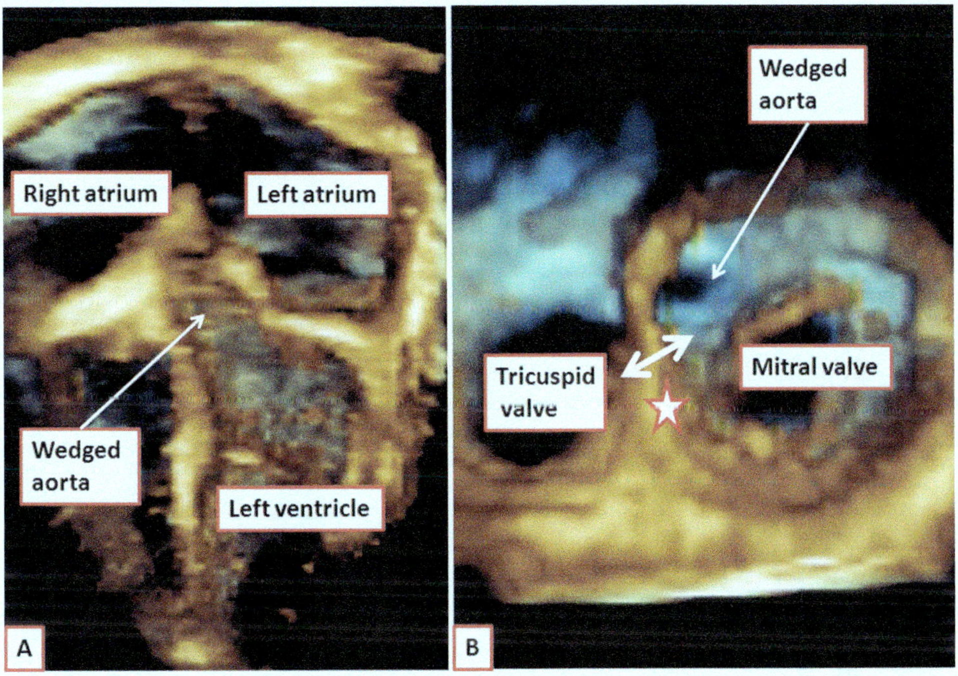

(Fig. 7-9B). The fold is distally continuous with the freestanding muscular infundibular sleeve. When viewed internally, the fold inserts between the limbs of the prominent muscular trabeculation known as either the septal band or the septomarginal trabeculation. As we will see, perimembranous defects open to the right ventricle between the limbs of the septomarginal trabeculation. It is only when the ventricular septum is deficient that it becomes possible to recognize the component parts of the supraventricular crest in their own right, the outlet septum, be it muscular (Fig. 7-5A and B) or fibrous (Fig. 7-5C) then interposing between the subaortic and subpulmonary outlets. The ventriculoinfundibular fold then remains recognizable because, as part of the inner heart curvature, it always interposes between the leaflets of an arterial valve and those of an atrioventricular valve.[11]

HOW TO INTERROGATE THE VENTRICULAR SEPTUM WITH 3DE

The advent of the 3D format has provided superior and unique views of the ventricular septum that historically were unachievable when using standard cross-sectional imaging. With the latter technique, it is difficult to interrogate the complex and spherical morphology of the ventricular septum because it requires the mental integration of multiple composite orthogonal views. In contrast, the 3D approach allows the visualization of the entire ventricular septum and is especially useful in delineating the static and dynamic shapes of defects, their spatial relationship to other cardiac structures, and the distance between multiple defects.[1,2]

Figure 7-8

3D image, taken in the four-chamber arrangement, showing the location of the membranous septum and revealing how the hinge of the septal leaflet of the tricuspid valve divides it into atrioventricular (white arrow) and interventricular (red arrow) components.

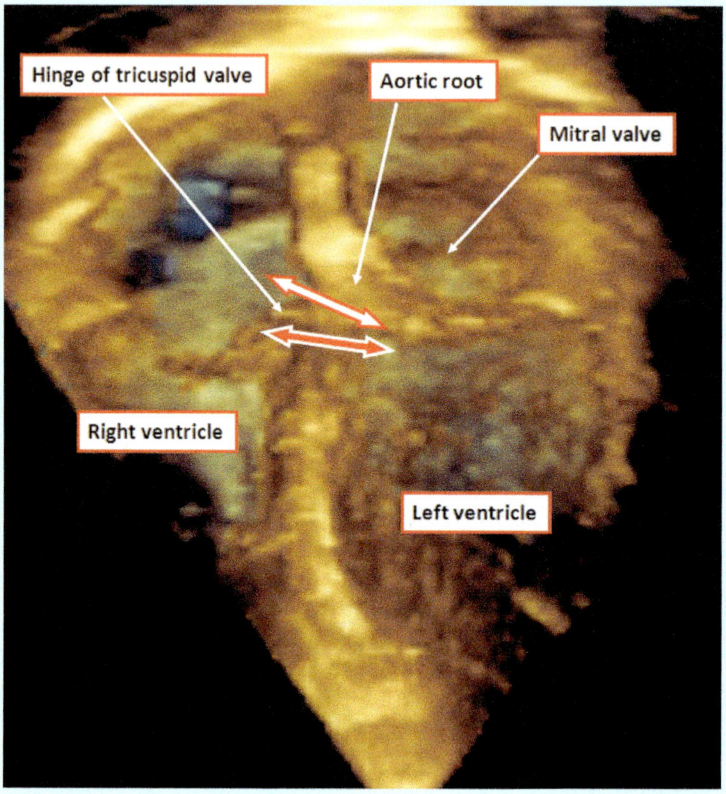

The ability to acquire real-time images and improved offline reconstruction have facilitated wider acceptance of this modality in the echocardiography laboratory, especially when making plans for either surgical or percutaneous closure.[2,12–15] Optimal preprocedural planning includes a complete and detailed transthoracic echocardiogram, which ideally consists of thorough cross-sectional imaging complemented by focused acquisitions in 3D. One of the primary merits of the 3D approach is the visualization of a structure in a dynamic mode from multiple views. One of the more useful views that may be achieved is the en face view of the ventricular septum. To attain this view, a full-volume acquisition is made from a standard apical position showing the four cardiac chambers. The lateral walls of the right and left ventricles are then cropped, leaving the ventricular septum in the middle. The image may then be rotated rightward to visualize the right ventricular aspect of the septum (Fig. 7-9B). Given that the view from the right ventricle is frequently obscured by overlying tissue or cardiac structures, the image can then be rotated through 180° so that it is viewed from the smooth-walled left ventricular surface. From the left ventricular view, visualization of the defect is generally unobstructed and the entire circumference of the defect may be seen, allowing accurate determination of its size and shape.[1,3] In these views, it is also possible to determine the precise location of the defect relative to the components of the ventricular septum or, if more than one septal defect is present, the spatial relationship of the defects to each other. Color Doppler may also be added to the images, assisting in the identification of all the defects that are present. Since data sets including color Doppler interrogation require longer acquisition times, and have lower frame rates, these sets are usually acquired with a notable decline in the quality of images. Thus, in our experience, the clinical utility of color Doppler interrogation is limited. Future advances in technology will likely improve this limitation.

Figure 7-9A and B

3D images showing (*A*) how the freestanding subpulmonary infundibulum (double-headed arrow) lifts the leaflets of the pulmonary valve away from the base of the heart. Because of the presence of this muscular sleeve, there is very little muscular outlet septum in the normal heart. Panel *B* shows that the greater part of the supraventricular crest is the inner heart curvature, interposed between the leaflets of the tricuspid and pulmonary valves.

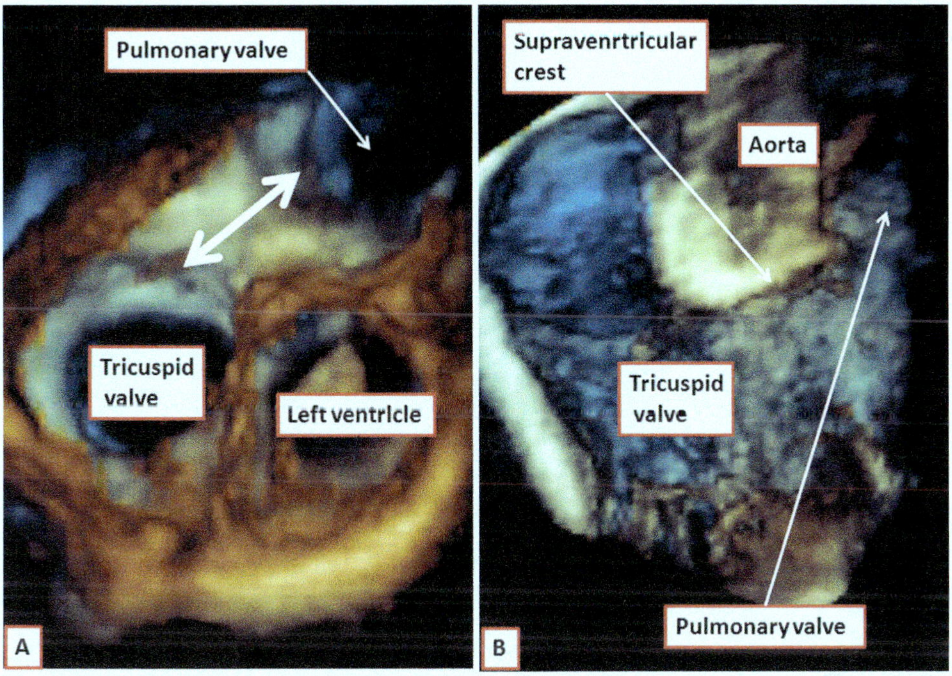

Ventricular septal defects versus holes between the ventricles

When describing the different types of ventricular septal defects, we define the phenotypic features as seen from the morphologically right ventricle. This creates potential problems if the hole then defined as the ventricular septal defect is also considered to represent interventricular communication, or hole between the ventricles. Many of the holes coexist with overriding of an arterial valve. In this situation, true interventricular communication is the plane represented by the continuation of the long axis of the ventricular septum to the undersurface of the closed arterial valve (Fig. 7-10). The true interventricular communication is not the hole that is closed by either the surgeon or the transcatheter interventionist to restore septal integrity. It is the right ventricular margin of the space between the leaflets of the overriding valve and the crest of the muscular septum that is closed so as to restore septal integrity. And it is this plane that, for those speaking Anglo-Saxon languages, is usually nominated as the ventricular septal defect. Presumably it is also this hole, rather than the plane separating the cavities of the right and left ventricles, that is described as the interventricular communication by those speaking languages such as French, Italian, Spanish, and Portuguese. Problems arise, however, should such usage be extended to patients with a double-outlet right ventricle. In this setting, it is the plane of space separating the cavities of the ventricles that, without question, is the interventricular communication. This hole is also the outlet for the morphologically left ventricle and cannot be closed during surgical repairs designed to restore biventricular communications unless an alternative outlet is provided for the left ventricle. In most surgical repairs, the hole between the ventricles is tunneled to one of the subarterial outlets. Most observers, nonetheless, describe the hole as the ventricular septal defect. If a comparison is made with isolated defects, the locus used by the surgeon to create the tunnel should be nominated as the ventricular septal defect (Fig. 7-11).

Figure 7-10

Computed tomographic image showing a four-chamber cut through a patient with marked overriding of the aortic valve, such that the aortic root is supported in its greater part by the right ventricle. The white arrow shows how the continuation of the long axis of the ventricular septum is the interventricular plane. The so-called ventricular septal defect closed by the surgeon in this setting, however, is shown by the gold arrow, which is the right ventricular entrance to the overriding aortic root. The yellow arrow shows the plane marking the outlet from the left ventricle.

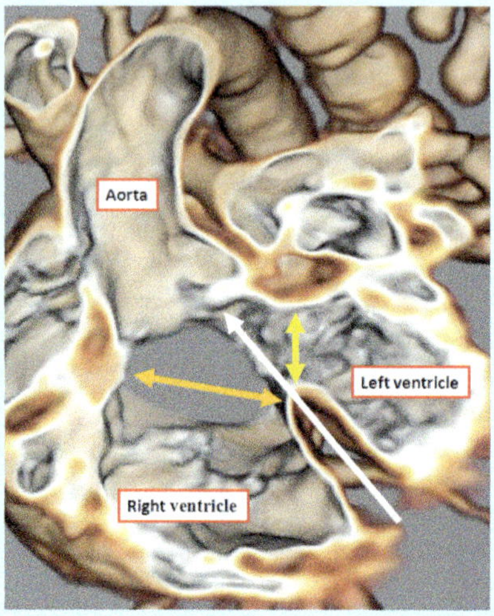

Figure 7-11

3D image showing a patient with double-outlet right ventricle, bilateral infundibulums (white arrow showing subaortic infundibulum), and subaortic defect. The yellow dashes outline the interventricular communication. This is not the hole closed by the surgeon to achieve biventricular repair. The locus for tunneling to achieve biventricular repair is shown by the green dashes. By analogy to the situation for isolated defects, this should be the plane defined as the ventricular septal defect.

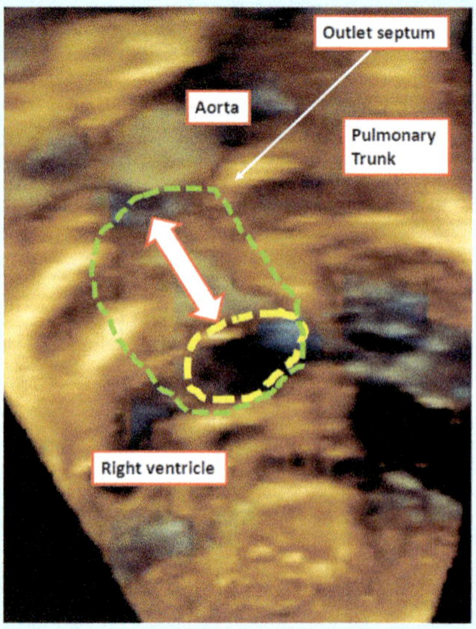

DIAGNOSING AND DESCRIBING VENTRICULAR SEPTAL DEFECTS

As we have discussed, the approach we use takes as its primary feature the structure of the borders of the defects as seen from the right ventricle. Over and above this feature, however, we have emphasized the need also to account for the way the defects open into the ventricle and any malalignment between the septal structures. It is now recognized that avoidance of the iatrogenic heart block, during either surgical repair[16] or interventional closure,[17] is of paramount importance when seeking the optimal therapeutic approach to closure, so it follows that providing knowledge of the site of the penetrating atrioventricular bundle should be one of the major tasks of the diagnostician. Since this information can be provided by knowing the phenotypic anatomy of the various defects,[18] it also follows that the establishment of the anatomic nature of the borders of the defects deserves recognition as the primary diagnostic feature.

Differentiating the holes that open to the inlet of the right ventricle

There are four phenotypically discrete holes that open toward the right ventricular inlet. The anatomic feature of the commonest type is the presence of fibrous continuity between the leaflets of the aortic, mitral, and tricuspid valves. Incorporated within this fibrous region is the atrioventricular component of the membranous septum, often with the remnant of the interventricular component of the membranous septum recognizable as a triangular fibrous flap reinforcing the posteroinferior margin of the defect. Such defects are perimembranous, having the components of the membranous septum as part of their perimeter (Fig. 7-12). Recognition of these features establishes the fact that the atrioventricular bundle is located posteroinferiorly relative to the defect (Fig. 7-13A).

Figure 7-12A and B

3D images showing how the components of the membranous septum (MS) form the posteroinferior margin of perimembranous defects opening into the inlet of the right ventricle. Panel *A* shows the view from the right ventricle, whereas panel *B* shows the left ventricular aspect. VSD, ventricular septal defect.

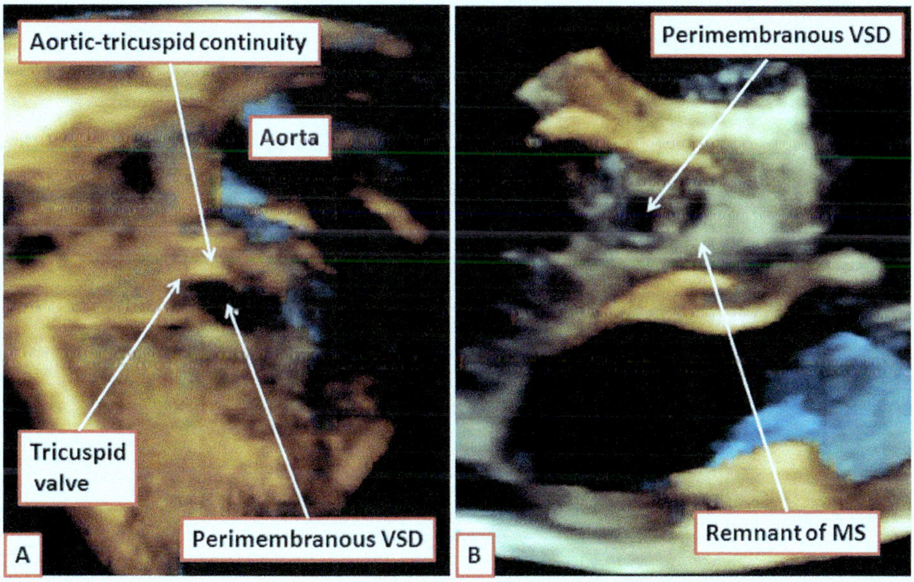

Figure 7-13A, B, and C

Three defects that open into the inlet of the right ventricle, showing how the location of the atrioventricular conduction axis (black dotted line) differs depending on the phenotype. Panel *A* shows a perimembranous defect, with the atrioventricular node (red oval) at the apex of the triangle of Koch. The axis is located posteroinferiorly. Panel *B* shows a muscular defect. The node is again at the apex of the triangle of Koch, but the axis is now located anterosuperiorly. Panel *C* shows the defect associated with the straddling and overriding of the tricuspid valve. A node is still present at the apex of the triangle of Koch (green oval), but it does not connect with the atrioventricular bundle. Instead, an anomalous node (red oval) is formed at the junction of the malaligned ventricular septum with the right atrioventricular junction.

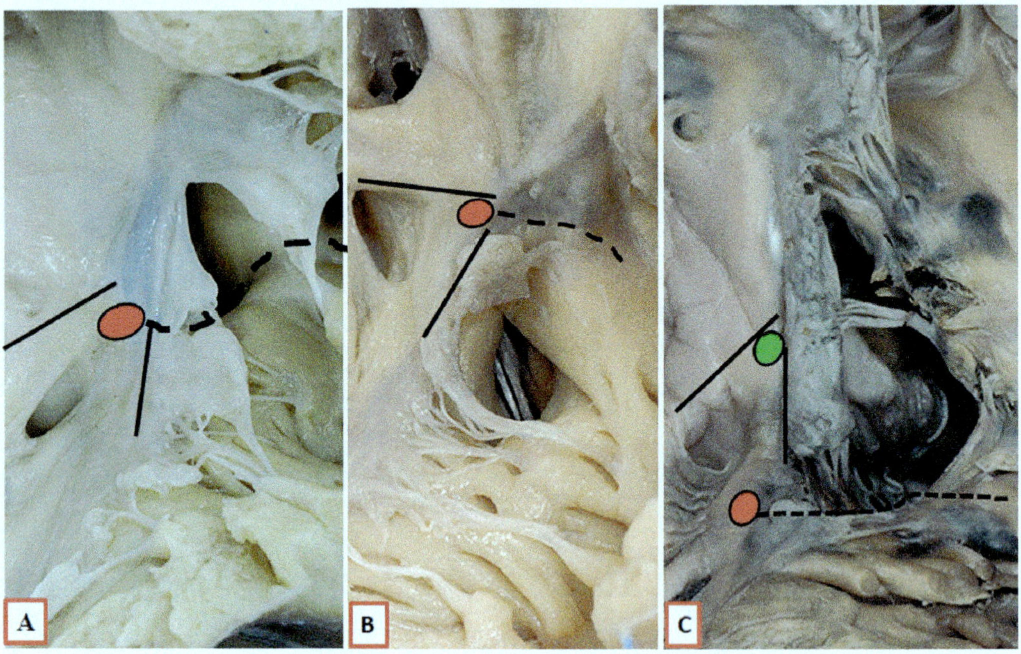

Muscular defects can also open to the inlet of the right ventricle (Fig. 7-14). Because of the integrity of the membranous septum in this setting, the atrioventricular conduction axis runs anterocephalad to the muscular inlet defect (Fig. 7-13B). Atrioventricular septal defects with exclusively ventricular shunting constitute another type of defect opening to the inlet of the right ventricle (Fig. 7-4A). These defects are similar to perimembranous defects in that they are bordered in part by fibrous tissue. The distinguishing echocardiographic feature is the presence of the common atrioventricular junction, along with the trifoliate left atrioventricular valve (Fig. 7-15). The atrioventricular conduction axis is positioned posteroinferiorly in atrioventricular septal defects, but the atrioventricular node is displaced markedly inferiorly, lying in a nodal triangle rather than the regular triangle of Koch.[19]

The final defect opening into the right ventricular inlet is the one associated with the straddling and overriding of the tricuspid valve (Fig. 7-4B). The diagnostic feature of this defect is malalignment between the atrial and ventricular septal structures. Not only does this feature permit echocardiographic recognition (Fig. 7-16), it also underscores the grossly abnormal location of the atrioventricular conduction axis, which arises from an anomalous atrioventricular node formed at the point of union between the malaligned ventricular septum and the right atrioventricular junction (Fig. 7-13C).[20]

Figure 7-14

3D image showing a muscular defect (double-headed arrow) opening into the inlet of the right ventricle. As can be seen, there is preservation of the offsetting of the hinges of the leaflets of the atrioventricular valves (red arrows).

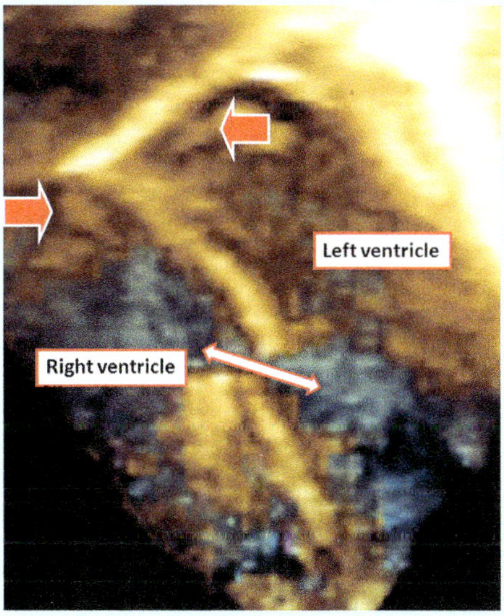

Figure 7-15

3D image showing the trifoliate left atrioventricular valve, the characteristic feature of patients with atrioventricular septal defect and common atrioventricular junction. The leaflets are the left ventricular components of the two leaflets bridging the ventricular septum (1, 2) and the mural leaflet (3), which guards less than one-third of the left half of the common junction. It would be necessary also to reconstruct the four-chamber plane so as to show that shunting across the atrioventricular septal defect is confined at the ventricular level when the bridging leaflets are attached to the underside of the atrial septum.

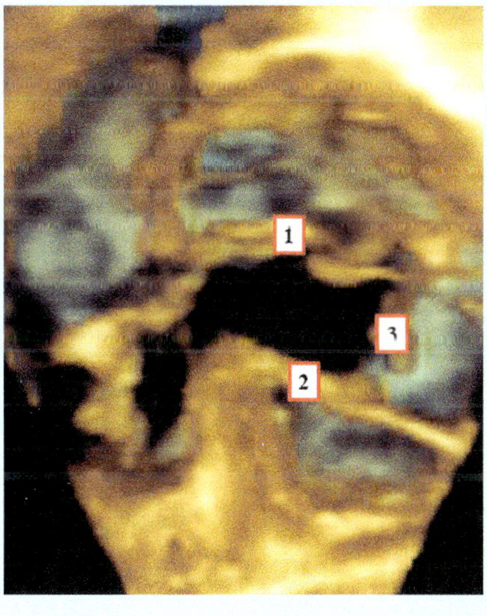

Figure 7-16

3D image showing malalignment between the atrial septum (white star with red border) and the muscular ventricular septum (red star with white border), this being the pathognomonic feature of the inlet defect found in the setting of the straddling and overriding of the tricuspid valve. Note that the mitral valve is supported by a discrete and separate left atrioventricular junction, showing that this is not an "atrioventricular canal" defect.

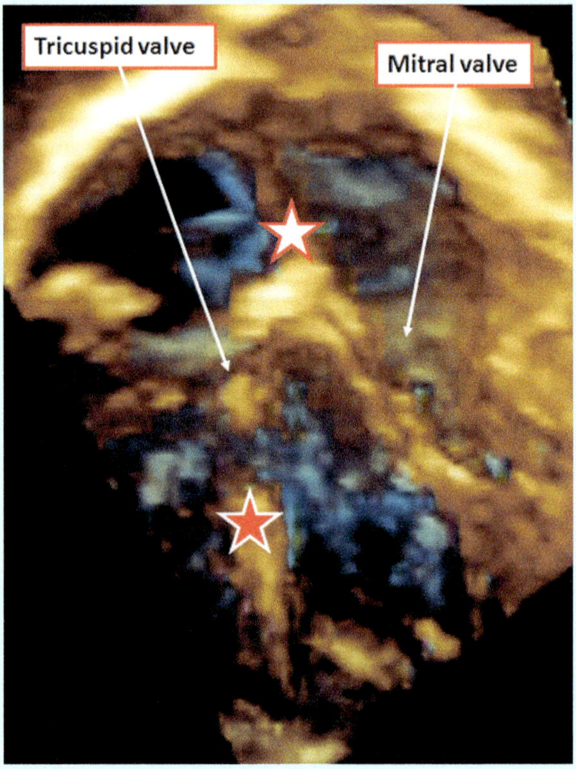

Holes opening into the right ventricle at the site of the membranous septum

Holes opening into the right ventricle at the site of the membranous septum are the commonest defects found in patients requiring therapeutic closure, although when taken overall muscular defects are probably the commonest holes between ventricles. The typical holes requiring closure open in the area usually filled by the interventricular component of the membranous septum. The holes requiring closure, however, occupy areas appreciably larger than the space usually filled by the interventricular component of the membranous septum.[2] As we have already seen when assessing such holes that open into the inlet of the right ventricle, the diagnostic feature is the presence of fibrous continuity between the leaflets of the aortic and tricuspid valves, with the fibrous area incorporating the components of the membranous septum as part of the anatomic border of the defect (Fig. 7-12). In all defects having this feature, apart from the ones associated with the straddling and overriding of the tricuspid valve, the atrioventricular bundle is related to the posteroinferior corner and will be found to the right hand of the surgeon operating through the orifice of the tricuspid valve (Fig. 7-13A). This is the case whether such defects, which open directly beneath the inner heart curvature, extend so as to open more into the inlet (Fig. 7-12) or open primarily into the outlet of the right ventricle (Fig. 7-17).

Figure 7-17

3D image showing the en face view of the ventricular septum from the right side, revealing fibrous continuity between the leaflets of the aortic and tricuspid valves, thus establishing the defect as being perimembranous. Note the malalignment between the muscular outlet septum and the remainder of the muscular septum, so that the defect opens into the outlet of the right ventricle.

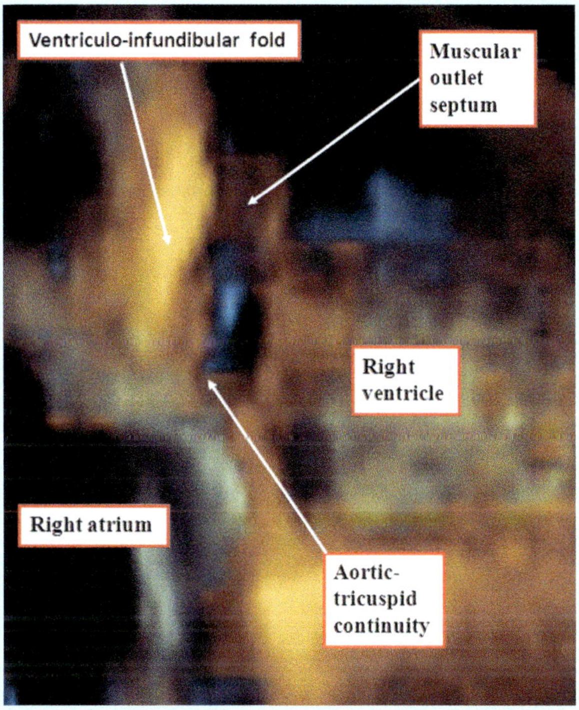

Defects opening into the outlet of the right ventricle

Defects with markedly different phenotypes can open in direct relationship to the ventricular outflow tracts. The commonest of these, once more, are the holes that possess fibrous continuity between the leaflets of the aortic and tricuspid valves as part of their border, thus making them perimembranous (Fig. 7-17). It is these defects that are often associated with either hypoplasia or malalignment of the muscular outlet septum, so that the leaflets of the aortic valve are supported in part by the right ventricle. When the outlet septum is malaligned with the remainder of the muscular septum, the defect opens into the right ventricle between the limbs of the septal band. This can be found with or without subpulmonary infundibular obstruction. In association with obstruction, this is tetralogy of Fallot (Fig. 7-5). When the pulmonary outflow tract is unobstructed, the entity is the so-called Eisenmenger defect.[21] In previous eras, these defects were recognized as being the ones most readily producing pulmonary hypertension. Nowadays, of course, the defect is closed on diagnosis so as to prevent the progression of pulmonary vascular changes. Irrespective of the presence or absence of subpulmonary stenosis, however, defects characterized by malalignment of the outlet septum can show subtly different phenotypic features. As already discussed, most frequently the defects are characterized by fibrous continuity in the posteroinferior rim between the leaflets of the aortic and tricuspid valves, making them perimembranous (Fig. 7-18). In a minority of cases, the posterocaudal limb of the septomarginal trabeculation will be found to have fused with the ventriculoinfundibular fold so that, when viewed from its right ventricular aspect, the defect has exclusively muscular borders. Defects can also open into the right ventricular outlet with exclusively muscular rims in the absence of malalignment between the muscular outlet

Figure 7-18

3D image showing the aortic and pulmonary valvar leaflets in fibrous continuity in the roof of a ventricular septal defect. This is the phenotypic feature of the doubly committed and juxta-arterial defect.

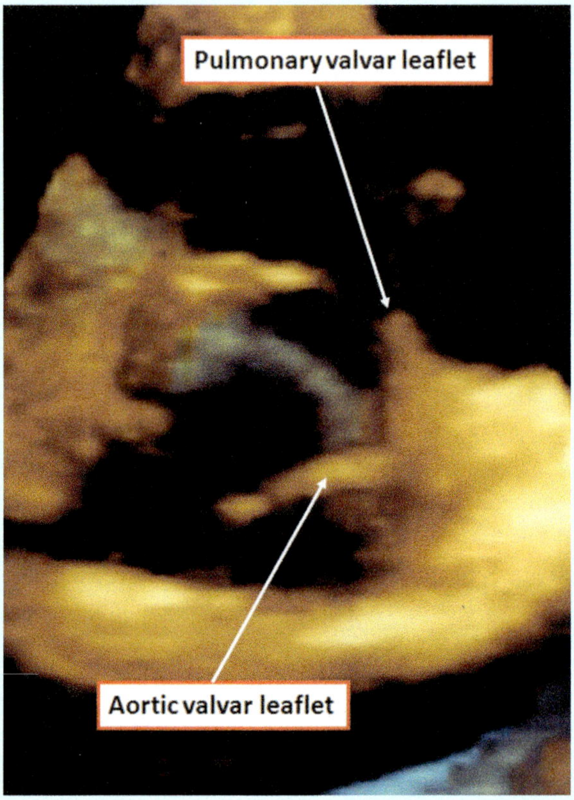

septum, although in this setting, the outlet septum itself is usually hypoplastic, and the muscular defect opens directly into the subpulmonary infundibulum (Fig. 7-2B).

There is then yet a third type of defect that opens into the outlet of the right ventricle. These are the holes exhibiting fibrous continuity between the leaflets of the aortic and pulmonary valves, making them doubly committed and juxta arterial (Fig. 7-3). The essential feature of these defects is the absence of the muscular subpulmonary infundibulum. This sleeve usually lifts the leaflets of the pulmonary valve away from the base of the heart; so, in its absence the arterial valvar leaflets are seen at the same level, this being the diagnostic echocardiographic feature (Fig. 7-18). It is sometimes possible to recognize a remnant of the outlet septum as a fibrous raphe on the ventricular aspect of the conjoined leaflets of arterial valves. Holes comparable to the doubly committed defect are also seen in the setting of common arterial trunk, although in such cases, self-evidently, it is then a common arterial valve, rather than separate aortic and pulmonary valves, which guards the common ventriculoarterial junction. Be there a common valve or separate aortic and pulmonary valves, it is most frequent to find doubly committed and juxta-arterial defects with a muscular rim formed posteroinferiorly due to the fusion of the posterocaudal limb of the septal band with the ventriculoinfundibular fold. In a small subset of patients, nonetheless, the defects can extend so as to be bordered by fibrous continuity between the leaflets of the arterial and atrioventricular valves, thus making them perimembranous. The significance of the muscular posteroinferior rim is that, when present, it covers the site of penetration of the atrioventricular conduction axis, that is, the atrioventricular bundle is less exposed during their closure.

Figure 7-19

3D image showing the aortic root in long axis from a patient with a perimembranous ventricular septal defect. There is prolapse of the right coronary leaflet of the aortic valve (arrow), which abuts the crest of the ventricular septum (star), and closes the defect.

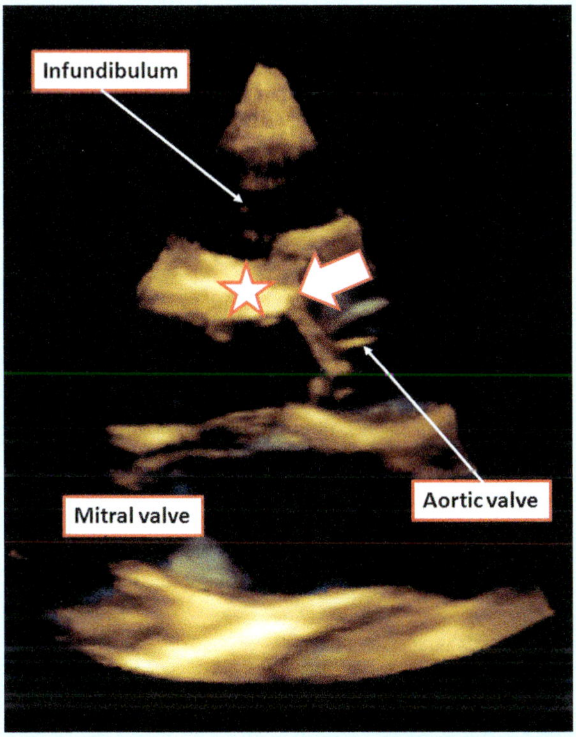

Associated lesions

The availability of 3DE interrogation now makes it possible to differentiate with total accuracy both the phenotypic features and the location of holes between ventricles. It also permits the diagnosis of associated lesions. Of these, perhaps the most important are prolapse of the leaflets of the aortic valve and ventricular outflow obstruction. Prolapsing aortic valvar leaflets are seen most frequently either with perimembranous defects opening into the outlet of the right ventricle (Fig. 7-19) or with doubly committed and juxta-arterial defects.[22,23]

Obstruction of the subpulmonary outflow tract is the essence of tetralogy of Fallot and, as we have seen, this is usually the consequence of anterocephalad malalignment of the muscular outlet septum (Fig. 7-4). We have also noted, however, that the outlet septum can be malaligned in the absence of subpulmonary obstruction. It is also the case, nonetheless, that obstruction can be acquired during life. 3DE interrogation is an excellent technique for establishing the changes that take place during the conversion of the so-called pink tetralogy to the situation with overt cyanosis. Obstruction can also be found in the left ventricular outflow tract, in many cases due to posterocaudal deviation of the muscular outlet septum (Fig. 7-6A). This lesion is typically associated with aortic coarctation or interruption. Coarctation is also seen in the setting of aortic overriding.[24] This combination should also be readily recognized using 3D interrogation. Obstruction of the left ventricular outflow tract in the setting of deficient ventricular septation can also be the consequence of the development of fibrous shelves in subaortic position, typically in association with a double-chambered right ventricle.[25]

Figure 7-20

3D image showing tissue tags derived from the leaflets of the tricuspid valve reducing the size of a perimembranous ventricular septal defect (VSD) opening into the inlet of the right ventricle. The defect is shown from the right ventricular aspect.

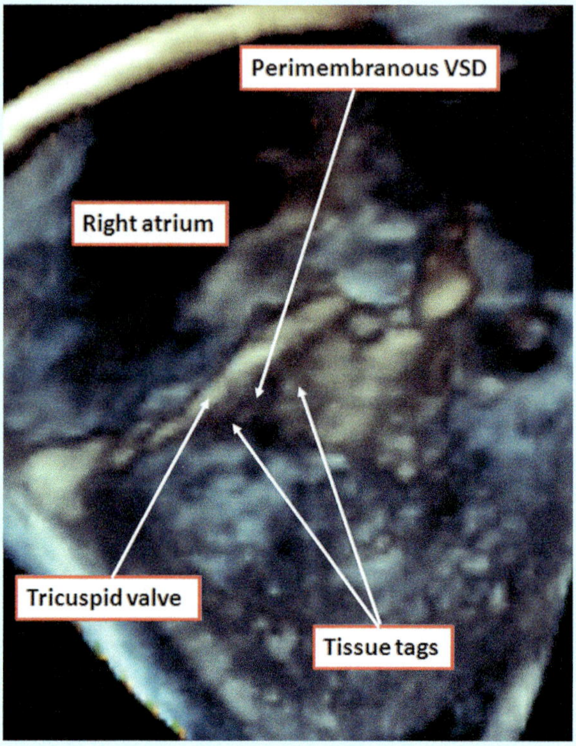

Assessing the size of a defect

3DE permits direct measurement of the size of holes in the ventricular septum and comparison of this size with the diameter of the aorta, this being one of the ways of determining whether a defect requires closure.

Spontaneous closure

Majority of the holes between ventricles undergo spontaneous diminution in size and, in many cases, complete spontaneous closure. 3DE now provides an ideal means of charting the natural history of the processes involved in spontaneous reduction in size and establishing whether or not there is complete closure of a defect. Majority of the defects undergoing spontaneous closure are small muscular ones, those identified as producing the "maladie de Roger." Many perimembranous defects also undergo spontaneous diminution in size, in this instance usually by the development of tissue tags from the adjacent leaflets of the tricuspid valve (Fig. 7-20), or plastering down of the septal leaflet of the valve across the defect.[26]

Interrogation will also reveal the defects that are most unlikely to close spontaneously, such as those with overriding of the aortic or tricuspid valves. Careful study will also reveal the cases that do close spontaneously despite the presence of straddling and overriding of the tricuspid valve. This apparently anomalous situation is seen when the straddling valve has dual orifices and the bridge of valvar tissue between the orifices is plastered down to the crest of the ventricular septum. This produces the situation of the so-called double-outlet right atrium, with one valvar orifice draining to the right ventricle and the other draining to the left ventricle, but seemingly in the absence of an interventricular communication. A comparable situation is found in double-outlet left atrium in the setting of discordant atrioventricular connections.[27]

SUMMARY

In the past, examination of autopsied specimens was taken as the gold standard for understanding the cardiac structure. Despite having the hearts in their hands, however, morphologists failed to reach consensus on how best to catagorize the holes between the ventricles. Perhaps this is because in autopsied hearts it is not always easy to recognize subtle features such as the presence of the sleeve of freestanding muscular subpulmonary infundibulum that lifts the pulmonary valvar leaflets away from the base of the ventricular mass. The ability provided by 3DE to dissect the heart during life has now changed the situation. As we have shown, using 3D interrogation it is possible to collate the features highlighted in previously disparate categorizations, identifying their similarities and also emphasizing their differences. Analyses of this type, which are now achievable during life, should lead to a more general acceptance of a unified system for the diagnosis and description of holes between ventricles.

REFERENCES

1. Kardon RE, Cao QL, Masani N, et al. New insights and observations in three-dimensional echocardiographic visualization of ventricular septal defects: experimental and clinical studies. *Circulation.* 1998;98:1307–1314.
2. Mercer-Rosa L, Seliem MA, Fedec A, et al. Illustration of the additional value of real-time 3-dimensional echocardiography to conventional transthoracic and transesophageal 2-dimensional echocardiography in imaging muscular ventricular septal defects: does this have any impact on individual patient treatment? *J Am Soc Echocardiogr.* 2006;19:1511–1519.
3. Hlavacek AM, Baker GH, Shirali GS. Innovation in three-dimensional echocardiography and cardiac computed tomographic angiography. *Cardiol Young.* 2009;19(suppl 2):35–42.
4. Friedman BA, Hlavacek A, Chessa K, et al. Clinico-morphological correlations in the categorization of holes between the ventricles. *Ann Pediatr Cardiol.* 2010;3:13–24.
5. Wells WJ, Lindesmith GG. Ventricular septal defect. In: Arciniegas E, ed. *Pediatric Cardiac Surgery.* Chicago, IL: Year Book Medical; 1985.
6. LaCorte MA, Fellows KE, Williams RG. Overriding tricuspid valve. Echocardiographic and angiographic features. 8 cases of ventricular septal defect of atrioventricular canal type. *Am J Cardiol.* 1976;37:911–919.
7. Anderson RH, Ho SY, Falcao S, et al. The diagnostic features of atrioventricular septal defect with common atrioventricular junction. *Cardiol Young.* 1998;8:33–49.
8. Van Praagh R, Geva T, Kreutzer J. Ventricular septal defects: how shall we describe, name and classify them? *J Am Coll Cardiol.* 1989;14:1298–1310.
9. Soto B, Becker AE, Moulaert AJ, et al. Classification of ventricular septal defects. *Br Heart J.* 1980;43:332–343.
10. Goor DA, Lillehei CW. *Congenital Malformations of the Heart.* New York, NY: Grune & Stratton; 1975.
11. Anderson RH, Becker AE, Van Mierop LHS. What should we call the "crista"? *Br Heart J.* 1977;39:856–859.
12. Andersen HO, de Leval MR, Tsang VT, et al. Is complete heart block after surgical closure of ventricular septum defects still an issue? *Ann Thorac Surg.* 2006;82:948–957.
13. Baker GH, Shirali G, Ringewald JM, et al. Usefulness of live three-dimensional transesophageal echocardiography in a congenital heart disease center. *Am J Cardiol.* 2009;103:1025–1028.
14. De Castro S, Caselli S, Papetti F, et al. Feasibility and clinical impact of live three-dimensional echocardiography in the management of congenital heart disease. *Echocardiography.* 2006;23:553–561.
15. Hlavacek AM, Crawford FA Jr, Chessa KS, Shirali GS. Real-time three-dimensional echocardiography is useful in the evaluation of patients with atrioventricular septal defects. *Echocardiography.* 2006;23:225–231.
16. Chen FL, Hsiung MC, Nanda N, et al. Real time three-dimensional echocardiography in assessing ventricular septal defects: an echocardiographic-surgical correlative study. *Echocardiography.* 2006;23:562–568.
17. Bentham JR, Gujral A, Adwani S, Archer N, Wilson N. Does the technique of interventional closure of perimembranous ventricular septal defect reduce the incidence of heart block? *Cardiol Young.* 2011;21:271–280.

18. Milo S, Ho SY, Wilkinson JL, Anderson RH. Surgical anatomy and atrioventricular conduction tissues of hearts with isolated ventricular septal defects. *J Thorac Cardiovasc Surg.* 1980;79:244–255.
19. Thiene G, Wenink ACG, Frescura C, et al. The surgical anatomy of conduction tissues in atrioventricular defects. *J Thorac Cardiovasc Surg.* 1981;82:928–937.
20. Milo S, Ho SY, Macartney FJ, et al. Straddling and overriding atrioventricular valves morphology and classification. *Am J Cardiol.* 1979;44:1122–1134.
21. Eisenmenger V. Die angeborenen Defecte der Kammerscheidewand des Herzens [in German]. *Z Klin Med.* 1897;32(Suppl):1–28.
22. Van Praagh R, McNamara JJ. Anatomic types of ventricular septal defect with aortic insufficiency. *Am Heart J.* 1968;75:604–619.
23. Tatsuno K, Konno S, Sakakibara S. Ventricular septal defect with aortic insufficiency. Angiographic aspects and a new classification. *Am Heart J.* 1973;85:13–21.
24. Smallhorn JF, Anderson RH, Macartney FJ. Morphological characterisation of ventricular septal defects associated with coarctation of aorta by cross-sectional echocardiography. *Br Heart J.* 1983;49:485–494.
25. Vogel M, Freedom RM, Brand A, et al. Ventricular septal defect and subaortic stenosis: an analysis of 41 patients. *Am J Cardiol.* 1983;52:1258–1263.
26. Anderson RH, Lenox CC, Zuberbuhler JR. Mechanisms of closure of perimembranous ventricular septal defects. *Am J Cardiol.* 1983;52:341–345.
27. Gnanapragasam JP, Houston AB, Anderson RH. Double outlet left atrium with co-existing double inlet left ventricle and discordant atrioventricular connections. *Cardiol Young.* 1991;1:155–157.

CHAPTER 8

THREE-DIMENSIONAL ECHOCARDIOGRAPHIC EVALUATION OF ATRIOVENTRICULAR SEPTAL DEFECT

Jeffrey F. Smallhorn, MBBS, FRACP, FRCP(C)

ABSTRACT

Three-dimensional echocardiography (3DE) provides an enhanced understanding of the morphological features of hearts with an atrioventricular septal defect (AVSD). The common features of hearts with this lesion are better defined by this technique, as are the associated risk factors that affect mortality and morbidity. 3DE confers an advantage in cases of inlet–outlet disproportion and in evaluating abnormal positioning of papillary muscles. 3DE comes into its own in assessing the nature of the atrioventricular valves and the "cleft" or what can be referred to as a zone of apposition between the bridging leaflets and in documenting "sprung" atrioventricular junction. It is also helpful in assessing abnormalities associated with AVSD, such as double-orifice left atrioventricular valve, abnormalities of the left ventricular outflow tract, and ventricular hypoplasia.

INTRODUCTION

Atrioventricular septal defect (AVSD) represents one of the lesions commonly encountered by echocardiographers. Two-dimensional echocardiography (2DE) is still the main mode of imaging used in both diagnosis and evaluation of this lesion.[1] 2DE has several limitations, and three-dimensional echocardiography (3DE) may provide improved diagnostic detail.[2,3] Those working with 3DE also have the opportunity to discover new applications, similar to what occurred when echocardiography developed from a predominant M-mode to two-dimensional technique. A close partnership with anatomic pathologists is also beneficial, as echocardiographers are now imaging the heart the way it really looks as opposed to examining slices without the benefit of depth perception.[4]

The transition from two to three dimensions is not straightforward and requires an in-depth understanding of the technology; its applications; and, importantly, its limitations. I believed that, because I knew 2DE very well, the transition would be simple; I was wrong. Although I have spent my academic life reviewing specimens from patients with AVSD, as well as performing and reviewing countless two-dimensional (2D) studies, it took me some time to appreciate the features of an AVSD in three-dimensional (3D) mode. I always felt that when I reviewed a 2D image I automatically translated it into three dimensions in my brain; I was wrong. There is a learning curve during which it is important to move back and forth between 2D and 3D images in any one study before it is possible to work solely in three dimensions. Once this step is achieved, untold treasures await the curious echocardiographer.

3D IMAGING

Limitless views can be created with 3DE; only some, however, are readily appreciated by the reviewer. As with 2DE, it is important to choose 3D imaging planes that make sense to the reviewer. Real-time 3DE overcomes the problem of stitch artifacts with full-volume data sets; however, this approach provides limited information. With a full-volume data set it is possible to work with a high frame rate, which is advantageous in patients with small hearts and high heart rates, where frame rate is everything. The other technique that can be used to overcome stitch artifacts is zoom mode, but this is applicable only to smaller patients and again suffers from slow frame rates. As a result, my preference is to sedate younger patients and work in a full-volume mode, with maximum line density. Challenges remain in examining neonates and infants as they breathe mainly with their diaphragms, resulting in pressure against the probe and in stitch artifacts. These problems can be minimized by acquiring 3D data sets at the beginning of the case in patients who are sedated. If this does not work, then reducing the number of acquired beats may help, as in some instances the acquisition is fast, occurring between respirations. The other option is to acquire the data sets in the operating department prior to surgery where the anesthetist can provide a breath hold, but this limits the amount of cropping that can be achieved before surgery. In general, once the surgeons are in the operating department their focus is on the operation and it may be difficult to obtain their full attention, whereas this is not the case if they can review the images separately prior to surgery. Some of these issues will be overcome in smaller children only when it becomes possible to obtain a single-cardiac-cycle, high-frequency, high-resolution data set.

The other issue is related to the imaging plane. In general, it is better to attempt to image the various structures in the axial plane, which provides superior imaging to its lateral counterpart. This works well for hearts with an AVSD, as the important structures can be imaged in the axial plane, which improves image quality and subsequent anatomic detail.

BASIC ANATOMY

Understanding the morphologic features of AVSDs is important when using 2DE, but this is even more important when using 3DE as we are finally imaging the structures as they exist in the heart.[4]

Certain features are common to all hearts with an AVSD regardless of whether they have an atrial or a ventricular communication.[1,4] This is an important concept as the echocardiographer will encounter hearts that have all the common features of an AVSD but have neither an atrial nor a ventricular level shunt. Many of these features can be appreciated on 2DE, whereas some are uniquely appreciated using 3D techniques. These common features include the following:

- Inlet–outlet disproportion
- Absence of the muscular atrioventricular septum
- Position of the papillary muscles
- Nature of the atrioventricular valves
- The presence of a cleft or zone of apposition between the bridging leaflets
- "Sprung" atrioventricular junction

Inlet–outlet disproportion

Inlet–outlet disproportion is seen as an inlet that is shorter than the outlet. Normally the inlet to outlet ratio is approximately 1, but in patients with an AVSD the ratio is greater than 1. This ratio also varies in specimens with an AVSD, as some are seen with far greater scooping out of the inlet septum. On 2DE, this can be best appreciated from the parasternal long or subcostal long-axis cut. 3DE permits the echocardiographer to determine the extent of scooping (Fig. 8-1). One of the best views for this is in a full-volume data set acquired from the parasternal long-axis view. The reviewer crops the image from the anterior, which is the "blue minimum," such that the interventricular septum is removed, and then rotates the image, such that the heart is imaged from above, or anteriorly. In this view, the two papillary muscles supporting the anterosuperior and posteroinferior bridging leaflets can be seen, as well as the cleft or zone of apposition between them. The two leaflets can be seen as they bridge the interventricular septum from their anterosuperior to posteroinferior locations. In this image, the extent of scooping of the interventricular septum can be appreciated, albeit with some minor adjustments to remove the two leaflets. A similar view can be obtained from the subcostal position; however, the transducer is farther away from the heart and the structures are imaged more in the lateral plane, reducing the image quality even further.

Absence of the muscular atrioventricular septum

Absence of the muscular atrioventricular septum is common to all forms of AVSD and results in the atrioventricular valves being at the same level. This abnormality is readily appreciated on 2DE, and its 3D counterpart does not confer any real advantage.

Position of the papillary muscles

The posterior medial papillary muscle in an AVSD is laterally rotated from its normal position such that the mural leaflet is smaller in comparison with the normal heart. Conversely, in the majority of cases the anterolateral muscle is in a similar location to the normal heart. Although both of these are readily seen on 2DE, a 3D view provides depth perception, particularly when the muscles are "abnormally located" or excessively hypertrophied (Fig. 8-2). 3DE also provides the echocardiographer with the ability to determine the precise location of the papillary muscles in 3D space and the ability to relate this to functional abnormalities of leaflets, chordae, and annulus. This approach will help in understanding why some of these patients are prone to developing long-term problems with chronic atrioventricular valve regurgitation.

Figure 8-1

Montage demonstrating the concept of inlet–outlet disproportion. The 2D image (left) shows the shorter inlet, as outlined by the two asterisks. The 3D image (right) is from the same patient and shows the scooped out area outlined by black dots, again with the shorter inlet. The video clip (Fig. 8-1 movie 1) shows the real-time 3DE features. This cut-plane was obtained from a parasternal long-axis view. LV, left ventricle.

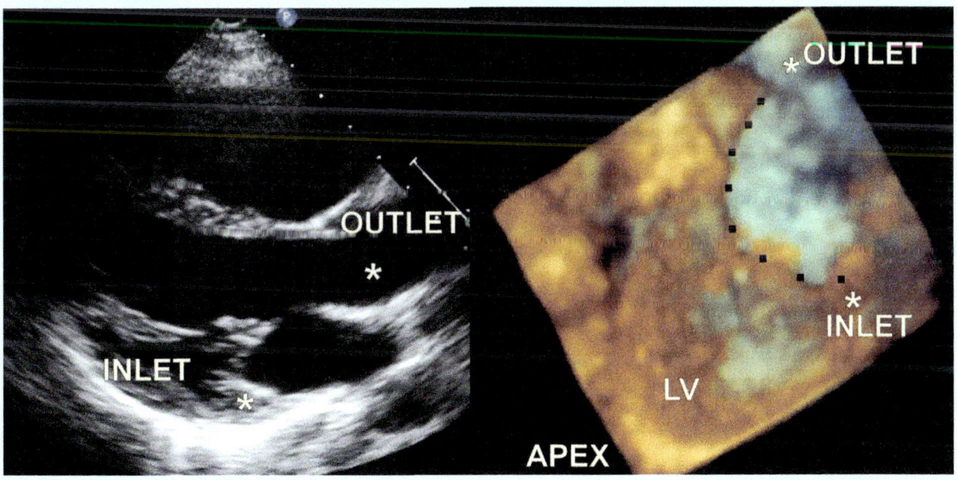

Figure 8-2

Papillary muscles as seen on 2DE and 3DE. Although they can be identified on 2DE (left), far more detail is obtained from the 3D image (right), as well as the associated chordal apparatus. Fig. 8-2 movie 1 shows the left ventricular papillary muscles in a two-dimensional perspective, whereas Fig.8-2 shows then as seen by RT3D echo. Note the additional detail by RT3D echo. ALPM, anterolateral papillary muscle; IBL, inferior bridging leaflet; PMPM, posteromedial papillary muscle; SBL, superior bridging leaflet.

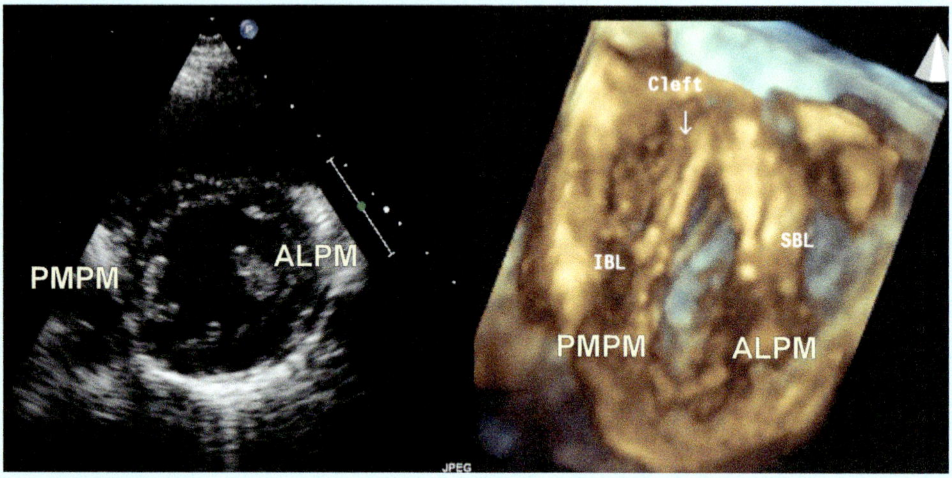

Nature of the atrioventricular valves and cleft or zone of apposition between the bridging leaflets

In assessing the nature of atrioventricular valves, 3DE comes into its own. Atrioventricular valve morphology in AVSDs in no way resembles a normal mitral valve. In most hearts with an AVSD, the left atrioventricular junction consists of three components: the mural leaflet, which extends from the anterolateral to posteromedial papillary muscle, and the two bridging leaflets, consisting of the anterosuperior and the posteroinferior leaflets (Fig. 8-3A and B). The extent of bridging differs from heart to heart, with varying degrees of attachment to the interventricular septum. In general, there is little correlation between the degree of bridging and leaflet attachment to the interventricular septum between the anterosuperior and posteroinferior leaflets. There is more likely to be an interventricular communication beneath the anterosuperior than the posteroinferior leaflet, which may have long-term implications with respect to chronic regurgitation.

Cleft or zone of apposition. It is appropriate to discuss the cleft or "zone of apposition" under the same heading, as this entity is an integral part of the valve leaflets. The cleft points to the interventricular septum, unlike a true cleft in the aortic or anterior leaflet of the normal mitral valve, where the direction is toward the left ventricular outflow tract (Fig. 8-3A and B). The other components that are important when evaluating the left atrioventricular valve are commissures.

Commissures. Commissures represent the zones of coaptation between the anterosuperior and posteroinferior leaflets and their mural counterparts (Figs. 8-3B and 8-4). Commissures are highly important in hearts with AVSDs, as they are in the normal mitral valve.

Atrioventricular valve orifice. Finally, the left atrioventricular valve in AVSDs may consist of a common or a partitioned orifice depending on the presence or absence of a connecting tongue of tissue

Figure 8-3A and B

A, The left atrioventricular valve leaflets as seen on 2DE. The 2D video clip (Fig. 8-3 movie 1) shows the cleft. *B*, This panel is from a patient with an AVSD and an intact interatrial septum, which is seen in the 2D panel. The 3D image is taken from below and shows the three leaflets and the cleft, as indicated by the black arrow. The video clip (Fig. 8-3 movie 2) shows the same features as the still image. AO, aorta; IBL, inferior bridging leaflet; LA, left atrium; LV, left ventricle; ML, mural leaflet; RV, right ventricle; SBL, superior bridging leaflet.

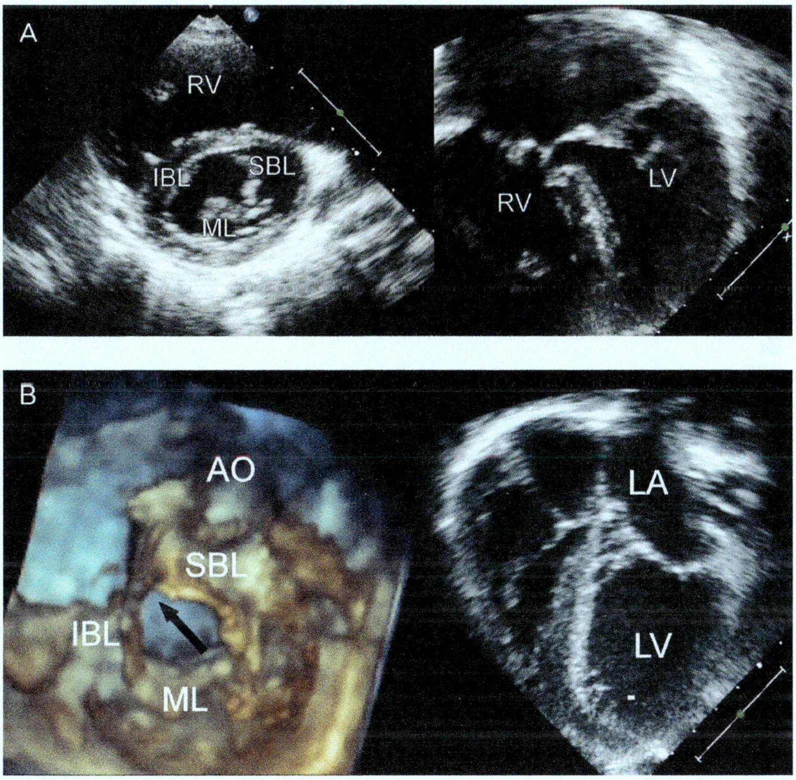

between the anterosuperior and posteroinferior bridging leaflets (Fig. 8-5A and B). Although 2DE can identify the leaflets and the zone of apposition, it does not do justice to the complex morphology of these structures. The evaluation of commissural abnormalities is also problematic using 2DE, both in the normal mitral valve and in the AVSD.

One of the best ways of imaging leaflets, cleft, and commissures is by obtaining a full-volume data set from the apical four-chamber view. Once obtained, the image can be cropped from above or below the left atrioventricular valve, yielding exquisite detail of all structures. The added advantage is that this image is acquired in the axial plane, which provides optimal resolution (Fig. 8-5A and B). These structures can be identified in the subcostal view in small children; however, the reconstructed images are imaged in a more lateral plane, which degrades image quality. The other image that is helpful is the one from the parasternal long-axis view, which can also image the left atrioventricular valve in the axial plane (Fig. 8-2). Nevertheless, we prefer the apical four-chamber view because it provides superior imaging of commissures. The view from the left ventricular aspect provides greater detail of the commissures, cleft, and extent of the connecting tongue between the two bridging leaflets (Fig. 8-4). This is in part because when leaflets coapt they bulge toward the low-pressure left atrium in systole. We know that the normal mitral valve has a degree of prolapse

Figure 8-4

3D image from a postoperative AVSD demonstrates the commissures (indicated by the asterisks) between the anterosuperior, posteroinferior, and mural leaflets. The cleft, which is indicated by the black arrow, has been sutured in this case. The video clip (Fig. 8-4 movie 1) demonstrates the same features in real time. AO, aorta; IBL, inferior bridging leaflet; LAVV, left atrioventricular valve; LVOT, left ventricular outflow tract; ML, mural leaflet; RV, right ventricle; SBL, superior bridging leaflet.

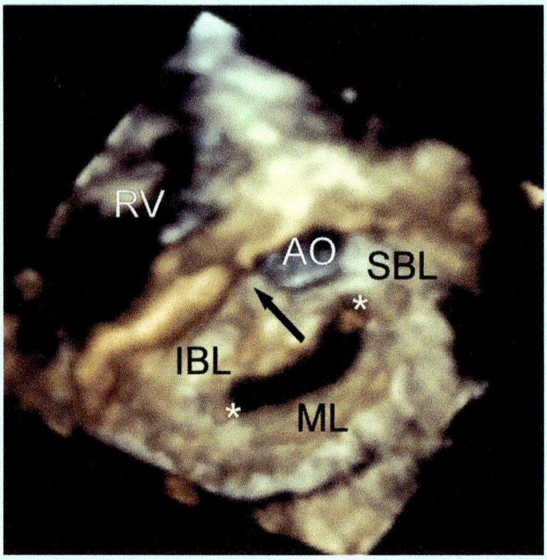

and tethering, and the same applies to the left atrioventricular valve in AVSDs. It can thus be more difficult to appreciate zones of coaptation between the leaflets in systole. Certainly the surgeons will immediately understand a cropped image displayed in a surgical view, but with minimal training they can fully appreciate the valve as seen from below. In fact, surgeons are very quick to understand the reconstructed images as they are what they see on a daily basis. The reconstructed images permit the reviewer to identify abnormalities of the leaflets and commissures, the extent of the cleft, and the relationship of the papillary muscles and their chordal structures to the leaflets.

Sprung atrioventricular junction

In all hearts with an AVSD, the aorta, rather than being wedged between the two components of the atrioventricular junction, is truly sprung. The ability to provide an image of this "unwedging" is unique to 3DE (Fig. 8-5A and B). This concept is best appreciated using an apical four-chamber view, with the atria removed and cropped from above. Here, the combined left and right atrioventricular annulus is elliptical in shape with the unwedged aorta positioned in front of it. Whether there is a common orifice or they are partitioned by a connecting tongue, the appearance is the same.

EVALUATION OF ASSOCIATED LESIONS IN HEARTS WITH AN AVSD

Once the fundamental morphology is appreciated in hearts with an AVSD, it is important to document associated abnormalities.

Figure 8-5A and B

A, Montage demonstrating the sprung atrioventricular junction as seen from above in a heart with an AVSD and partitioned orifices. Note the unwedged position of the aorta and the connecting tongue (black arrow) between the superior and inferior bridging leaflets. *B*, 3D image viewed from above, demonstrating a sprung atrioventricular junction, as well as a common atrioventricular valve with no connecting tongue between the superior and inferior bridging leaflets. The paler interventricular septum is seen beneath the two bridging leaflets. The video clip (Fig. 8-5 movie 1) shows the same features as the still image. ANT, anterior; AO, aorta; CAVV, common atrioventricular valve; IBL, inferior bridging leaflet; LAVV, left atrioventricular valve; POST, posterior; RAVV, right atrioventricular valve; RV, right ventricle; SBL, superior bridging leaflet.

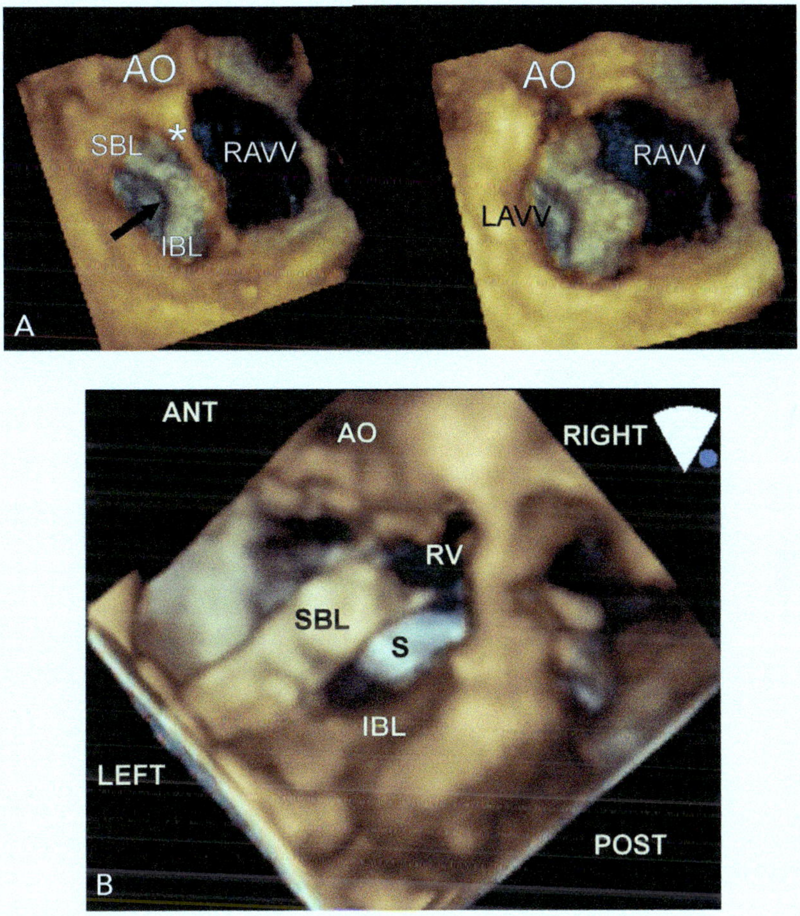

Interatrial communication

Most patients with an AVSD have a primum defect as the result of a lack of fusion of the mesenchymal cap and the endocardial cushions. Others, particularly younger children, have a true secundum atrial septal defect, due to a deficiency in the primary septum (Fig. 8-6). We do not use the term *primum atrial septal defect* to describe the more inferior interatrial communication as it does not represent a defect in the true atrial septum. In some hearts, there is no interatrial communication, as both the septum secundum and the bridging leaflets, which are fused with the inferior margin of the remnants of the mesenchymal cap (Fig. 8-6), are intact.

Figure 8-6

Montage demonstrating the 3DE appearance of a primum atrial defect as imaged from the right side of the heart. Note the different sizes during systole and diastole. There is also an area of dropout in the vicinity of the primum atrial septum, which is common using the 3D technique. The video clip (Fig. 8-6 movie 1) shows the 2D image of the primum defect. ANT, anterior; AVV, atrioventricular valve; POST, posterior; PRIM, primum atrial defect; RA, right atrium; RV, right ventricle.

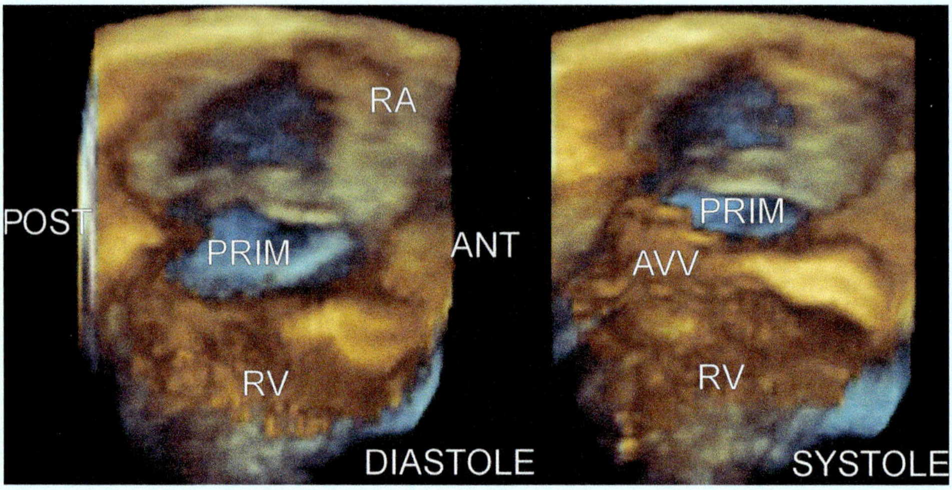

A primum defect is readily identified on 2DE from the subcostal, precordial, and apical views (Fig. 8-3A), so in general 3DE does not add a great deal. The only potential advantage is that on 3DE it is possible to identify the total extent of a defect; however, this probably has little clinical relevance (Fig. 8-6). The size and number of interatrial communications can be seen from both the same views as on 2DE. One of the limitations of 3DE is that the resolution is not as good, owing to lower frame rates. Therefore, because the atrial septum is a thin structure, it is more likely to have dropout on 3DE (Fig. 8-6). This is further compounded by the fact that the atrial septum can be imaged only in the lateral plane, where resolution is suboptimal.

One associated lesion is double-outlet atrium, which usually involves the right atrium owing to the deviation of the interatrial septum to the left side. In extreme cases, this defect can result in restrictive interatrial communication, with associated pulmonary venous and subsequently pulmonary arterial hypertension (Fig. 8-7). This association is readily diagnosed using either 2D or 3D techniques.

Interventricular communication

The interventricular communication in AVSDs sits beneath the anterosuperior and/or posteroinferior bridging leaflets. The size of the defect depends on the extent of attachment of the leaflets to the crest of the interventricular septum. The leaflets may be completely adhered to the septum, or may be partially connected by chordae, between which the interventricular communication exists (Figs. 8-3A and B), or they may be freely floating with a large defect (Fig. 8-5B). The presence or size of the defect varies between the two bridging leaflets. An interventricular communication is more likely to be found beneath the anterosuperior than the posteroinferior bridging leaflets. This entity may well have implications with respect to long-term left atrioventricular valve dysfunction. Although 2DE and color Doppler techniques provide excellent imaging of interventricular communications prior to repair, 3DE is probably superior in the postoperative period when there is residual interventricular shunting. The latter technique permits precise identification of the site and often anatomic size of the defect, which is helpful if additional surgical intervention is necessary. Part of the added benefit of 3DE is that a postoperative interventricular communication is frequently involved with an abnormal component of the atrioventricular valve in the same region, with associated regurgitation, making identification of what is a shunt and what is a regurgitation difficult using 2D techniques (Fig. 8-8A–C).

Abnormalities of the atrioventricular valve

Abnormalities of the atrioventricular valve can be divided into abnormalities at the leaflets, chordae, and papillary muscles. Leaflet dysplasia is a frequent mechanism of left atrioventricular valve regurgitation. The leaflets appear thickened and in some cases deficient. This defect results in abnormal zones of coaptation with their counterpart leaflets and subsequent regurgitation. Such abnormalities are more frequently seen in hearts with an absent or a small interventricular communication. The assessment of leaflet size and dysplasia is still subjective; however, 3DE will provide an improved understanding compared to its 2D counterpart.[5–8] One of the advantages of 3DE is that the leaflets can be seen as a whole, and more subtle abnormalities can be appreciated (Fig. 8-9A). Not infrequently, the mural leaflet has scallops in it that are difficult to see using 2DE. Commissural length can be identified on 3DE (Fig. 8-9B). Those with shorter, or malformed, commissures are best imaged from a data set acquired from the four-chamber view, with cropping from below and above. Although the leaflets can be imaged in a data set obtained from the parasternal long-axis or subcostal view, lateral resolution still degrades the quality of the images.

Figure 8-7

Montage from a patient with an AVSD with deviation of the atrial septum to the left, such that there is a double-outlet right atrium with a restrictive interatrial communication as indicated by the color Doppler jet. The video clip (Fig. 8-7 movie 1) shows the double-outlet right atrium in real time. LA, left atrium; LV, left ventricle; RA, right atrium.

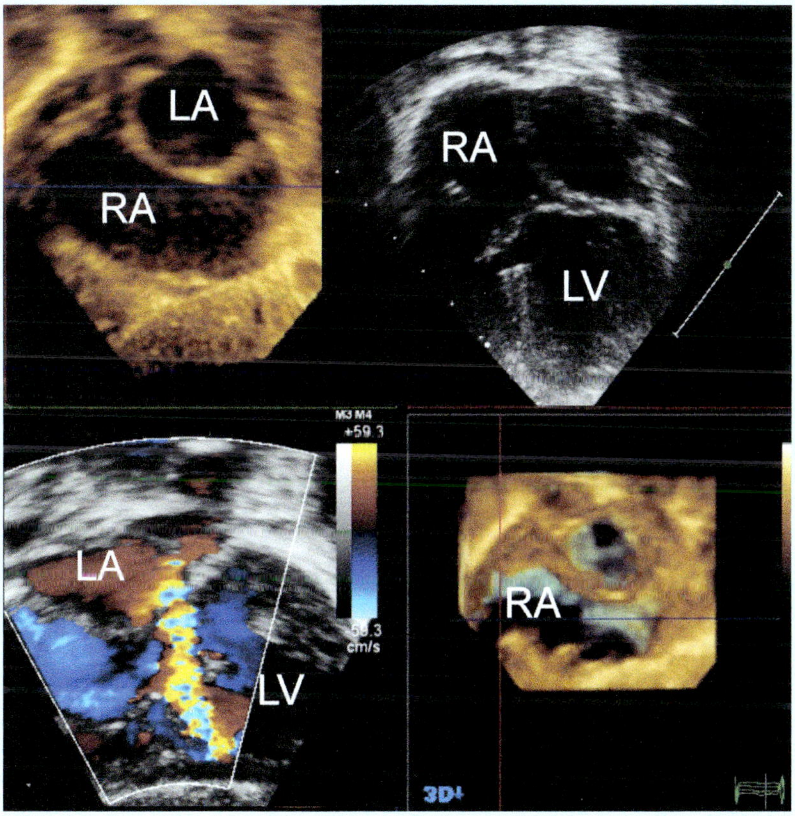

Figure 8-8A, B and C

A, Image from a postoperative patient with AVSD who had significant associated residual left atrioventricular valve regurgitation, as well as a residual interventricular communication. The residual interventricular communication is imaged from the right side and is indicated by the black arrow. This is also seen in the video clip (Fig. 8-8 movie 1). *B*, Montage demonstrating the en face view of the left atrioventricular valve and that seen from the left ventricular aspect in the same patient. A small residual cleft is indicated by the asterisk, and partial dehiscence of the superior bridging leaflet is indicated by the black arrow. The video clip (Fig. 8-8 movie 2) shows the left atrioventricular valve in the en face or surgical view. *C*, Montage showing the color Doppler signals from the same case. The 2D image shows significant left atrioventricular valve regurgitation and an interventricular communication. The 3D image shows the precise location of the residual regurgitant lesions (asterisk and plus sign) as well as the residual interventricular communication (minus sign). Movie 3 shows the regurgitation. ANT, anterior; AO, aorta; IBL, inferior bridging leaflet; LA, left atrium; LV, left ventricle; LVOT, left ventricular outflow tract; POST, posterior; RA, right atrium; RAVV, right atrioventricular valve; RV, right ventricle; SBL, superior bridging leaflet.

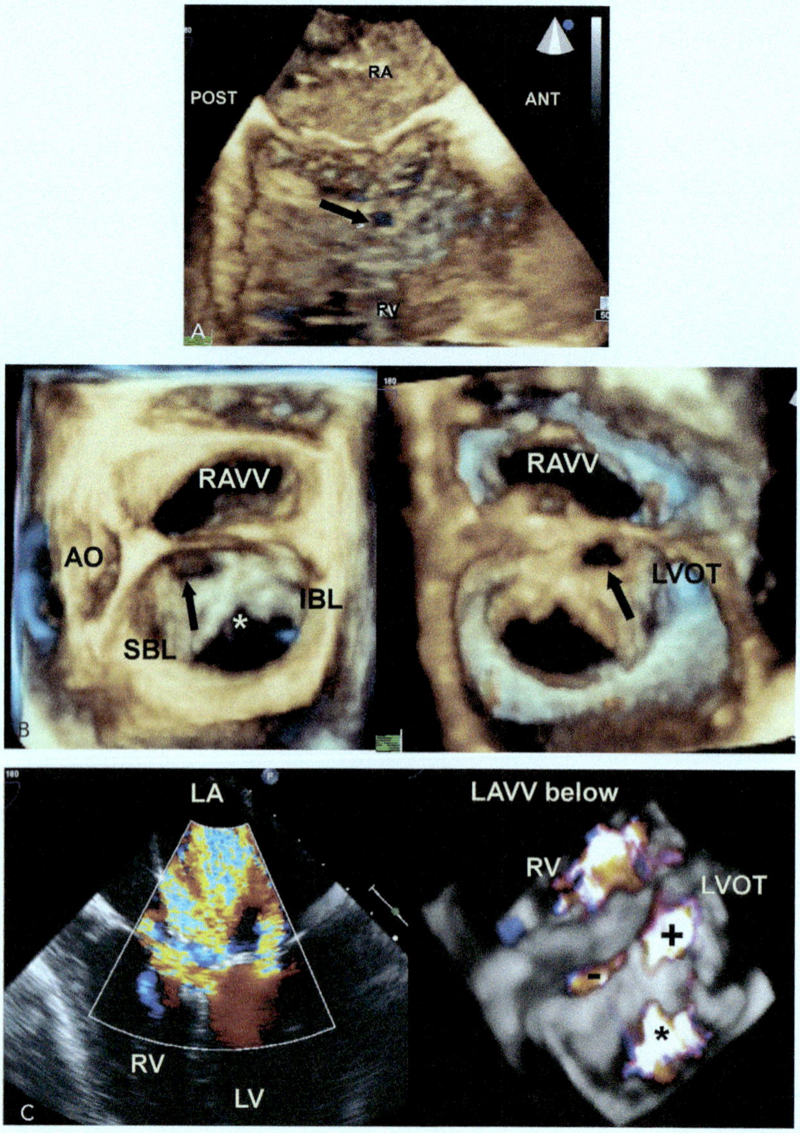

Figure 8-9A and B

A, Montage showing the left atrioventricular valve in a patient with leaflet dysplasia. The en face view of the left atrioventricular valve demonstrates the thickened dysplastic leaflets, whereas the 2D image is less convincing. Figure 8-9 movie 1 shows the same image in real time. *B*, Two images from the same case demonstrating the abnormal leaflets, as well as the poorly formed commissures as indicated by the asterisks in the right-hand panel. Note the cleft is eccentric, as shown by the black arrows. The video clips (Fig. 8-9 movies 2 and 3) show the same features. Fig. 8-9 movie 4 shows the 2D and 3D images obtained using this mode. The color Doppler video clips (Fig. 8-9 movies 5 and 6) demonstrate the significant regurgitation in this case. AO, aorta; IBL, inferior bridging leaflet; LAVV, left atrioventricular valve; LFT, left; LV, left ventricle; ML, mural leaflet; RT, right; RV, right ventricle; SBL, superior bridging leaflet.

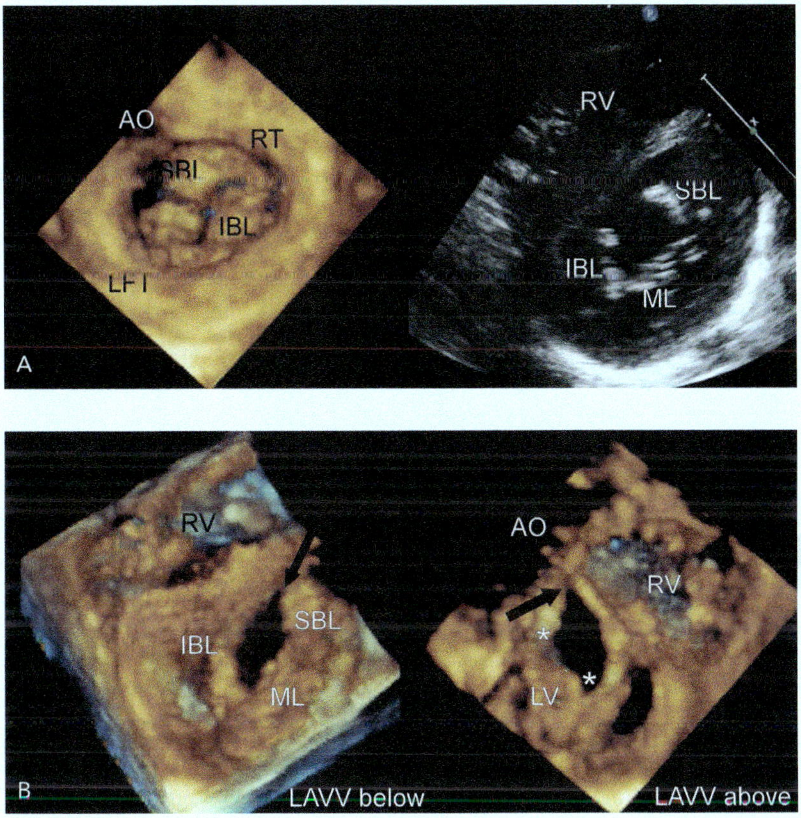

Data dropout can be a significant problem that results in loss of confidence in the use of this technique. In general, if the 2D image is of good quality when the data set is acquired then the same applies to the reconstructed image. A good way to ensure quality is to image the atrioventricular valves in the X-plane image first, with the two planes at right angles to each other. Using the multiplanar reconstruction mode to navigate through the structures in both 2D and 3D modes is also helpful. If all components of the leaflets can be seen in both, then invariably the final rendered image is relatively complete. The most common site of dropout in such images is the attachment of the leaflets to the annulus, as this is the thinnest part of the leaflet, providing the weakest signal with current 3DE techniques. Conversely, the strongest signals are usually derived from the zones of coaptation, which are the regions where most regurgitation occurs. As described later, color Doppler can help to resolve this limitation of pure imaging.

Double-orifice left atrioventricular valve

Double-orifice left atrioventricular valve is one of the most important associations to recognize, because it has significant surgical implications.[9,10] More commonly, the secondary orifice involves the posteroinferior mural component of the valve, rather than its more anterior counterpart. The second orifice may be very small or may be the same size as the other orifice. Frequently, both have some chordal support, although in some patients it may appear more like a leaflet perforation. A double orifice has significant surgical implications, as it is difficult for the surgeon to repair one that is regurgitant. This is particularly significant if the regurgitant orifice is the larger one. Although there are many 2DE descriptions of a double-orifice left atrioventricular valve in AVSDs, retrospective reviews of reliability indicate that many of the smaller orifices have been missed in the past.[11] This is most likely because seeing some of the smaller orifices can be difficult, particularly if the valve leaflets are thickened. Although 3DE provides superior imaging of the left atrioventricular valve, it is unclear whether this technique will improve the routine detection of double-orifice valves (Fig. 8-10). I suspect that the answer is yes, particularly if en face views are used.

Color flow Doppler assessment of regurgitation

Color flow Doppler is an essential component of atrioventricular valve evaluation. This application can accurately pinpoint the sites of regurgitation, determine the number and size of the jets, and resolve the problem of what represents dropout. The latter is straightforward, because if there appears to be a deficiency in the valve leaflets, but no associated regurgitation, this identifies dropout.

Once again, the four-chamber view is the best imaging plane to evaluate atrioventricular valve regurgitation. This view provides optimal image and color Doppler resolution because the data are acquired in the axial plane. The limitation of combining color Doppler with imaging is the degradation of the 3D image with current techniques. To overcome this, we use the image acquired at the same time as the color Doppler acquisition as purely a roadmap for the location of the regurgitant jets, using a full-volume image without color, but in the identical position for valve morphology.

To determine the size of vena contracta, which correlates closely with the volume of regurgitation, we obtain an "Oreo cookie" view of the jet. This view is achieved by cropping from above and below in a plane that is at right angles to the regurgitant jet (Figs. 8-8 and 8-9). This overcomes the problem of overestimation of vena contracta size, as the jet and the subsequent vortices are removed from the image. If there are multiple regurgitant jets, then they can be summated.

Although obtaining good data from combined 2D and color Doppler imaging is possible, the technique is inferior to 3DE. Determining the number of jets is frequently difficult, in particular as many may run along a commissure and appear as multiple jets, whereas in fact they are one continuous jet. It can also be difficult to pinpoint the location of a regurgitant jet on 2D color Doppler, as well as relate it to valve pathology.[6,7]

Surgeons are beginning to rely on 3D assessment of atrioventricular valve morphology and function prior to valve repair as it provides more accurate information.[8] Further, data support the notion that 3DE provides superior assessment of sites of atrioventricular valve regurgitation when compared with 2DE.[7] This is important because the surgical assessment of atrioventricular valve regurgitation is based on saline testing, which is nonphysiological and performed on a flaccid heart. Color Doppler assessment can also be achieved in the parasternal long-axis and subcostal views; however, once again, lateral resolution can hamper image quality.

Cleft (zone of apposition)

The cleft (zone of apposition) is considered an important component of the left-sided atrioventricular valve in AVSDs, but it is one that probably has achieved higher status than it deserves. Although in some patients the cleft is the site of regurgitation, others have a large cleft preoperatively but no associated regurgitation. Therefore, other mechanisms must be associated with a cleft in the left atrioventricular valve and regurgitation. These mechanisms are most likely related to leaflet dysplasia, tethering, and deficiency. The cleft is readily seen from the left ventricular aspect. 3DE permits an evaluation of its length, as well as an assessment of the connecting tongue. Although the cleft usually points toward the center of the right ventricle (Figs. 8-2 and 8-3A and B), in some cases it is eccentric, pointing more toward the left ventricular outflow tract. This defect is usually associated with an abnormality of the superior bridging leaflet, particularly leaflet deficiency (Figs. 8-9 and 8-11).

Figure 8-10

This three-dimensional image demonstrates a double orifice left atrioventricular valve in an atrioventricular septal defect as seen from the left ventricular aspect (Fig. 8-10 movie 1). Note that in this case orifice 1 is smaller than orifice 2. Fig. 8-10 movie 1 shows the double orifice left atrioventricular valve as seen from the left ventricular aspect.

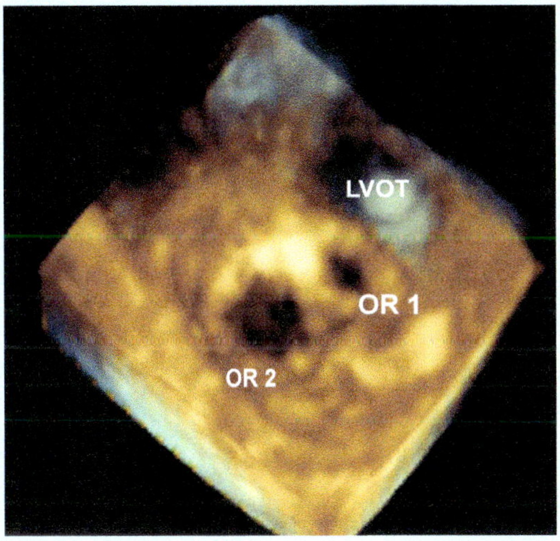

Figure 8-11A and B

A, Patient with a dysplastic left atrioventricular valve with deficiency of the superior bridging leaflet such that the cleft is eccentric, pointing more toward the left ventricular outflow tract (black arrow). The 3D video clip (Fig. 8-11 movie 1) shows the eccentric cleft, whereas the 2D video clip (Fig. 8-11 movie 2) is less clear. *B*, Image from the same patient showing the features as seen from below. Note the small superior bridging leaflet and the eccentric cleft. There is also an accessory tissue tag in the left ventricular outflow tract (white arrows identify the structures indicated by the associated labels). Note in the associated 2D video clip that the eccentric nature of the cleft is not fully appreciated. AO, aorta; AOV, aortic valve; IBL, inferior bridging leaflet; LAVV, left atrioventricular valve; ML, mural leaflet; PM, papillary muscles; RA, right atrium; RAVV, right atrioventricular valve; SBL, superior bridging leaflet.

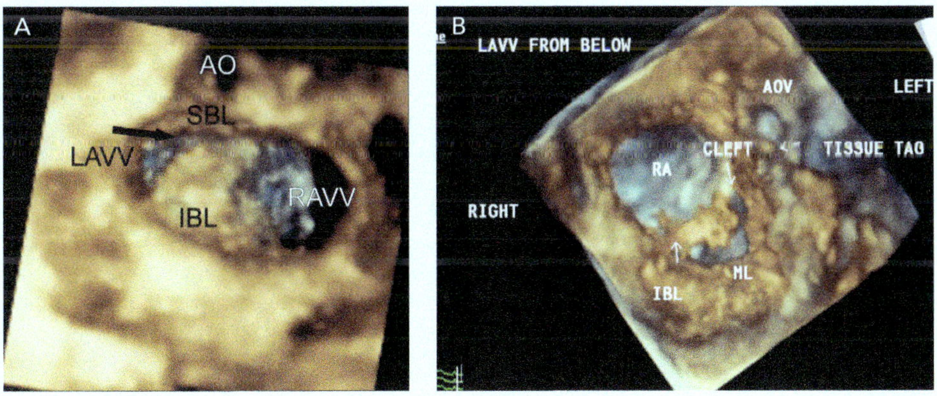

Abnormalities of the papillary muscles and chordae

The very location of papillary muscles in AVSDs places the leaflets at a disadvantage.[12] Unlike the normal mitral valve, where the chordal apparatus and papillary muscles are situated such that the force on the leaflets is almost at right angles, in hearts with AVSDs the pull is at more of an angle, which potentially places abnormal stress on the leaflets during systole (Fig. 8-2).[13] It is also not infrequent to encounter shortened chordae, which are less forgiving, potentially displacing and tethering the leaflets before, and especially after, repair.[14] As the cleft is closed in almost all cases with an AVSD, this abnormality has the potential to result in leaflet tethering, particularly in patients with shortened chordae. Tethering usually results in associated regurgitation, which causes annular and ventricular dilatation, placing further tension on the leaflets. Although the papillary muscles and chordae can be imaged on 2DE, more subtle abnormalities are difficult to appreciate. There is scant literature to support the role of imaging chordal apparatus by 2DE, either in the normal heart or in hearts with an AVSD.

3DE provides a unique opportunity to delve into this area in considerable detail. Not only can the number of papillary muscles be seen but also can their size and relationship to other structures be appreciated, particularly when there are concerns about left ventricular outflow tract obstruction. Shortened chordae can be identified, as well as their impact on leaflet mobility (Fig. 8-9B). Using more detailed quantitative methods, the spatial relationship of papillary muscles and their chordal connections can be determined through 3D imaging. This requires exporting the data sets to systems that can determine the spatial coordinates of the annulus, leaflets, chordae, and papillary muscles.[15,16] In general, we have used the apical four-chamber view to obtain these data, as it provides optimal imaging due to the axial orientation. Although we prefer quantitative imaging, excellent data can be obtained from the parasternal long-axis view, with the image cropped from above (Fig. 8-2). This provides a view of the leaflets and the chordae, both of which are imaged in the axial plane. Subcostal imaging can be of additional help, but control of respiration is important in smaller patients to avoid significant stitch artifacts.

A solitary papillary muscle is readily recognized on 2DE; however, 3DE helps in determining the length of the zone of apposition and its relationship to any associated regurgitation (Fig. 8-12). Although some patients have a solitary papillary muscle, others have a dominant one that supports most of the valve leaflets, with a secondary smaller muscle that may have some minor chordal attachments. In general, this results in an abnormal mural leaflet and is invariably treated as though there were only a single papillary muscle.

Abnormalities of the left ventricular outflow tract

Abnormalities of the left ventricular outflow tract represent one of the most important associated lesions in AVSD. The left ventricular outflow tract is prone to obstruction owing to the sprung atrioventricular junction, which results in a more elongated left ventricular outflow tract.[11,17] The mechanisms may be relatively simple, or multiple and complex. Some abnormalities will be present at the first evaluation, whereas others in the form of fibromuscular subaortic stenosis may occur over time, occasionally many years after the initial repair. More complex mechanisms of obstruction include accessory left atrioventricular valve tissue, chords, and papillary muscles. Some patients have diffuse hypoplasia of the left ventricular outflow tract, resulting in tunnel stenosis. When the lesion is more complex, in particular with accessory chords and papillary muscles, it is important to be sure that these accessory chords do not represent major support mechanisms of the valve leaflets. Differentiating primary support apparatuses from secondary is important, as in general the latter can be removed without disrupting the left atrioventricular valve. Surgical resection is invariably performed through the aortic root, which provides limited visualization, emphasizing the importance of an accurate preoperative evaluation by echocardiography.

2DE is adequate for patients with fibromuscular stenosis (Fig. 8-13A), though 3DE demonstrates the extent of the obstruction and provides a more detailed assessment of the relationship to the aortic valve (Fig. 8-13B). Several imaging planes can be used when applying 3DE. A full-volume data set in the parasternal long-axis view can be used to image the outflow tract in two ways. First, a surgical view

Figure 8-12

Image of the left atrioventricular valve as seen from below, demonstrating a single papillary muscle, and the long cleft between the superior and inferior bridging leaflets. The video clip shows the same features (Fig. 8-12 movies 1 and 2). The white arrows point to the cleft and the commissure. AO, aorta; COMM, commissure; IBL, inferior bridging leaflet; LAVV, left atrioventricular valve; RV, right ventricle; SBL, superior bridging leaflet.

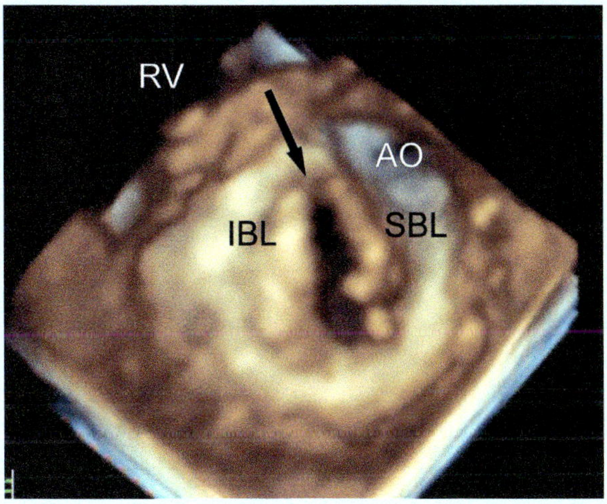

is obtained by cropping the image from above the aortic valve and orientating it in the surgical plane (Fig. 8-13B). Surgeons find this view informative as it demonstrates the relationship of the abnormal structures in the left ventricular outflow tract to the aortic valve leaflets, but this view is limited when sorting out complex mechanisms of obstruction. What is more helpful using 3DE is to image the left ventricular outflow tract in its long axis and crop from the outer to the inner margin. This procedure enables the echocardiographer to image structures in the left ventricular outflow tract and, more importantly, to visualize their relationship to the left atrioventricular and aortic valve leaflets (Fig. 8-14). These views are of particular value when deciding whether accessory chordal tissue or papillary muscles represent primary or secondary support apparatuses. The advantage of this view is that the structures are imaged in the axial plane, providing optimal resolution. Acquiring a data set from the apical view, and cropping from the left ventricular aspect, can also provide images in the axial plane and is particularly good for imaging the extent of fibromuscular subaortic stenosis. The main limitation of this method is related to the distance from the area of interest, particularly in older patients, which limits optimal resolution. The subcostal view is useful in smaller children; however, the left ventricular outflow tract is imaged in a more lateral plane, which hampers optimal resolution. Stitch artifacts can be a greater problem, unless respiration is controlled. Transesophageal 3DE is a useful adjunct in patients who meet the current weight criteria for adult 3DE probes and provides optimal 2D and 3D imaging of the left ventricular outflow tract.

Ventricular hypoplasia

Determining whether there is associated ventricular hypoplasia is important in AVSD. Left ventricular hypoplasia is invariably associated with other abnormalities of the "left side," such as a single papillary muscle, stenotic left atrioventricular valve, or left ventricular outflow tract obstruction. In this setting, the associated lesions, rather than the absolute size of the left ventricle, often dictate the management strategy. Conversely, right ventricular hypoplasia can be more subtle. Commonly the right ventricular inflow and outflow tracts are adequate in size, and the apical trabecular zone is attenuated. In this setting, an absolute volume measurement is useful. 3DE is clearly superior to 2DE when assessing absolute chamber size. The main limiting factor relates to image quality; however, early reports are encouraging with respect to this application of 3DE. How big is big enough for the right ventricle is still unclear; however, with the use of an associated fenestrated atrial septum, or bidirectional cavopulmonary shunt in those with low pulmonary vascular resistance, a biventricular, or one-and-a-half ventricular, repair can be achieved in many cases.

Figure 8-13A and B

A, 2D images of left ventricular outflow tract obstruction due to a fibromuscular ridge. The image on the left views the left ventricular outflow tract in the long axis with a thin slice, whereas the one on the right is from multiplanar reconstruction, with a thicker cut. Note more detail of the extent of the ridge. *B*, Two images from the same patient imaging the left ventricular outflow tract from the left ventricular aspect in the left panel and through the aorta in a simulated surgical view in the right panel. In the left panel, a small residual cleft is seen, along with the fibromuscular ridge, which extends onto the superior bridging leaflet. The right panel shows the full extent of the fibromuscular ridge, which is crescent shaped. The video clips (Fig. 8-13 movies 1 and 2) show these features in real time. AO, aorta; LA, left atrium; LAVV, left atrioventricular valve; RV, right ventricle; SUB-AS, subaortic stenosis.

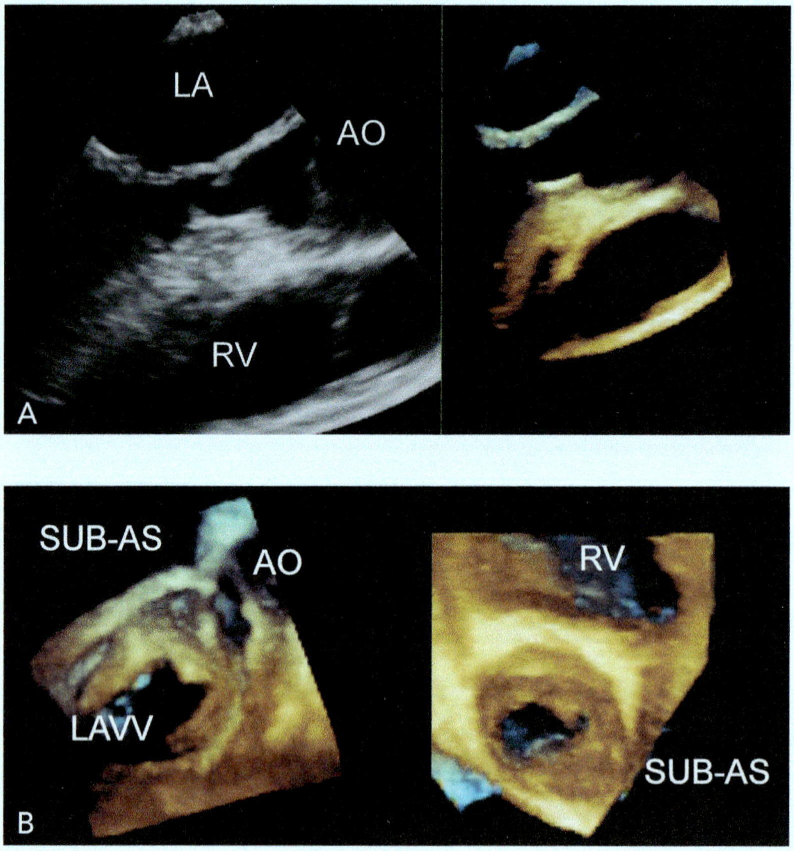

Figure 8-14

Two images from a patient with AVSD and complex left ventricular outflow tract obstruction due to accessory tissue and papillary muscle (arrows). The latter did not provide support to the left atrioventricular valve, so it was removed at surgery. The video clip (Fig. 8-14 movie 1) shows the accessory papillary muscle and the accessory chords in the left ventricular outflow tract as seen from the side. Movie 2 is from the same case, acquired in a long-axis plane and then rotated such that it is imaged in an axial plane from above, with the interventricular septum removed. ACC, accessory; AO, aorta; AOV, aortic valve; LA, left atrium; LV, left ventricle; PM, papillary muscle; RV, right ventricle.

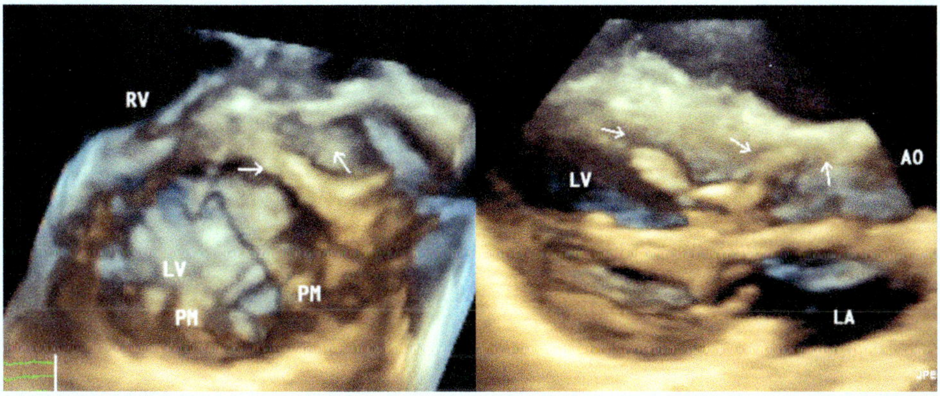

REFERENCES

1. Smallhorn JF. Cross-sectional echocardiographic assessment of atrioventricular septal defect: basic morphology and preoperative risk factors. *Echocardiography*. 2001;18(5):415–432.
2. Hlavacek AM, Crawford FA Jr, Chessa KS, Shirali GS. Real-time three-dimensional echocardiography is useful in the evaluation of patients with atrioventricular septal defects. *Echocardiography*. 2006;23(3):225–231.
3. van den Bosch AE, Ten Harkel DJ, McGhie JS, et al. Surgical validation of real-time transthoracic 3D echocardiographic assessment of atrioventricular septal defects. *Int J Cardiol*. 2006;112(2):213–218.
4. Mahle WT, Shirali GS, Anderson RH. Echo-morphological correlates in patients with atrioventricular septal defect and common atrioventricular junction. *Cardiol Young*. 2006;16(suppl 3):43–51.
5. van den Bosch AE, van Dijk VF, McGhie JS, et al. Real-time transthoracic three-dimensional echocardiography provides additional information of left-sided AV morphology after AVSD repair. *Int J Cardiol*. 2006;106(3):360–364.
6. Takahashi K, Guerra V, Roman KS, et al. Three-dimensional echocardiography improves the understanding of the mechanisms and site of left atrioventricular valve regurgitation in atrioventricular septal defect. *J Am Soc Echocardiogr*. 2006;19(12):1502–1510.
7. Takahashi K, Mackie AS, Rebeyka IM, et al. Two-dimensional versus transthoracic real-time three-dimensional echocardiography in the evaluation of the mechanisms and sites of atrioventricular valve regurgitation in a congenital heart disease population. *J Am Soc Echocardiogr*. 2010;23(7):726–734.
8. Barrea C, Levasseur S, Roman K, et al. Three-dimensional echocardiography improves the understanding of left atrioventricular valve morphology and function in atrioventricular septal defects undergoing patch augmentation. *J Thorac Cardiovasc Surg*. 2005;129(4):746–753.
9. Hoohenkerk GJ, Wenink AC, Schoof PH, et al. Results of surgical repair of atrioventricular septal defect with double-orifice left atrioventricular valve. *J Thorac Cardiovasc Surg*. 2009;138(5):1167–1171.
10. Shuhaiber JH, Ho SY, Rigby M, Sethia B. Current opinions and outcomes for the management of atrioventricular septal defect. *Eur J Cardiothorac Surg*. 2009;35(5):891–900.
11. Sittiwangkul R, Ma RY, McCrindle BW, et al. Echocardiographic assessment of obstructive lesions in atrioventricular septal defect. *J Am Coll Cardiol*. 2001;38(1):253–261.

12. Ando M, Takahashi Y. Variations of atrioventricular septal defects predisposing to regurgitation and stenosis. *Ann Thorac Surg.* 2010;90(2):614–621.
13. Kanani M, Elliott M, Cook A, et al. Late incompetence of the left atrioventricular valve after repair of atrioventricular septal defects: the morphologic perspective. *J Thorac Cardiovasc Surg.* 2006;132(3):640–646.
14. Bharucha T, Sivaprakasam MC, Haw MP, et al. The angle of the components of the common atrioventricular valve predicts outcome of surgical correction in patients with atrioventricular septal defect and common atrioventricular junction. *J Am Soc Echocardiogr.* 2008;21(10):1099–1104.
15. Roman KS, Nii M, Macgowan CK, et al. The impact of patch augmentation on left atrioventricular valve dynamics in patients with atrioventricular septal defects: early and midterm follow-up. *J Am Soc Echocardiogr.* 2006;19(11):1382–1392.
16. Takahashi K, Inage A, Rebeyka IM, et al. Real-time 3-dimensional echocardiography provides new insight into mechanisms of tricuspid valve regurgitation in patients with hypoplastic left heart syndrome. *Circulation.* 2009;120(12):1091–1098.
17. Lim DS, Ensing GJ, Ludomirsky A, et al. Echocardiographic predictors for the development of subaortic stenosis after repair of atrioventricular septal defect. *Am J Cardiol.* 2003;91(7):900–903.

CHAPTER

9

LEFT-SIDED HEART OBSTRUCTIVE LESIONS

Leng Jiang, MD; CuiZhen Pan, MD

ABSTRACT

Left-sided heart obstructive lesions encompass a series of obstructions starting in the pulmonary vein and stretching to the proximal descending aorta. The combination of two-dimensional and Doppler echocardiography has formed the cornerstone of cardiac imaging in the evaluation of these obstructive lesions. Three-dimensional echocardiography (3DE) has potential advantages because it can provide precise anatomic diagnoses and display unique en face imaging of the obstructive lesions. This chapter describes congenital left-sided heart obstructive lesions and reviews the incremental utility of 3DE in imaging them.

INTRODUCTION

Left-sided heart obstructive lesions encompass a series of obstructions starting in the pulmonary vein and stretching to the proximal descending aorta. These lesions can be divided into left ventricular inflow (LVIF) obstruction and left ventricular outflow tract (LVOT) obstruction. The former includes pulmonary vein stenosis (PVS), cor triatriatum, supravalvular mitral ring (SVMR), congenital mitral valve stenosis, and parachute mitral valve (PMV) deformity. The latter includes subvalvular aortic valve stenosis (sub-AS), aortic valve stenosis (secondary to bicuspid or unicuspid valve), supravalvular aortic stenosis (SVAS), and coarctation of the aorta (CoA) (Table 9-1). These obstructive lesions may present alone or in combination, as in the Shone complex, which is characterized by multiple levels of obstruction to blood flow into and out of the left ventricle and in the aorta. The classic picture of the Shone complex includes mitral stenosis with a PMV, sub-AS, bicuspid aortic valve, and CoA.[1] Left-sided heart obstructive lesions may also be associated with other cardiac defects. Some lesions, such as subvalvular aortic membrane, may arise late after the initial cardiac operation. Early accurate imaging diagnosis has made successful surgical or interventional management possible. Regular follow-up visits with these patients, particularly including imaging techniques, are mandatory.

The combination of two-dimensional echocardiography (2DE) and Doppler echocardiography has formed the cornerstone of cardiac imaging in evaluating these obstructive lesions. Alternative cardiac imaging modalities, such as cardiac magnetic resonance imaging (CMRI) and cardiac computed tomography (CT), can offer complementary information in selected patient groups. These modalities are particularly valuable for better visualization of the thoracic aorta, coronary arteries, and venous return.

Three-dimensional echocardiography (3DE) has gone through dramatic developments over the past few decades, from reconstructed wire-frame static images[2–6] to real-time dynamic volumetric imaging.[7–10]

Table 9-1 Left-sided heart obstructive lesions

LVIF obstruction	Left ventricular outflow obstruction
PVS	Sub-AS
Cor triatriatum	Aortic valve stenosis
SVMR	Unicuspid valve
Mitral valve stenosis	Bicuspid valve
PMS	SVAS
	CoA

Abbreviations: CoA, coarctation of the aorta; LVIF, left ventricular inflow; PMS, parachute mitral valve; PVS, pulmonary vein stenosis; sub-AS, subvalvular aortic valve stenosis; SVAS, supravalvular aortic stenosis; SVMR, supravalvular mitral ring.

The current second-generation real-time three-dimensional echocardiography (RT3DE) using the novel fully sampled matrix array transducer enables instantaneous three-dimensional (3D) data acquisition and display, thus circumventing many of the disadvantages of the primitive 3D reconstruction methods, and improves the accuracy of cardiac chamber volume measures.[11–21] These processes are beneficial to patients with congenital heart disease, because appropriate timing for intervention is based on accurate determination of the hemodynamics. The multiplanar review mode enables the review of cardiac structure in infinite planes, providing more information than conventional 2DE. Contemporary RT3DE has been used to evaluate various congenital heart diseases and has proved valuable because it enhances the visualization of morphological abnormalities and their complex relationships.[22–30] RT3DE has been shown to have potential advantages over 2DE for evaluating congenital left-sided heart obstructive lesions because it provides better anatomic evaluation and displays unique en face views of the obstructive lesions.

We describe the individual congenital left-sided heart obstructive lesions and review the clinical application and incremental utility of 3DE in imaging these obstructions. With future refinement in 3DE imaging resolution and volume rates and further experience with its application, RT3DE will evolve as an important integral part of a routine echocardiographic examination, with ultimate success and widespread clinical application.

LEFT VENTRICULAR INFLOW OBSTRUCTION

Congenital LVIF obstruction is rare. It can manifest as a congenital mitral apparatus abnormality (mitral valve stenosis, double-orifice mitral valve [DOMV], or PMV) or may be caused by an abnormal left atrial membrane (cor triatriatum or SVMR) or PVS.[31–33] Different forms of LVIF obstruction can coexist or be associated with additional LVOT obstruction, as seen in the Shone complex.[1]

All of the LVIF obstructive lesions share common pathophysiological characteristics: obstruction of blood flow between the pulmonary venous system and the left ventricle, leading to pulmonary venous and pulmonary arterial hypertension. As a result, clinical manifestations of these lesions are similar. The exact obstructive anatomic abnormality is often not clear even after complete invasive cardiac catheterization and cineangiographic examination.[31–33] M-mode echocardiography is also of limited value in defining the obstructive anatomic abnormality because it is one dimensional.[34–36] 2DE is routinely used to define LVIF obstructive lesions.[34–36] 3DE has proved to be feasible and useful, providing incremental anatomic data,[37,38] as well as accurate chamber volume quantification for assessing the consequence of an obstruction.[11–21]

CONGENITAL MITRAL VALVE STENOSIS

Congenital mitral valve stenosis is a rare condition, found on postmortem examination in 0.6% of patients with congenital heart disease.[31–33] Although it is a rare entity, it takes several forms, with deformities in the valve leaflets and/or subvalvular apparatus. The deformities can occur alone or in combination. Mitral stenosis is often associated with other cardiac abnormalities, especially obstructive lesions. Severe mitral valve hypoplasia or atresia can result in a hypoplastic left ventricle.

Congenital mitral stenosis is usually detected in infancy if the stenosis or associated heart lesions are severe. Hemodynamically significant mitral stenosis usually results in left atrial enlargement, pulmonary venous congestion, and right ventricular enlargement. Echocardiography is the method of choice in the diagnosis of mitral stenosis. 2DE provides direct visualization of the mitral valve apparatus, leaflet motility, and left atrial/right-sided heart enlargement.[35–36] Doppler technique provides useful hemodynamic data, including transmitral pressure gradients, valve area, and pulmonary arterial systolic pressure.[36] Transesophageal echocardiography is used when the quality of transthoracic echocardiography is suboptimal, particularly in adults, or when there is a need to assess left atrial appendage thrombus to guide cardioversion or intervention. RT3DE, either transthoracic or transesophageal, has been shown to provide further insight into the complex valvular malformation, aiding in preoperative planning.[22–24,37,38] Three subtypes of congenital mitral stenosis include leaflet fusion, DOMV, and PMV.

Mitral leaflet fusion

With the fusion of commissures, leaflets move as a single unit with a limited opening, leading to the obstruction of blood flow to the left ventricle. The subvalvular apparatus is often abnormal, thickened, and shortened or even lacking chordae tendineae. At the extremity, papillary muscles are directly inserted into the leaflets, forming a mitral arcade.

Espinola-Zavaleta et al.[37] applied transesophageal RT3DE to five adults with congenital mitral stenosis. Using a volume-rendered display of the appropriate cut-plane from 3D data sets, they were able to clarify the underlying anatomic characteristics of mitral apparatus abnormalities, including mitral arcade, DOMV, accessory mitral tissue, cleft mitral valve, and unicuspid mitral valve. Some of the abnormalities were not detected by a routine transesophageal 2DE examination. Thus, the various 3D projections helped to discern congenital mitral valve anomalies, particularly the extent and spatial location of the deformities. Seliem et al.[38] reported that transthoracic 3DE, although it did not change the basic diagnosis made using conventional 2DE in 41 patients with congenital atrioventricular valve abnormalities, did play an incremental role by providing better delineation of the morphological features of leaflets, subvalvular abnormalities, and the mechanism and origin of regurgitation.

Figure 9-1 is a transthoracic RT3DE image showing a congenital mitral stenosis of the leaflet fusion type. The image was obtained from a 14-year-old girl with exertional shortness of breath and significant systolic and diastolic murmur on physical examination. A 2DE examination showed a membranous ventricular septal defect as well as mitral stenosis. RT3DE with narrow-angle mode clearly demonstrates typical congenital mitral stenosis with fused leaflets and chordae tendineae. A small membranous ventricular septal defect is also visualized. The left atrium is enlarged, so three pulmonary veins are visible in this picture. The right panel is the en face view of the small mitral orifice. As illustrated, the fusion of the leaflets in congenital mitral stenosis is different from that in rheumatic mitral stenosis, where the abnormality involves the free edge of the leaflets more than the body, presenting diastolic doming of the anterior leaflet with a "hockey stick" appearance and immobility of the posterior leaflet.

The ability of RT3DE to obtain an en face view, depicted in Figure 9-2, is unique, which can have a significant impact on the assessment of mitral stenosis severity. 2DE and Doppler-based methods, although commonly used, have limitations. Direct planimetry of the mitral orifice area (MOA) is highly dependent on the orientation and location of the plane imaged.[39] The MOA delivered from pressure half-time method is influenced by multiple factors, such as hemodynamic variables, left ventricular hypertrophy, and associated valvular disease.[36,40–42] Several studies[43–47] have demonstrated that 3DE planimetry of MOA performed en

Figure 9-1A, B and C

3D transthoracic images showing congenital mitral stenosis during systole (left panel, A) and diastole (middle and right panels, B and C). The right panel (C) is a unique en face view of the mitral orifice (MO) cropped from 3D data sets.

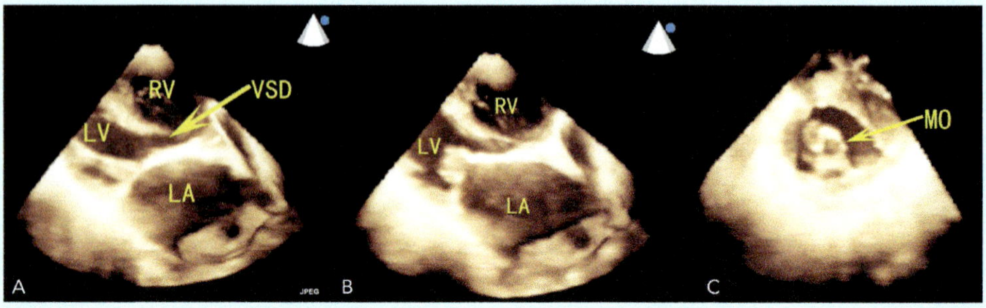

Figure 9-2

A unique cut-plane through the stenotic mitral orifice can be obtained by cropping the coronal and sagittal planes from 3D data sets. This process allows excellent definition of the smallest orifice area in diastole for quantification.

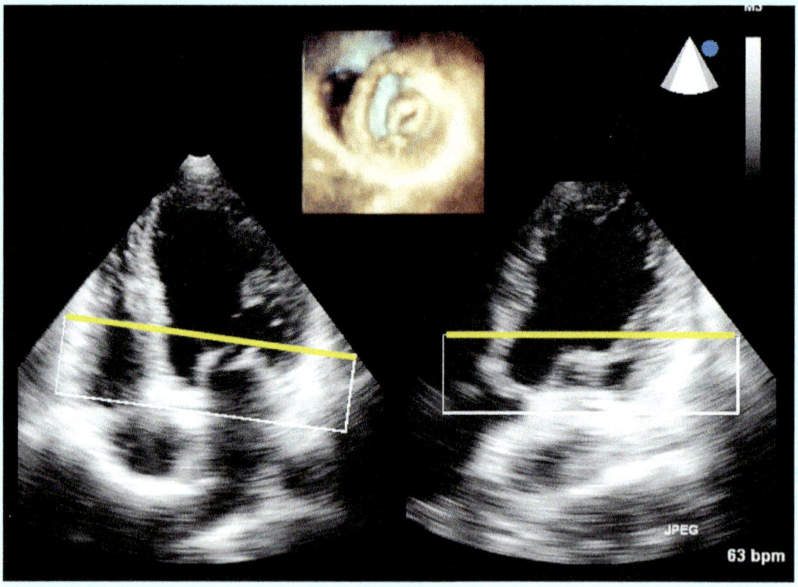

face was better than 2DE and Doppler-based methods when compared with invasively determined MOA. Zamorano et al.[46] examined 80 consecutive patients with mitral stenosis and found that results from RT3DE planimetry had the best agreement with catheter-derived MOA results among all the currently available methods, with small average differences and limits of agreement (0.08 cm^2 [–0.48 to 0.6 cm^2]) and low inter- and intraobserver variabilities. Although all of these validation studies were performed in patients with rheumatic mitral stenosis, it should be possible to extend this technique to congenital mitral stenosis. Studying congenital mitral stenosis might be easier because there is usually less interference from leaflet calcification. However, an anatomic evaluation of the MOA by planimetry may not suffice if there is significant subvalvular fusion or stenosis.

Double-Orifice Mitral Valve

DOMV is an uncommon anomaly. There are three subtypes: (1) the mitral valve opening is divided by an abnormal tissue creating an accessory hole; (2) an extra opening occurs in the mitral valve leaflet; or (3) there are two mitral valves, each with its own annulus, leaflets, chordae tendineae, and papillary muscles (duplicate valves). The accessory hole is the most common subtype, and the duplicate type is the least common. The leaflets may be normal in function but can be significantly stenotic or regurgitant secondary to leaflet thickening, fusing, cleft, perforation, or flailing. DOMV can occur as an isolated anomaly, but associated heart defects, such as atrioventricular septal defect (AVSD), ventricular septal defect, CoA, and interrupted aortic arch, are common.

2DE, either transesophageal or transthoracic, is useful in the diagnosis. However, imaging DOMV by 2DE can be difficult owing to the nonplanar relationship between the orifices and the annulus. Recent case reports have demonstrated that 3DE helped in a more detailed evaluation of the structural abnormality of DOMV.[36,48–52] These studies found that RT3DE was particularly useful for the appropriate orientation of DOMV by multiplanar review. It provided better visualization of the valve than conventional 2DE, including supplemental information on the central bridging tissue and the spatial relationship of the leaflets with submitral structures. In a series of five patients, Lu et al.[48] found that the addition of RT3DE provided a more accurate pathoanatomic definition of DOMV, including the width and depth of the cleft, degree of fibrosis and edge retraction, presence of accessory chordae, and origin and mechanism of the regurgitant jet. In one patient with known rheumatic mitral stenosis, 3DE revealed a congenital DOMV, which was confirmed at surgery. Figure 9-3 shows two examples of RT3DE imaging of DOMV. The image on the left shows a rare duplicate type of DOMV obtained from a 28-year-old woman with a partial AVSD. The DOMV has two

Figure 9-3A and B

3D echocardiographic en face images of DOMV from the left ventricular perspective, revealing the presence of two valve orifices. Left, Two separate symmetrical mitral orifices with a knot-like appearance. A cleft is visible on the anterior leaflet of the left orifice (arrow). Right, Eccentric-type DOMV with bridging tissue in the middle and unequally sized orifices. A smaller accessory orifice is seen on the left and a larger one on the right (arrows). (Left panel courtesy of Q. Lu and X. F. Wang, Union Hospital, Tongji Medical College, Huazhong University of Science and Technology, Wuhan, China.)

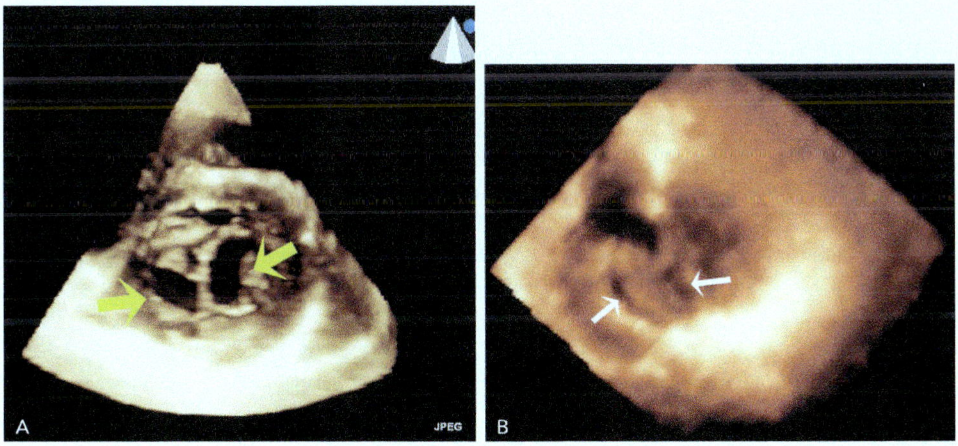

separate symmetrical mitral orifices, giving it a knot-like appearance. The right panel shows a DOMV of the eccentric type, with a central bridging tissue and unequally sized orifices.

Parachute Mitral Valve

PMV is a rare congenital anomaly of the mitral apparatus, characterized by the insertion of chordae tendineae into a single papillary muscle.[1,31,53] In most instances, PMV is associated with other congenital cardiac anomalies, particularly as seen in the Shone complex. Most cases are seen in infants or children; PMV as an isolated anomaly in adults is rare.[54,55]

Diagnosis of PMV in adults is often made by transthoracic 2DE[34–36,54–56] or transesophageal 2DE.[57] Typically, the posteromedial papillary muscle or pair of muscles is present and gives origin to the chordae. The anterolateral papillary muscle and chordae are missing and are replaced by bands of muscle. The chordae are thick and short, and all attach to the single papillary muscle. RT3DE can provide better visualization of the papillary muscle by multiplanar review[58] and is valuable in the evaluation of this entity.[36–59]

CONGENITAL LEFT ATRIAL MEMBRANES

An abnormal membrane in the left atrium can cause LVIF obstruction. Cor triatriatum is a rare congenital anomaly, accounting for 0.1% of cases of congenital heart disease.[31,32,60] The two main forms of LVIF obstruction are cor triatriatum and SVMR, although other variants exist. In this entity, the left atrial membrane bisects the atrium into two chambers: one superior dorsal chamber receives pulmonary venous return, and one inferior ventral chamber has contact with the mitral valve and contains the atrial appendage and the atrial septum that bears the fossa ovalis. The septation can significantly vary in shape, size, and opening. There are great variations in the anatomy. The accessory left atrial chamber can receive only a portion of the pulmonary venous return (subtotal cor triatriatum). The remainder of the pulmonary veins may, directly or indirectly, connect to the left atrium, right atrium, coronary sinus, or systemic veins. The septation can be in the right atrium (cor triatriatum dextrum). Particularly in children, cor triatriatum may be associated with other cardiac lesions, such as atrial septal defects, persistent left superior vena cava, unroofed coronary sinus, ventricular septal defects, and CoA.[60]

Clinical manifestations depend mainly on the size of the opening in the membrane and the presence of associated cardiac defects. The diagnosis is usually achieved by 2DE, which has great advantages over single-dimensional M-mode echocardiography, and is superior to angiography.[34–36,61–63] On 2DE imaging, the cor triatriatum membrane is characteristically located upstream from the left atrial appendage, which differentiates it from an SVMR. Color flow helps to delineate the communication between the two chambers. Transesophageal echocardiography can help when the transthoracic window is suboptimal. However, with these techniques it may be difficult to clarify some of the morphological details of the membrane and its attachment; thus, small openings in the membrane or coexisting lesions can be missed.[62–65] Both transthoracic and transesophageal 3DE have been used to characterize cor triatriatum.[64–72] Many elegantly illustrated case reports have proved the incremental value of RT3DE in the evaluation of cor triatriatum and associated lesions. Detailed membrane fenestration shape and size can be well visualized on an en face view, which is complementary to conventional 2DE.[68] Mercer-Rosa et al.[69] reported on four patients with cor triatriatum in whom the diagnosis was correctly made using transthoracic 2DE. However, RT3DE with a matrix array transducer led to the cancellation of planned surgical intervention in one case, because the membrane was only a broad band crossing the left atrium. Figure 9-4 is an RT3DE image of cor triatriatum obtained from a 55-year-old man who had mild exertional dyspnea. A left atrial membrane that divides the left atrium into two chambers is clearly demonstrated. A single centrally located orifice is well visualized on the membrane.

Baweja et al.[64] were able to make a definitive diagnosis of cor triatriatum associated with a common atrium, an extremely rare entity, using RT3DE. The lesions mimicked a classical partial AVSD and were undiagnosed by transthoracic or transesophageal 2DE. Figure 9-5 presents a similar case, obtained from a 53-year-old woman who had dyspnea, heart murmur, and an enlarged heart. 2DE showed a common atrium with severe mitral regurgitation. Transthoracic RT3DE demonstrated the complete lack of an atrial septum

Figure 9-4

3D transthoracic echocardiogram showing a membrane dividing the left atrium (LA) into a superior dorsal chamber (S-LA) and an inferior ventral chamber (I-LA) with a single central orifice (arrow) connecting the two chambers. LV, left ventricle.

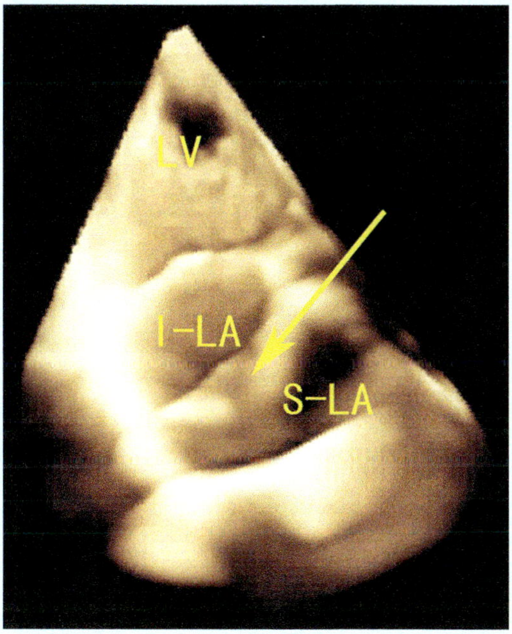

Figure 9-5A and B

3D transthoracic echocardiogram (left panel) demonstrating a rare congenital abnormality with a cor triatriatum membrane in a common atrium. There is a hole on the membrane (asterisk) connecting the uniatrium (UA). Three pulmonary veins (small white arrows) are clearly seen entering the superior chamber. In addition, there is a classic cleft mitral valve (right panel).

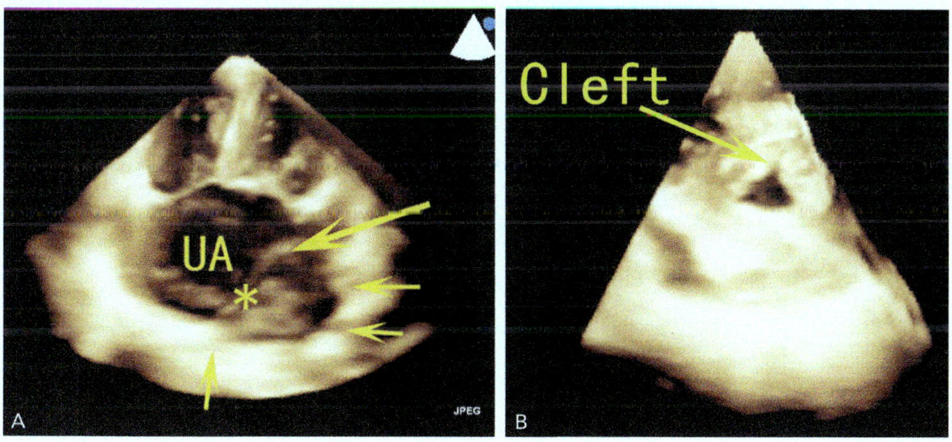

Figure 9-6A and B

3D transthoracic echocardiogram (left panel) showing a partial anomalous pulmonary venous connection, with the right pulmonary vein (RPV) going to the coronary sinus (CS). This anomaly was confirmed on a CT angiographic image (right panel).

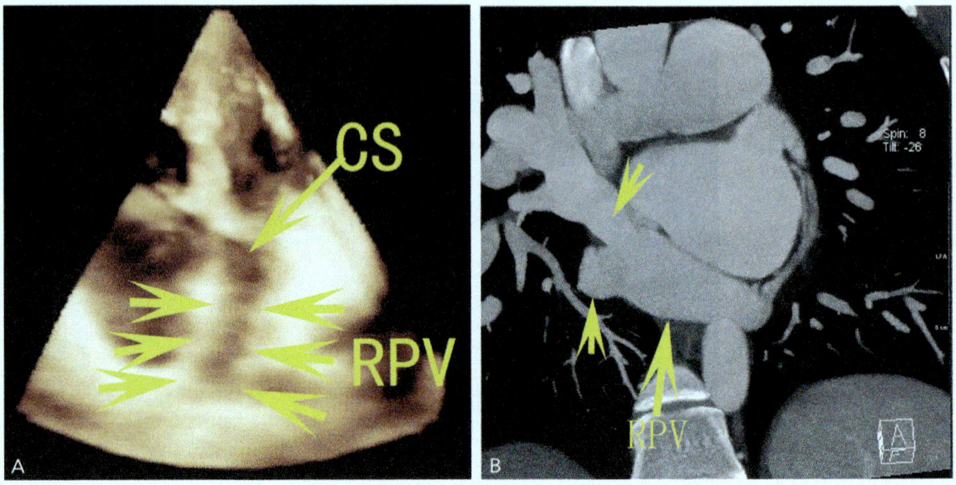

and the presence of a cor triatriatum membrane with a hole communicating with the common atrium. Three pulmonary veins are clearly seen entering the superior chamber. In addition, there is a classic cleft mitral valve (right panel). All of these findings were confirmed during open heart surgery.

Anomalous pulmonary venous return is one of the commonly associated cardiac anomalies, which can be a challenge to examine using 2DE. However, the diagnosis of subtotal cor triatriatum is important for preoperative evaluation. RT3DE offers an advantage over 2DE because one can view the infinite cut-planes from the complete 3D data set. Figure 9-6 shows a partial anomalous pulmonary venous connection on transthoracic RT3DE, with the right pulmonary veins connecting to the coronary sinus. This anomaly was confirmed on CT angiography (right panel).

SVMR is distinguished from cor triatriatum by its position inferior to the left atrial appendage. It is much rarer than cor triatriatum. SVMR can occur in isolation but often coexists with other cardiac anomalies, such as AVSDs or other left-sided obstructive lesions.[31,36,73,74]

Diagnosis is mainly made using 2DE, showing a linear echo in the left atrium just above the mitral valve. This proximity to the mitral valve differentiates SVMR from cor triatriatum. In real time, the SVMR membrane characteristically moves toward the mitral valve orifice in diastole and away from the mitral valve in systole. However, the exact attachments of the membrane can be extremely difficult to evaluate by 2DE.[36,75] Novero et al.[75] described an 8-month-old infant with SVMR and complete AVSD. Both lesions were diagnosed on conventional 2DE, but the morphology of the SVMR was more accurately delineated by RT3DE. The entire circumference of the obstructive ring was well visualized from both left atrial and left ventricular perspectives; thus, the authors were able to accurately evaluate the size and shape of the ring orifice and the proximity of surrounding structures to the ring. These anatomic details aid in preoperative planning.

CONGENITAL PULMONARY VEIN STENOSIS

Congenital PVS is rare, seen mostly in young children with or without other forms of congenital heart defects. The stenosis can progress with time, which may be due to the proliferation of abnormal myofibroblastic cells.[76,77] PVS may also be secondary to anomalous pulmonary vein surgery in children or acquired by mediastinal neoplasms or fibrosis in adults.[78] It can also be a complication after radiofrequency ablation for atrial fibrillation.[78,79]

The timing and severity of symptoms in patients with PVS depend on the number of pulmonary veins involved and the severity of obstruction to individual veins. The prognosis of PVS is guarded, although improvement has been achieved with new surgical and interventional catheter procedures. Diligent follow-up visits are warranted because repeat procedures are often needed.[78,80,81]

Conventional 2DE is often the initial diagnostic tool. In young children, transthoracic 2DE can be used to visualize almost all of the pulmonary veins because the acoustic windows are often good. Color Doppler facilitates the diagnosis by delineating turbulent flow at the stenotic site. Continuous-wave Doppler helps to define functionally significant obstructions by showing characteristic monophasic flow patterns and increased flow velocities (>1.6 m/s).[34,78,82,83] However, the diagnostic value of 2DE Doppler can be limited if the acoustic window is suboptimal, particularly in adults. CMRI and multidetector CT angiography are excellent tools for a detailed analysis of the pulmonary veins. However, the long acquisition time (and thus the tendency to create artifacts) with CMRI and the ionizing radiation with CT angiography are concerns.[78] Jing-Jing et al.[84] reported their initial experience with transthoracic RT3DE in a 3-year-old girl who had left upper PVS. RT3DE clearly delineated the lesion, which was confirmed by CMRI and surgery.

LEFT VENTRICULAR OUTFLOW TRACT OBSTRUCTIONS

LVOT obstruction occurs in six of 10,000 live births or in 7% of patients with congenital heart disease.[85] It encompasses a series of stenotic lesions from the LVOT to the descending portion of the aorta. These obstructive lesions may present alone or in combination.[86] All types of LVOT obstructions impose increased afterload on the left ventricle, leading to circulatory failure in the neonatal period if the obstruction is critical or progressing with left ventricular hypertrophy, dilatation, and eventual failure.[86] Accurately defining the exact anatomy of an obstruction and its severity is essential for clinical decision making. Physical examination, electrocardiography, and chest radiography are routine parts of the clinical evaluation, but they often do not yield specific results. Cardiac imaging, therefore, plays a critical role in the clinical evaluation. 2DE is the imaging modality of choice for defining LVOT obstructions. It is the most widely used tool for initial diagnosis and serial follow-up assessments.[87–89] Transesophageal echocardiography is useful, particularly in adults with a suboptimal acoustic window.[90] Color Doppler helps to delineate the obstructive site, and continuous-wave Doppler provides pressure gradients across the obstruction.[87–90] 3DE has shown advantages over conventional 2DE[51,91,92] by providing better spatial orientation and visualization of the obstructive lesion. Dall'Agata et al.[92] applied RT3DE in 13 patients with LVOT obstructions, including subvalvular (eight), valvular (13), and supravalvular (one) obstructions. Four of the patients had complex obstructions. The authors found that 3DE was suitable for the analysis of all of the subvalvular and supravalvular obstructions and for 77% of the valvular obstructions. Operative findings revealed an accuracy of 100% for subvalvular and supravalvular obstructions and 90% for valvular obstructions. The study concluded that RT3DE was feasible and accurate for analyzing LVOT obstructions. Particularly, generation of nonconventional cross-sectional views allowed better definition of the extent and severity of obstructive lesions.

VALVULAR AORTIC STENOSIS

Congenital aortic valve abnormalities, such as unicuspid, bicuspid, malformed tricuspid, or even quadricuspid valves, can cause valvular aortic stenosis (VAS). VAS is by far the most common type of LVOT obstructive lesions; it accounts for 70% of the obstructions.[85] Critical stenosis with congestive heart failure is rare in infancy; it may be seen in those with a unicuspid valve. The majority of patients with a congenital aortic valve abnormality present with no stenosis or only mild stenosis early in life, but VAS does progress over time.[85,86]

Bicuspid aortic valve is the most common type of congenital aortic valve malformation and the most common congenital cardiovascular abnormality, with an estimated incidence of 1%–2% of the population.[85,86,93] Bicuspid aortic valve can be inherited, and familial clustering has been observed.[86,93] A majority of patients with a bicuspid aortic valve do not develop symptoms until middle age or later. Associated cardiovascular anomalies are common; approximately 6% of cases have a coexisting aortic coarctation. Conversely, as many as 40%–75% of patients with a coarctation have a bicuspid aortic valve.[93] Dilated ascending aorta is common, even in cases with a normally functioning bicuspid aortic valve.[85,86,93] Histological studies have demonstrated that the aortic tissue structure is invariably abnormal in patients with a bicuspid aortic valve, with changes similar to those seen in Marfan syndrome.[93] Complications include aortic valve stenosis or insufficiency, endocarditis, aortic aneurysm, and dissection. The latter is infrequent but dreaded.[85,86,93]

2DE is routinely used for the evaluation of VAS,[93–99] providing morphological information. Bicuspid aortic valve classically has two cusps, usually one larger and one smaller. A raphe (false commissure) is frequently present. Bicuspid aortic valve commonly occurs with a horizontal commissure: the leaflets are oriented anteriorly and posteriorly, the raphe is on the anterior leaflet, and both coronary arteries arise from the same sinus above the anterior leaflet. Less commonly, a bicuspid aortic valve has a vertical commissure: the leaflets are oriented to the right and left, the raphe is on the right leaflet, and the coronary arteries arise from the sinuses above each leaflet. A bicuspid aortic valve with a vertical commissure is reported to have a high incidence of valvular dysfunction.[97] Rarely, the leaflets are symmetrical or there is no raphe, known as a "pure" bicuspid valve.[93] A bicuspid aortic valve can usually be identified by transthoracic 2DE if an adequate acoustic window is available. The reported sensitivities and specificities are more than 90%.[93,95] Transesophageal echocardiography can further improve visualization of a bicuspid aortic valve.[96] A unicuspid aortic valve has a single asymmetrical commissure. The circumference of the valve and the ascending aorta is often reduced. 2DE is diagnostic but can be challenging. The sensitivity and specificity achieved with transthoracic echocardiography are reported to be 27% and 50%, respectively, and with transesophageal echocardiography 75% and 86%, respectively.[98] Malformed tricuspid aortic valves often have unequally sized cusps with various commissural fusions. A quadricuspid aortic valve has four cusps that can be unequally sized. It has a higher prevalence in patients with persistent truncus arteriosus (25%) but may be an incidental finding on a 2DE examination, although many of these patients develop aortic incompetence later in life.[99]

3DE has shown its feasibility and utility in defining various types of congenital aortic valve malformations,[100–107] including bicuspid,[100,101,105,107] unicuspid,[102] and quadricuspid valves.[103,104,106] Figure 9-7 is a transthoracic RT3DE image of a bicuspid aortic valve at systole (left panel) and diastole (right panel).

Figure 9-7A and B

3D transthoracic images: a bicuspid aortic valve viewed en face from an aortic perspective during systole (left panel) and diastole (right panel). The anterior (A) and posterior (P) leaflets are symmetrical; no raphe is identified, consistent with the rare form of pure bicuspid valve. (Image courtesy of L. He and X. F. Wang, Union Hospital, Tongji Medical College, Huazhong University of Science and Technology, Wuhan, China.)

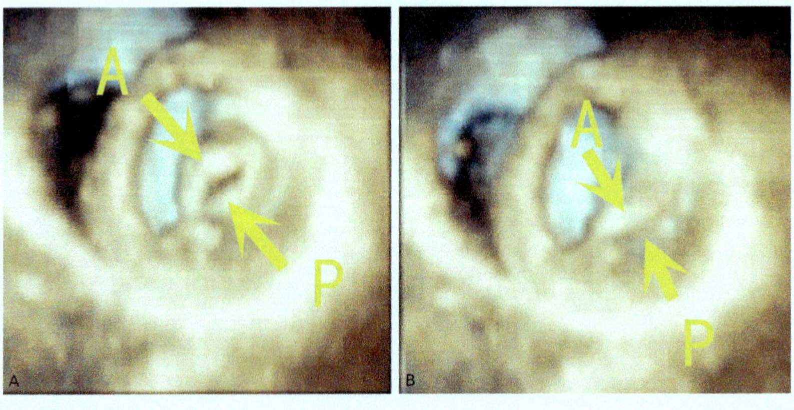

Figure 9-8A and B

3D transthoracic images: a stenotic unicuspid aortic valve (UAV) viewed en face from the aortic perspective during systole (left panel). The right panel shows the UAV (yellow arrow) seen at the time of surgery. The aorta is open, and its walls are retracted with sutures. LA, left atrium; RA, right atrium; RVOT, right ventricular outflow tract.

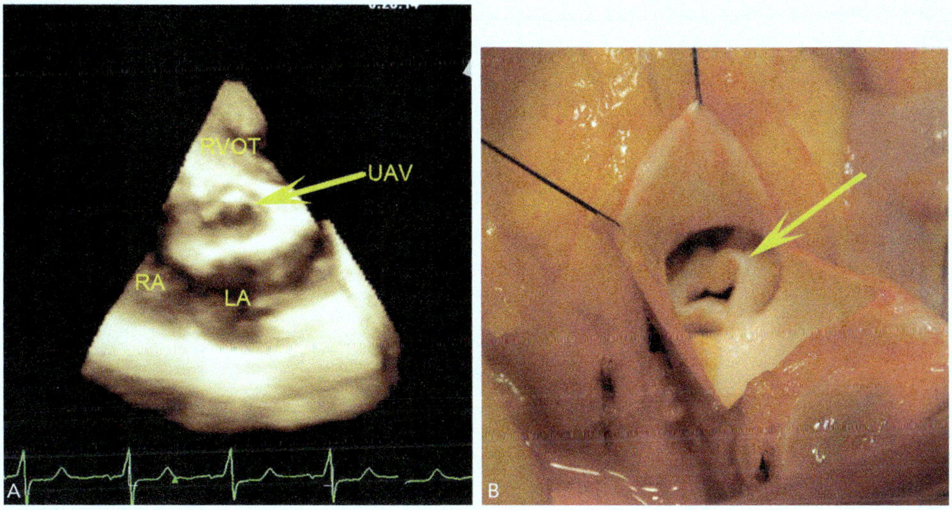

In this case, the anterior (A) and posterior (P) leaflets are symmetrical and no raphe is identified. The image is consistent with a rare form of pure bicuspid valve. Figure 9-8 is a transthoracic RT3DE image from a 13-year-old boy with severe symptoms from a stenotic unicuspid aortic valve (left panel). The mean gradient was 47 mmHg, and the valve area was 0.78 cm^2. The morphology of the unicuspid valve shown on transthoracic RT3DE corresponded well with that seen at surgery (right panel).

The accuracy of 3DE in qualitative assessment of the morphology of the aortic valve has been well documented. Sadagopan et al.,[100] in their prospective cross-sectional observational study, demonstrated that transthoracic 3DE could be used to measure the diameter of the aortic valve orifice, number of aortic valve cusps, and sites of leaflet fusion, all of which closely corresponded with the surgical findings. Espinola-Zavaleta et al.[105] reported good correlations between transthoracic 3DE imaging results and anatomic findings in the assessment of size and features of the cusps, fusion of the commissures, and the presence of thickening and calcification of congenital bicuspid aortic valve in 14 patients and 20 autopsy specimens. Case reports have repeatedly shown that important valve morphology delineated by transthoracic RT3DE was missed by prior 2DE studies.[102,103,108,109] Because of its excellent definition of anatomic details, transthoracic RT3DE has recently been used to screen patients referred for transcatheter aortic valve implantation.[107] Data from 3D imaging for transcatheter aortic valve implantation may also impact further device design, because 3DE allows accurate quantification of the in vivo anatomy and deformation of the aortic root.[110] RT3DE was also used for epicardial imaging in the operating department and reported to be superior to transesophageal 2DE in depicting the morphology of aortic cusp lesions and the LVOT spatial relationships with the mitral apparatus and aortic root and the mitral leaflets.[111]

Another area of active interest is improvement in quantification of the severity of VAS using 3DE. Mean gradients obtained using Doppler echocardiography have proved comparable to catheter-delivered measures. However, challenges are often encountered. Underestimation can happen when the beam is not parallel to the velocity jet, when patients have a low cardiac output, or when a nonrestrictive ventricular septal defect shunts the flow to the right ventricle. Overestimation may also occur in patients with high cardiac output, coexisting

LVOT stenosis, and a small aortic root that may be associated with significant recovery of pressure.[112,113] In these circumferences, measurement of the aortic valve orifice may be more reliable. Direct planimetry of the aortic valve orifice has been used on the 2DE short-axis view by transesophageal[114,115] or even by transthoracic echocardiography with harmonic imaging.[116] However, imaging an aortic valve orifice using 2DE can be challenging, often because of an oblique cross section. Multiplanar RT3DE has the advantage of obtaining a perpendicular cut-plane right through the valve orifice. Studies have shown that planimetry of the aortic valve orifice on RT3DE agrees well with the catheter-derived measures and has better reproducibility.[117–119] However, planimetric assessment of an anatomic aortic valve orifice may overestimate an effective aortic valve orifice in the stenotic bicuspid aortic valve because of the eccentricity of the jet and the larger aortic root, which is associated with less pressure recovery.[120,121]

The continuity equation has been routinely used to calculate effective aortic valve orifice; however, these results have been challenged by recent RT3DE studies that have demonstrated the eccentricity of LVOT. Thus, incorrectly assuming a round LVOT geometry when calculating an aortic valve orifice may lead to significant underestimation.[122,123] Furthermore, calculating the aortic valve orifice using the continuity equation yielded RT3DE color Doppler–derived LVOT stroke volume that was more accurate than that obtained using conventional 2DE, which is based on geometric assumptions of LVOT area.[123,124] Alternatively, on the basis of the continuity equation, using stroke volume directly measured by RT3DE as a substitute for Doppler-derived stroke volume improves the accuracy of the aortic valve orifice calculation compared with the invasive Gorlin formula.[125,126]

SUBVALVULAR AORTIC VALVE STENOSIS

Sub-AS is an uncommon type of LVOT obstruction. It may take different forms, such as a discrete fibrous or muscular ridge; circumferential fibromuscular ring; or long, diffuse, and tunnel-like muscular narrowing. The obstruction can be focal or diffuse.[127,128] The discrete type of sub-AS is the one most frequently encountered (90%).[129] Sub-AS can be an isolated congenital lesion associated with other cardiac defects, or it can be acquired.[130] The associated cardiac defects occur in 40%–60% of patients.[128,129] The two most frequently associated lesions are perimembranous ventricular septal defect and CoA. Other associated lesions are AVSDs, patent ductus arteriosus, bicuspid aortic valve, or double-outlet right ventricle. Aortic regurgitation is common (>50%), which may be related to the sub-AS downstream turbulent flow.[131] Acquired sub-AS is usually a secondary lesion appearing years after a surgical repair of other cardiac defects.[129,130] Progression of sub-AS in childhood or adulthood and recurrence of sub-AS after successful surgical excision occur frequently.[129,132] Altered shear stress secondary to subtle LVOT abnormalities was proposed to be the trigger for cell proliferation, leading to the development or progression of sub-AS.[133]

Echocardiography is usually the only diagnostic tool used in the diagnosis, follow-up, and presurgical evaluation of sub-AS lesions. The morphology of an LVOT obstruction, such as a discrete membrane or a diffuse narrowing, can be well delineated on 2DE.[86–88] Transesophageal echocardiography may help to better visualize the anatomy, particularly in adults. Color Doppler flow mapping can show flow acceleration and turbulence at the obstruction. Continuous-wave Doppler is used to measure the peak instantaneous gradient across the lesion to quantify the degree of obstruction. It usually is accurate when the sub-AS is discrete, but it may not be accurate when the lesion is long or exhibits tunnel-like narrowing because of the use of the modified Bernoulli equation. CMRI is a useful alternative noninvasive imaging tool to define the anatomy and to quantify flow velocity.

The availability of 3DE allows more accurate diagnosis and more detailed analysis of sub-AS lesions. RT3DE has been used to find missed or misdiagnosed discrete subvalvular membranes, resulting in a change in the surgical plan.[134,135] Different anatomic types of sub-AS can be well illustrated by either transthoracic or transesophageal 3DE, such as a remnant crescent, a broken fibrotic subaortic membrane, double subvalvular membranes, and a circumferential obstruction.[136,137] The exact site and full extent of sub-AS can be well defined by RT3DE, and the findings on 3DE correlate well with surgical findings.[136–141] Because it provides a multiplanar review of the infinite planes from the full 3D data sets, RT3DE is particularly useful in offering a comprehensive analysis for identifying other associated lesions[140,141] and for displaying an en face view

Figure 9-9A and B

3D transthoracic images demonstrating a thick discrete fibrous ring located 1.5 cm below the aortic valve (yellow arrows). The aortic annulus is small, and the aortic valve is thickened. AV, aortic valve; LA, left atrium; LV, left ventricle; RA, right atrium; RV, right ventricle.

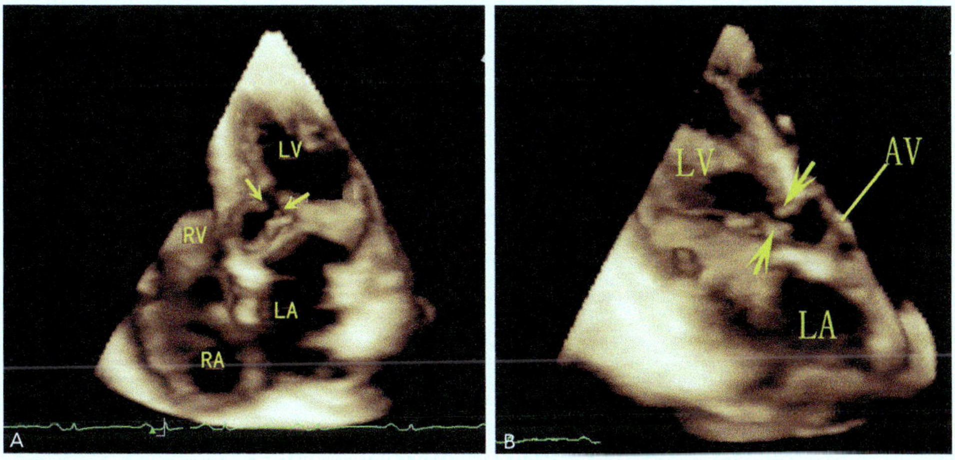

of the obstruction.[141–143] Thus, the stenotic area of the obstruction and its dynamic changes can be accurately quantified.[141,143] On the basis of a larger orifice measured on the en face view, transthoracic RT3DE permitted the correct identification of a significant sub-AS erroneously diagnosed by Doppler, providing important information for clinical decision making.[143]

Because the associated left ventricular structural abnormality may play a role in the progression and recurrence of discrete sub-AS, Bharucha et al.[141] were able to quantify intracardiac geometry in a group of 16 consecutive patients with sub-AS using multiplanar review analysis of the RT3DE data sets. They found that the aortoseptal angle was significantly decreased in patients with sub-AS compared with normal subjects. The finding of a steeper aortoseptal angle in patients with sub-AS agreed with the findings from a previous report[144] and supported the "altered shear stress" concept. It is also demonstrated that measuring intracardiac geometry as the aortoseptal angle on RT3DE images is feasible and may be more accurate because the multiplanar review allows one to find the correct plane to analyze.

We illustrate transthoracic 3DE imaging of sub-AS in Figure 9-9. This image was obtained from a 55-year-old woman with severe exertional dyspnea and chest pain. A thick discrete fibrous ring (d = 10 mm) was clearly seen 1.5 cm below the aortic valve. The aortic annulus was small (d = 17 mm), and the aortic valve was thick. The patient also had a small membranous septal aneurysm consistent with a spontaneously closed ventricular septal defect (not shown). Continuous-wave Doppler measured a peak pressure gradient of 72 mmHg. Doppler color flow mapping showed mild aortic regurgitation. The patient underwent successful surgical repair, and all of the RT3DE findings were confirmed at surgery.

SUPRAVALVULAR AORTIC STENOSIS

SVAS is the rarest form of LVOT obstruction. There are at least two anatomic forms: an hourglass deformity and a diffuse narrowing. A discrete membranous stenosis that may be a variant of the hourglass deformity is also occasionally reported.[145–148] The classic SVAS starts at the sinotubular junction and often involves the entire ascending aorta. All forms of SVAS tend to progress. SVAS may occur as part of Williams syndrome, which is characterized by SVAS, intellectual impairment, and distinct facial features.[149,150] It may also be inherited as an autosomal dominant trait or manifest as a sporadic anomaly. A mutation in the elastin gene has been identified, which leads to elastin arteriopathy.[151] Pulmonary artery stenosis, either of the main pulmonary artery or of branch arteries, is common, occurring in about 50% of patients. Involvement of the aortic arch, descending aorta (coarctation), and peripheral arterial system (such as carotid, cerebral, renal, and iliac artery) can occur but is rare.[147–150] Coronary artery stenosis can result from focal or diffuse narrowing, accelerated atherosclerosis, or obstruction by redundant aortic valve leaflets.[152] Aortic valve abnormalities occur in 50% of patients. The aortic valve leaflets can be thickened, redundant, restricted, or partially adherent to the stenosing supravalvular ridge. Resultant aortic stenosis or regurgitation is the most frequent reason for reoperation.[147,148] Congenital bicuspid aortic valve and sub-AS may also coexist.

The diagnosis of SVAS was traditionally made by cardiac catheterization with invasive angiography. Many noninvasive imaging modalities are now available for the diagnosis and quantification of SVAS. CMRI and CT angiography provide excellent display of the ascending aorta and can accurately delineate the extent of SVAS. Transthoracic 2DE is useful for detecting the narrowing of the proximal ascending aorta.[86–88] Transesophageal echocardiography is superior to transthoracic echocardiography for imaging the lesions.[153] It is particularly useful for evaluating the aortic valve–related mechanism of coronary artery ostial obstruction associated with SVAS. However, visualization of the full extent of the ascending aorta is often challenging, especially the distal portion. Nevertheless, 3DE (especially transesophageal) has been reported to be successful in the evaluation of patients with SVAS.[92,154,155] In preliminary studies, transesophageal RT3DE has proved its incremental role in relation to 2DE, because it can fully delineate the semilunar configuration of SVAS on an en face view of the lesion as opposed to just a ridge as seen on 2DE individual views.[155]

Figure 9-10 is a transthoracic RT3DE image from a 16-year-old young man with Williams syndrome. The ascending aorta was diffusely narrowed starting at the level of the sinotubular junction (left panel). The narrowest internal dimension of the lesion measured only 8 mm; continuous-wave Doppler delivered a peak pressure gradient of 120 mmHg, indicating severe obstruction. The RT3DE findings were confirmed at surgery, as shown in the right panel. The pathology report described intimal hypertrophy with disorganization of the elastin fibers within the media of the ascending aortic wall.

Figure 9-10A and B

3D transthoracic image showing congenital SVAS (left panel, A, yellow arrows). The ascending aorta is diffusely narrowed starting at the level of the sinotubular junction. The surgical findings (right panel, B, yellow arrows) are comparable to the RT3DE findings. LA, left atrium; LV, left ventricle; RV, right ventricle.

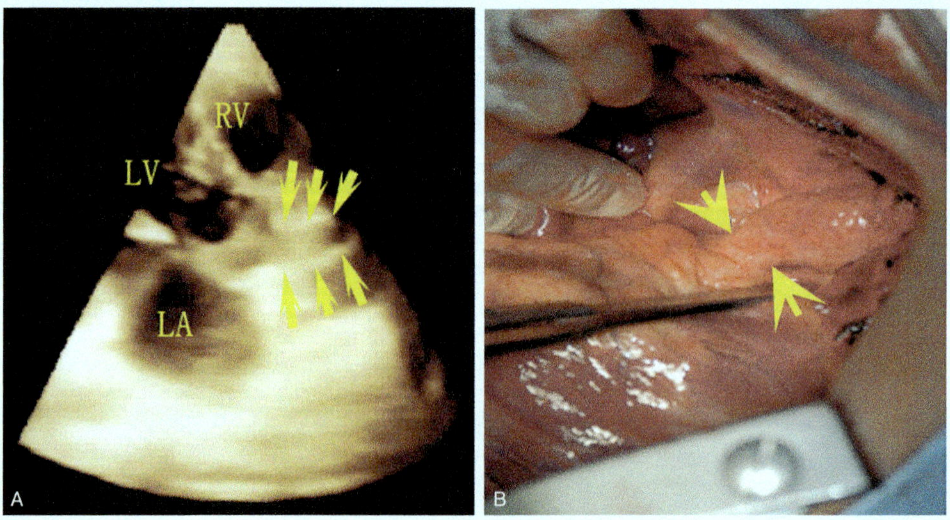

AORTIC COARCTATION

CoA is a relatively common malformation, accounting for 6%–8% of all congenital heart defects. Its prevalence is increased in certain disorders, such as Turner syndrome (>10%). A majority of cases occur sporadically, and familial recurrence is rare.[156] CoA is typically a discrete narrowing of the thoracic aorta just distal to the left subclavian artery. However, the constriction can be proximal to the left subclavian artery, involving the arch or isthmus. A more diffuse form may present, involving a long segment as tubular hypoplasia. CoA is a diffuse arteriopathy.[157,158] Cystic changes in the aortic media have been described in the paracoarctation segments and the ascending aorta.[159] CoA is frequently associated with a bicuspid aortic valve. Other associated cardiac lesions can occur, such as ventricular septal defect, patent ductus arteriosus, all forms of aortic stenoses, and PMV stenosis (Shone complex).[1] Intracranial aneurysms can be detected in up to 10% of the cases.

Clinically, heart failure may occur in neonates and infants, especially in those with other associated cardiac defects. Otherwise, these conditions are usually asymptomatic, especially in children beyond infancy or in adults. Heart murmur, hypertension, and delayed or diminished femoral pulses should lead one to clinically suspect the disease. A chest radiograph may show the characteristic "3" sign of the aorta and rib notching secondary to extensive collateral formation.

Traditionally, invasive catheterization and angiography of the aorta have been used to evaluate CoA. Contemporary CMRI and CT angiography with 3D reconstruction are now becoming the preferred tools to define the degree and extent of CoA as well as collaterals. Transthoracic two-dimensional echocardiography and Doppler echocardiography are useful noninvasive imaging modalities for the initial evaluation of the presence of CoA. From the suprasternal view, 2DE may show the narrowed segment at the distal aortic arch and isthmus and the dilation in the proximal and distal regions.[160,161] High-quality 2DE with color Doppler mapping can establish the diagnosis of CoA, especially in infants and children.[160–162] Left ventricular size, wall thickness and function, and associated lesions can be well assessed. Continuous-wave Doppler[161,163] can enhance diagnostic sensitivity by demonstrating the presence of classic continuing diastolic anterograde flow (diastolic runoff) in the descending aorta. It also provides a peak instantaneous pressure gradient across the CoA site; however, this often overestimates the severity of CoA due to significant pressure recovery and the use of a simplified Bernoulli equation.[164] It can also underestimate the lesion if the ultrasound beam does not align to the jet. Moreover, gradients ascertained either by catheter or by Doppler can be unreliable when extensive collaterals are present. Therefore, accurate anatomic imaging of the lesion is more valuable.

3DE may improve the spatial appreciation of CoA. Studies in vitro and in vivo, using either a multiplanar transesophageal probe[165] or an intravascular ultrasound,[166] were able to successfully achieve 3D reconstruction of CoA. The reconstructed images corresponded well with the actual anatomic specimens, with high reproducibility. Clinically, RT3DE with wide-angle acquisition from the suprasternal notch can image the CoA lesion as long as the acoustic window is optimal. **Figure 9-11** presents a transthoracic RT3DE image from a 46-year-old woman with CoA. A long, narrow segment of the descending aorta (yellow arrows) and dilated proximal and distal segments are well delineated. The length of the lesion is 30 mm, with the narrowest dimension of 6 to 7 mm. Continuous-wave Doppler showed a peak gradient of 64 mmHg, indicating severe CoA.

However, visualization and quantification of CoA by the transthoracic approach, with either 2DE or 3DE, are often challenging, particularly in adults. Scohy et al.[167] applied RT3DE with an intrathoracic approach (epicardial imaging) for perioperative evaluation of CoA lesions. With online multiplanar review, they were able to comprehensively view extensive morphological details and quantify the cross-sectional area of the CoA segment preoperatively and the anastomosis after repair. In three of nine surgical procedures, intraoperative 3DE provided additional information to support surgical decision making. One patient underwent a reanastomosis procedure on the basis of findings showing a small cross-sectional area after the first anastomosis, one patient was surgically retreated for a thrombus in the descending aorta, and one patient avoided unnecessary redo after 3DE showed an adequate anastomosis area despite a significant brachial ankle pressure difference measured postoperatively. The authors concluded that RT3DE is a feasible and useful imaging modality for intraoperative assessment of CoA lesions and repairs. The results are encouraging, and the role of RT3DE is continuing to evolve.

Figure 9-11

Real-time transthoracic 3D image with wide-angle acquisition from the suprasternal notch, showing CoA. The long narrow segment of the descending aorta (yellow arrows) and the dilated proximal and distal segments are well delineated.

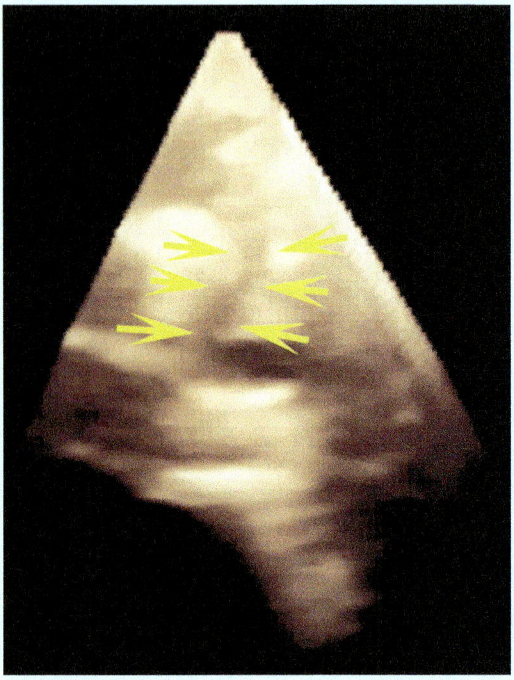

REFERENCES

1. Shone JD, Sellers RD, Anderson RC, et al. The developmental complex of "parachute mitral valve," supravalvular ring of left atrium, subaortic stenosis, and coarctation of aorta. *Am J Cardiol.* 1963;11:714–725.
2. King DL, Harrison MR, King DL Jr, et al. Improved reproducibility of left atrial and left ventricular measurements by guided three-dimensional echocardiography. *J Am Coll Cardiol.* 1992;20(5):1238–1245.
3. Siu SC, Rivera JM, Guerrero JL, et al. Three-dimensional echocardiography. In vivo validation for left ventricular volume and function. *Circulation.* 1993;88(4 Pt 1):1715–1723.
4. Jiang L, Siu SC, Handschumacher MD, et al. Three-dimensional echocardiography. In vivo validation for right ventricular volume and function. *Circulation.* 1994;89(5):2342–2350.
5. Jiang L, Vazquez de Prada JA, Handschumacher MD, et al. Three-dimensional echocardiography: in vivo validation for right ventricular free wall mass as an index of hypertrophy. *J Am Coll Cardiol.* 1994;23(7):1715–1722.
6. Gopal AS, Schnellbaecher MJ, Shen Z, et al. Freehand three–dimensional echocardiography for determination of left ventricular volume and mass in patients with abnormal ventricles: comparison with magnetic resonance imaging. *J Am Soc Echocardiogr.* 1997;10(8):853–861.
7. Franke A, Kuhl HP. Second-generation real-time 3D echocardiography: a revolutionary new technology. *Medicamundi.* 2003;47:34–40.
8. Sugeng L, Weinert L, Thiele K, Lang RM. Real-time three-dimensional echocardiography using a novel matrix array transducer. *Echocardiography.* 2003;20(7):623–635.
9. Lang RM, Mor-Avi V, Sugeng L, et al. Three-dimensional echocardiography: the benefits of the additional dimension. *J Am Coll Cardiol.* 2006;48(10):2053–2069.
10. Hung J, Lang R, Flachskampf F, et al. 3D echocardiography: a review of the current status and future directions. *J Am Soc Echocardiogr.* 2007;20(3):213–233.

11. Schmidt MA, Ohazama CJ, Agyeman KO, et al. Real-time three-dimensional echocardiography for measurement of left ventricular volumes. *Am J Cardiol.* 1999;84(12):1434–1439.
12. Lee D, Fuisz AR, Fan PH, et al. Real-time 3-dimensional echocardiographic evaluation of left ventricular volume: correlation with magnetic resonance imaging—a validation study. *J Am Soc Echocardiogr.* 2001;14(1):1001–1009.
13. Kühl HP, Schreckenberg M, Rulands D, et al. High-resolution transthoracic real-time three-dimensional echocardiography: quantitation of cardiac volumes and function using semi-automatic border detection and comparison with cardiac magnetic resonance imaging. *J Am Coll Cardiol.* 2004;43(11):2083–2090.
14. Arai K, Hozumi T, Matsumura Y, et al. Accuracy of measurement of left ventricular volume and ejection fraction by new real-time three-dimensional echocardiography in patients with wall motion abnormalities secondary to myocardial infarction. *Am J Cardiol.* 2004;94(5):552–558.
15. Jenkins C, Bricknell K, Hanekom L, Marwick TH. Reproducibility and accuracy of echocardiographic measurements of left ventricular parameters using real-time three-dimensional echocardiography. *J Am Coll Cardiol.* 2004;44(4):878–886.
16. Corsi C, Lang RM, Veronesi F, et al. Volumetric quantification of global and regional left ventricular function from real-time three-dimensional echocardiographic images. *Circulation.* 2005;112(8):1161–1170.
17. Riehle TJ, Mahle WT, Parks WJ, et al. Real-time three-dimensional echocardiographic acquisition and quantification of left ventricular indices in children and young adults with congenital heart disease: comparison with magnetic resonance imaging. *J Am Soc Echocardiogr.* 2008;21(1):78–83.
18. van den Bosch AE, Robbers-Visser D, Krenning BJ, et al. Real-time transthoracic three-dimensional echocardiographic assessment of left ventricular volume and ejection fraction in congenital heart disease. *J Am Soc Echocardiogr.* 2006;19(1):1–6.
19. Niemann PS, Pinho L, Balbach T, et al. Anatomically oriented right ventricular volume measurements with dynamic three-dimensional echocardiography validated by 3 Tesla magnetic resonance imaging. *J Am Coll Cardiol.* 2007;50(17):1668–1676.
20. Lu X, Nadvoretskiy V, Bu L, et al. Accuracy and reproducibility of real-time three-dimensional echocardiography for assessment of right ventricular volumes and ejection fraction in children. *J Am Soc Echocardiogr.* 2008;21(1):84–89.
21. Soriano BD, Hoch M, Ithuralde A, et al. Matrix-array 3-dimensional echocardiographic assessment of volumes, mass, and ejection fraction in young pediatric patients with a functional single ventricle: a comparison study with cardiac magnetic resonance. *Circulation.* 2008;117(14):1842–1848.
22. Acar P, Abadir S, Paranon S, et al. Live 3D echocardiography with the pediatric matrix probe. *Echocardiography.* 2007;24(7):750–755.
23. Bharucha T, Roman KS, Anderson RH, Vettukattil JJ. Impact of multiplanar review of three-dimensional echocardiographic data on management of congenital heart disease. *Ann Thorac Surg.* 2008;86(3):875–881.
24. Seliem MA, Fedec A, Szwast A, et al. Atrioventricular valve morphology and dynamics in congenital heart disease as imaged with real-time 3-dimensional matrix-array echocardiography: comparison with 2-dimensional imaging and surgical findings. *J Am Soc Echocardiogr.* 2007;20(7):869–876.
25. Marx GR, Su X. Three-dimensional echocardiography in congenital heart disease. *Cardiol Clin.* 2007;25(2):357–365.
26. Shirali GS. Three-dimensional echocardiography in congenital heart defects. *Ann Pediatr Cardiol.* 2008;1(1):8–17.
27. Nanda NC, Miller AP. Real time three-dimensional echocardiography: specific indications and incremental value over traditional echocardiography. *J Cardiol.* 2006;48(6):291–303.
28. Simpson JM. Real-time three-dimensional echocardiography of congenital heart disease using a high frequency paediatric matrix transducer. *Eur J Echocardiogr.* 2008;9(2):222–224.
29. Del Pasqua A, Sanders SP, de Zorzi A, et al. Impact of three-dimensional echocardiography in complex congenital heart defect cases: the surgical view. *Pediatr Cardiol.* 2009;30(3):293–300.
30. Bonnichsen CR, Anavekar NS, Connolly HM. Three dimensional echocardiography in adult congenital heart disease. *Curr Cardiovasc Imaging Rep.* 2010;3(5):294–302.
31. Collins Nakai RL, Rosenthal A, Castaneda AR, et al. Congenital mitral stenosis. A review of 20 years' experience. *Circulation.* 1977;56(6):1039–1047.
32. Moore P, Adatia I, Spevak PJ, et al. Severe congenital mitral stenosis in infants. *Circulation.* 1994;89(5):2099–2106.
33. McElhinney DB, Sherwood MC, Keane JF, et al. Current management of severe congenital mitral stenosis: outcomes of transcatheter and surgical therapy in 108 infants and children. *Circulation.* 2005;112(5):707–714.
34. Snider B, Roge CL, Schiller BN, Silverman HN. Congenital left ventricular inflow obstruction evaluated by two-dimensional echocardiography. *Circulation.* 1980;61(4):848–855.
35. Vitarelli A, Landolina G, Gentile R, et al. Echocardiographic assessment of congenital mitral stenosis. *Am Heart J.* 1984;108(3 Pt 1):523–531.
36. Banerjee A, Kohl T, Silverman NH. Echocardiographic evaluation of congenital mitral valve anomalies in children. *Am J Cardiol.* 1995;76(17):1284–1291.

37. Espinola-Zavaleta N, Vargas-Barron J, Keirns C, et al. Three-dimensional echocardiography in congenital malformations of the mitral valve. *J Am Soc Echocardiogr.* 2002;15(5):468–472.
38. Martin RP, Rakowski H, Kleiman JH, et al. Reliability and reproducibility of two-dimensional echocardiographic measurement of stenotic mitral valve orifice area. *Am J Cardiol.* 1979;43(3):560–568.
39. Nakatani S, Masuyama T, Kodama K, et al. Value and limitations of Doppler echocardiography in the quantification of stenotic mitral valve area: comparison of the pressure half-time and the continuity equation methods. *Circulation.* 1988;77(1):78–85.
40. Karp K, Teien D, Bjerle P, Eriksson P. Reassessment of valve area determinations in mitral stenosis by the pressure half-time method: impact of left ventricular stiffness and peak diastolic pressure difference. *J Am Coll Cardiol.* 1989;13(3):594–599.
41. Flachskampf FA, Weyman AE, Gillam L, et al. Aortic regurgitation shortens Doppler pressure half-time in mitral stenosis: clinical evidence, in vitro simulation and theoretic analysis. *J Am Coll Cardiol.* 1990;16(2):396–404.
42. Chen Q, Nosir YF, Vletter WB, et al. Accurate assessment of mitral valve area in patients with mitral stenosis by three-dimensional echocardiography. *J Am Soc Echocardiogr.* 1997;10(2):133–140.
43. Binder TM, Rosenhek R, Porenta G, et al. Improved assessment of mitral valve stenosis by volumetric real-time three-dimensional echocardiography. *J Am Coll Cardiol.* 2000;36(4):1355–1361.
44. Sugeng L, Weinert L, Lammertin G, et al. Accuracy of mitral valve area measurements using transthoracic rapid freehand 3-dimensional scanning: comparison with noninvasive and invasive methods. *J Am Soc Echocardiogr.* 2003;16(12):1292–1300.
45. Zamorano J, Cordeiro P, Sugeng L, et al. Real-time three-dimensional echocardiography for rheumatic mitral valve stenosis evaluation: an accurate and novel approach. *J Am Coll Cardiol.* 2004;43(11):2091–2096.
46. Sugeng L, Coon P, Weinert L, et al. Use of real-time 3-dimensional transthoracic echocardiography in the evaluation of mitral valve disease. *J Am Soc Echocardiogr.* 2006;19(4):413–421.
47. Lu Q, Lu X, Xie M, et al. Real-time three-dimensional echocardiography in assessment of congenital double orifice mitral valve. *J Huazhong Univ Sci Technolog Med Sci.* 2006;26(5):625–628.
48. Abdullah M, Pearce K, Palmer N, Chenzbraun A. Double orifice mitral valve with dysplastic tricuspid valve and intact interatrial septum: a three-dimensional echocardiographic study. *Eur J Echocardiogr.* 2008;9(4):598–599.
49. Anwar AM, McGhie JS, Meijboom FJ, Ten Cate FJ. Double orifice mitral valve by real-time three-dimensional echocardiography. *Eur J Echocardiogr.* 2008;9(5):731–732.
50. Aggarwal G, Schlosshan D, Arronis C, et al. Images in cardiovascular medicine. Real-time 3-dimensional transesophageal echocardiography in the evaluation of a patient with concomitant double-orifice mitral valve, bicuspid aortic valve, and coarctation of the aorta. *Circulation.* 2009;120(22):e277–e279.
51. Tandon R, Takkar S, Kumbhkarni S, et al. A rare case of double orifice mitral valve with perimembranous ventricular septal defect: application of three-dimensional echocardiography for clinical decision making. *Ann Pediatr Cardiol.* 2010;3(1):87–89.
52. Marino BS, Kruge LE, Cho CJ, et al. Parachute mitral valve: morphologic descriptors, associated lesions, and outcomes alter biventricular repair. *J Thorac Cardiovasc Surg.* 2009;137:385–393.e4.
53. Hakim FA, Kendall CB, Alharthi M, et al. Parachute mitral valve in adults—a systematic overview. *Echocardiography.* 2010;27(5):581–586.
54. Motoda H, Murata M, Iwanaga S, et al. Parachute mitral valve incidentally diagnosed in an adult patient with hypertension. *J Echocardiogr* 2010;8:28–29.
55. Popescu BA, Jurcut R, Serban M, et al. Shone's syndrome diagnosed with echocardiography and confirmed at pathology. *Eur J Echocardiogr.* 2008;9(6):865–867.
56. Almeida S, Cotrim C, Miranda R, et al. The role of echocardiography in assessing parachute mitral valve [in English, Portuguese]. *Rev Port Cardiol.* 2009;28(3):335–339.
57. Arat N, Gölbasi Z, Ilkay E, et al. Live three-dimensional transthoracic echocardiography in the assessment of the papillary muscle abnormality with mitral regurgitation. *Anadolu Kardiyol Derg.* 2007;7(4):459.
58. Baird CW, Bengur AR, Bensky A, Watts LT. Congenital absence of posteromedial papillary muscle and anterior mitral leaflet chordae: the use of three-dimensional echocardiography and approach in complex pediatric mitral valve disease. *J Thorac Cardiovasc Surg.* 2010;139(4):e75–e77.
59. Godoy I, Tantibhedhyangkul W, Karp R, Lang R. Images in cardiovascular medicine. Cor triatriatum. *Circulation.* 1998;98(24):2781.
60. Ostman–Smith I, Silverman NH, Oldershaw P, et al. Cor triatriatum sinistrum. Diagnostic features on cross sectional echocardiography. *Br Heart J.* 1984;51(2):211–219.
61. Sadiq M, Sreeram N, Silove ED. Congenitally divided left atrium: diagnostic pitfalls in cross-sectional echocardiography. *Int J Cardiol.* 1995;48(1):99–101.
62. Buchholz S, Jenni R. Doppler echocardiographic findings in 2 identical variants of a rare cardiac anomaly, "subtotal" cor triatriatum: a critical review of the literature. *J Am Soc Echocardiogr.* 2001;14(8):846–849.

63. Baweja G, Nanda NC, Kirklin JK. Definitive diagnosis of cor triatriatum with common atrium by three-dimensional transesophageal echocardiography in an adult. *Echocardiography.* 2004;21(3):303–306.
64. Abadir S, Acar P. Live 3D transthoracic echocardiography for assessment of cor triatriatum sinister. *Echocardiography.* 2008;25(10):1147–1148.
65. Tantibhedhyangkul W, Godoy I, Karp R, Lang RM. Cor triatriatum in a 70-year-old woman: role of transesophageal echocardiography and dynamic three-dimensional echocardiography in diagnostic assessment. *J Am Soc Echocardiogr.* 1998;11(8):837–840.
66. Melzer C, Bartel T, Müller S, et al. Dynamic three-dimensional echocardiography in the assessment of cor triatriatum. *Clin Cardiol.* 1997;20(1):82–83.
67. Jacobs A, Weinert LC, Goonewardena S, et al. Three-dimensional transthoracic echocardiography to evaluate cor triatriatum in the adult. *J Am Soc Echocardiogr.* 2006;19(4):468.e1–468.e4.
68. Mercer-Rosa L, Fedec A, Gruber P, Seliem M. Cor triatriatum sinister with and without left ventricular inflow obstruction: visualization of the entire supravalvular membrane by real-time three-dimensional echocardiography. Impact on clinical management of individual patient. *Congenit Heart Dis.* 2006;1(6):335–339.
69. Lee YS, Kim KS, Lee JB, et al. Cor triatriatum dexter assessed by three-dimensional echocardiography reconstruction in two adult patients. *Echocardiography.* 2007;24(9):991–994.
70. Pericas P, Rodríguez-Fernández A, Melis G, et al. Real-time three-dimensional transesophageal echocardiographic imaging of cor triatriatum and persistent left superior vena cava. *J Am Soc Echocardiogr.* 2011;24(6):706.e1–706.e3.
71. Hamdan R, Mirochnik N, Celermajer D, et al. Cor Triatriatum Sinister diagnosed in adult life with three dimensional transesophageal echocardiography. *BMC Cardiovasc Disord.* 2010;10:54.
72. Stretton TB, Fentem PH. Stenosis of the left atrioventricular canal. *Br Heart J.* 1962;24:237–240.
73. Toscano A, Pasquini L, Iacobelli R, et al. Congenital supravalvar mitral ring: an underestimated anomaly. *J Thorac Cardiovasc Surg.* 2009;137(3):538–542.
74. Novero LJ, Rosenkranz ER, Kardon RE. Supravalvar mitral ring with complete atrioventricular septal defect: a case report and three-dimensional echocardiography evaluation. *J Am Soc Echocardiogr.* 2010;23(7):792.e1–792.e2.
75. Edwards JE. Congenital stenosis of pulmonary veins: pathologic and developmental considerations. *Lab Invest.* 1960;9:46–66.
76. Bini RM, Cleveland DC, Ceballos R, et al. Congenital pulmonary vein stenosis. *Am J Cardiol.* 1984;54(3):369–375.
77. Latson LA, Prieto LR. Congenital and acquired pulmonary vein stenosis. *Circulation.* 2007;115(1):103–108.
78. Dong J, Vasamreddy CR, Jayam V, et al. Incidence and predictors of pulmonary vein stenosis following catheter ablation of atrial fibrillation using the anatomic pulmonary vein ablation approach: results from paired magnetic resonance imaging. *J Cardiovasc Electrophysiol.* 2005;16(8):845–852.
79. Devaney EJ, Chang AC, Ohye RG, Bove EL. Management of congenital and acquired pulmonary vein stenosis. *Ann Thorac Surg.* 2006;81(3):992–995.
80. Minich LL, Tani LY, Breinholt JP, et al. Complete follow-up echocardiograms are needed to detect stenosis of normally connecting pulmonary veins. *Echocardiography.* 2001;18(7):589–592.
81. Tan CW, Munfakh N, Helmcke F, et al. Congenital bilateral pulmonary venous stenosis in an adult: diagnosis by Echo-Doppler. *Catheter Cardiovasc Interv.* 2000;49(3):328–330.
82. Smallhorn JF, Pauperio H, Benson L, et al. Pulsed Doppler assessment of pulmonary vein obstruction. *Am Heart J.* 1985;110(2):483–486.
83. Jing-Jing Y, Wei-ze X, Qiang S, et al. Real time three-dimensional transthoracic echocardiography evaluation in a patient with congenital pulmonary vein stenosis. *Echocardiography.* 2010;27(9):E109–E111.
84. Arnold R, Kitchiner D. Left ventricular outflow obstruction. *Arch Dis Child.* 1995;72(2):180–183.
85. Aboulhosn J, Child JS. Left ventricular outflow obstruction: subaortic stenosis, bicuspid aortic valve, supravalvar aortic stenosis, and coarctation of the aorta. *Circulation.* 2006;114(22):2412–2422.
86. Weyman AE. Cross sectional echocardiographic assessment of aortic obstruction. *Acta Med Scand Suppl.* 1979;627:120–136.
87. Weyman AE, Feigenbaum H, Hurwitz RA, et al. Localization of left ventricular outflow obstruction by cross-sectional echocardiography. *Am J Med.* 1976;60(1):33–38.
88. Tworetzky W, McElhinney DB, Brook MM, et al. Echocardiographic diagnosis alone for the complete repair of major congenital heart defects. *J Am Coll Cardiol.* 1999;33(1):228–233.
89. Marelli AJ, Child JS, Perloff JK. Transesophageal echocardiography in congenital heart disease in the adult. *Cardiol Clin.* 1993;11(3):505–520.
90. Salustri A, Spitaels S, McGhie J, et al. Transthoracic three-dimensional echocardiography in the adult patient with congenital heart disease. *J Am Coll Cardiol.* 1995;26(3):759–767.
91. Dall'Agata A, Cromme-Dijkhuis AH, Meijboom FJ, et al. Use of three-dimensional echocardiography for analysis of outflow obstruction in congenital heart disease. *Am J Cardiol.* 1999;83(6):921–925.

92. Siu SC, Silversides CK. Bicuspid aortic valve disease. *J Am Coll Cardiol.* 2010;55(25):2789–2800.
93. Radford DJ, Bloom KR, Izukawa T, et al. Echocardiographic assessment of bicuspid aortic valves. Angiographic and pathological correlates. *Circulation.* 1976;53(1):80–85.
94. Brandenburg RO, Tajikh AJ, Edwards WD, et al. Accuracy of 2-dimensional echocardiographic diagnosis of congenitally bicuspid valve: echocardiographic-anatomic correlation in 115 patients. *Am J Cardiol.* 1983;51(9):1469–1473.
95. Espinal M, Fuisz AR, Nanda NC, et al. Sensitivity and specificity of transesophageal echocardiography for determination of aortic valve morphology. *Am Heart J.* 2000;139(6):1071–1076.
96. Beppu S, Suzuki S, Matsuda H, et al. Rapidity of progression of aortic stenosis in patients with congenital bicuspid aortic valves. *Am J Cardiol.* 1993;71(4):322–327.
97. Chu JW, Picard MH, Agnihotri AK, Fitzsimons MG. Diagnosis of congenital unicuspid aortic valve in adult population: the value and limitation of transesophageal echocardiography. *Echocardiography.* 2010;27(9):1107–1112.
98. Tutarel O. The quadricuspid aortic valve: a comprehensive review. *J Heart Valve Dis.* 2004;13(4):534–537.
99. Sadagopan SN, Veldtman GR, Sivaprakasam MC, et al. Correlations with operative anatomy of real time three-dimensional echocardiographic imaging of congenital aortic valvar stenosis. *Cardiol Young.* 2006;16(5): 490–494.
100. Singh P, Dutta R, Nanda NC. Live/real time three-dimensional transthoracic echocardiographic assessment of bicuspid aortic valve morphology. *Echocardiography.* 2009;26(4):478–480.
101. Buchner S, Kobuch R, Luchner A, Debl K. Diagnosis of unicommissural unicuspid aortic valve stenosis by different imaging modalities. *J Cardiovasc Med (Hagerstown).* 2011;12(5):347–348.
102. Burri MV, Nanda NC, Singh A, Panwar SR. Live/real time three-dimensional transthoracic echocardiographic identification of quadricuspid aortic valve. *Echocardiography.* 2007;24(6):653–655.
103. Nucifora G, Badano LP, Iacono MA, et al. Congenital quadricuspid aortic valve associated with obstructive hypertrophic cardiomyopathy. *J Cardiovasc Med (Hagerstown).* 2008;9(3):317–318.
104. Espinola-Zavaleta N, Muñoz-Castellanos L, Attié F, et al. Anatomic three-dimensional echocardiographic correlation of bicuspid aortic valve. *J Am Soc Echocardiogr.* 2003;16(1):46–53.
105. Armen TA, Vandse R, Bickle K, Nathan N. Three-dimensional echocardiographic evaluation of an incidental quadricuspid aortic valve. *Eur J Echocardiogr.* 2008;9(2):318–320.
106. Unsworth B, Malik I, Mikhail GW. Recognizing bicuspid aortic stenosis in patients referred for transcatheter aortic valve implantation: routine screening with three-dimensional transoesophageal echocardiography. *Heart.* 2010;96(8):645.
107. Nanda NC, Roychoudhury D, Chung SM, et al. Quantitative assessment of normal and stenotic aortic valve using transesophageal three-dimensional echocardiography. *Echocardiography.* 1994;11(6):617–625.
108. Malagoli A, Barbieri A, Modena MG. Bicuspid aortic valve regurgitation: quantification of anatomic regurgitant orifice area by 3D transesophageal echocardiography reconstruction. *Echocardiography.* 2008;25(7):797–798.
109. Schoenhagen P, Hill A. Transcatheter aortic valve implantation and potential role of 3D imaging. *Expert Rev Med Devices.* 2009;6(4):411–421.
110. De Castro S, Salandin V, Cavarretta E, et al. Epicardial real-time three-dimensional echocardiography in cardiac surgery: a preliminary experience. *Ann Thorac Surg.* 2006;82(6):2254.
111. Niederberger J, Schima H, Maurer G, Baumgartner H. Importance of pressure recovery for the assessment of aortic stenosis by Doppler ultrasound. Role of aortic size, aortic valve area, and direction of the stenotic jet in vitro. *Circulation.* 1996;94(8):1934–1940.
112. Bahlmann E, Cramariuc D, Gerdts E, et al. Impact of pressure recovery on echocardiographic assessment of asymptomatic aortic stenosis: a SEAS substudy. *JACC Cardiovasc Imaging.* 2010;3(6):555–562.
113. Stoddard MF, Hammons RT, Longaker RA. Doppler transesophageal echocardiographic determination of aortic valve area in adults with aortic stenosis. *Am Heart J.* 1996;132(2 Pt 1):337–342.
114. Tribouilloy C, Leborgne L, Rey JL, et al. Can Doppler echocardiography help to avoid cardiac catheterization in the surgical decision-making in isolated left heart valve diseases? [in French]. *Arch Mal Coeur Vaiss.* 1996;89(12):1607–1616.
115. Brasch AV, Luo H, Khan SS, et al. Effect of harmonic imaging for planimetry on transthoracic echocardiography on visualization of the aortic valve. *Am J Cardiol.* 2001;88(9):1047–1049.
116. Menzel T, Mohr-Kahaly S, Kölsch B, et al. Quantitative assessment of aortic stenosis by three-dimensional echocardiography. *J Am Soc Echocardiogr.* 1997;10(3):215–223.
117. Ge S, Warner JG Jr, Abraham TP, et al. Three-dimensional surface area of the aortic valve orifice by three-dimensional echocardiography: clinical validation of a novel index for assessment of aortic stenosis. *Am Heart J.* 1998;136(6):1042–1050.

118. Goland S, Trento A, Iida K, et al. Assessment of aortic stenosis by three-dimensional echocardiography: an accurate and novel approach. *Heart*. 2007;93(7):801–807.
119. Bernard Y, Meneveau N, Vuillemenot A, et al. Planimetry of aortic valve area using multiplane transoesophageal echo-cardiography is not a reliable method for assessing severity of aortic stenosis. *Heart*. 1997;78(1):68–73.
120. Donal E, Novaro GM, Deserrano D, et al. Planimetric assessment of anatomic valve area overestimates effective orifice area in bicuspid aortic stenosis. *J Am Soc Echocardiogr*. 2005;18(12):1392–1398.
121. Doddamani S, Bello R, Friedman MA, et al. Demonstration of left ventricular outflow tract eccentricity by real time 3D echocardiography: implications for the determination of aortic valve area. *Echocardiography*. 2007;24(8):860–866.
122. Poh KK, Levine RA, Solis J, et al. Assessing aortic valve area in aortic stenosis by continuity equation: a novel approach using real-time three-dimensional echocardiography. *Eur Heart J*. 2008;29(20):2526–2535.
123. De Simone R, Glombitza G, Vahl CF, et al. Three-dimensional color Doppler flow reconstruction and its clinical applications. *Echocardiography*. 2000;17(8):765–771.
124. Gutiérrez-Chico JL, Zamorano JL, Prieto-Moriche E, et al. Real-time three-dimensional echocardiography in aortic stenosis: a novel, simple, and reliable method to improve accuracy in area calculation. *Eur Heart J*. 2008;29(10):1296–1306.
125. Veronesi F, Corsi C, Mor-Avi V, et al. Quantification of aortic valve stenosis using transesophageal real-time 3D echocardiographic images. *Comput Cardiol*. 2009;36:37–40.
126. Choi JY, Sullivan ID. Fixed subaortic stenosis: anatomical spectrum and nature of progression. *Br Heart J*. 1991;65(5):280–286.
127. Maginot KR, Williams RG. Fixed subaortic stenosis. *Prog Pediatr Cardiol*. 1994;3(3):141–149.
128. Oliver JM, González A, Gallego P, et al. Discrete subaortic stenosis in adults: increased prevalence and slow rate of progression of the obstruction and aortic regurgitation. *J Am Coll Cardiol*. 2001;38(3):835–842.
129. Leichter DA, Sullivan I, Gersony WM. "Acquired" discrete subvalvular aortic stenosis: natural history and hemodynamics. *J Am Coll Cardiol*. 1989;14(6):1539–1544.
130. Feigl A, Feidl D, Lucas RV Jr, Edwards JE. Involvement of the aortic valve cusps in discrete subaortic stenosis. *Pediatr Cardiol*. 1984;5(3):185–190.
131. Wright GB, Keane JF, Nadas AS, et al. Fixed subaortic stenosis in the young: medical and surgical course in 83 patients. *Am J Cardiol*. 1983;52(7):830–835.
132. Cape EG, Vanauker MD, Sigfússon G, et al. Potential role of mechanical stress in the etiology of pediatric heart disease: septal shear stress in subaortic stenosis. *J Am Coll Cardiol*. 1997;30(1):247–254.
133. Maréchaux S, Juthier F, Banfi C, et al. Illustration of the echocardiographic diagnosis of subaortic membrane stenosis in adults: surgical and live three-dimensional transoesophageal findings. *Eur J Echocardiogr*. 2011;12:E2.
134. Tanaka H, Kawai H, Tatsumi K, et al. Accessory mitral valve associated with aortic and mitral regurgitation and left ventricular outflow tract obstruction in an elderly patient: a case report. *J Cardiol*. 2007;50(1):65–70.
135. Ge S, Warner JG Jr, Fowle KM, et al. Morphology and dynamic change of discrete subaortic stenosis can be imaged and quantified with three-dimensional transesophageal echocardiography. *J Am Soc Echocardiogr*. 1997;10(7):713–716.
136. Kelpis TG, Ninios VN, Dardas PS, Pitsis AA. Subaortic stenosis in an adult caused by two discrete membranes: a three-dimensional transesophageal echocardiographic visualization. *Ann Thorac Surg*. 2009;88(5):1703.
137. Agrawal GG, Nanda NC, Htay T, et al. Live three-dimensional transthoracic echocardiographic identification of discrete subaortic membranous stenosis. *Echocardiography*. 2003;20(7):617–619.
138. Misra A, McCulloch M, Gangopadhyay S, et al. Images in cardiology: remarkable correlation of subaortic membrane visualization by three-dimensional echocardiography and at surgery. *Clin Cardiol*. 2005;28(7):356.
139. Vogel M, Ho SY, Anderson RH, Redington AN. Transthoracic 3-dimensional echocardiography in the assessment of subaortic stenosis due to a restrictive ventricular septal defect in double inlet left ventricle with discordant ventriculoarterial connections. *Cardiol Young*. 1999;9:549–555.
140. Bharucha T, Ho SY, Vettukattil JJ. Multiplanar review analysis of three-dimensional echocardiographic datasets gives new insights into the morphology of subaortic stenosis. *Eur J Echocardiogr*. 2008;9(5):614–620.
141. Miyamoto K, Nakatani S, Kanzaki H, et al. Detection of discrete subaortic stenosis by 3-dimensional transesophageal echocardiography. *Echocardiography*. 2005;22(9):783–784.
142. Bandarupalli N, Faulkner M, Nanda NC, Pothineni KR. Erroneous diagnosis of significant obstruction by Doppler in a patient with discrete subaortic membrane: correct diagnosis by 3D-transthoracic echocardiography. *Echocardiography*. 2008;25(9):1004–1006.
143. Kleinert S, Geva T. Echocardiographic morphometry and geometry of the left ventricular outflow tract in fixed subaortic stenosis. *J Am Coll Cardiol*. 1993;22(5):1501–1508.

144. O'Connor WN, Davis JB Jr, Geissler R, et al. Supravalvular aortic stenosis. Clinical and pathologic observations in six patients. *Arch Pathol Lab Med.* 1985;109(2):179–185.
145. Flaker G, Teske D, Kilman J, et al. Supravalvular aortic stenosis. A 20-year clinical perspective and experience with patch aortoplasty. *Am J Cardiol.* 1983;51(2):256–260.
146. Sharma BK, Fujiwara H, Hallman GL, et al. Supravalvular aortic stenosis: a 29-year review of surgical experience. *Ann Thorac Surg.* 1991;51(6):1031–1039.
147. Stamm C, Kreutzer C, Zurakowski D, et al. Forty-one years of surgical experience with congenital supravalvular aortic stenosis. *J Thorac Cardiovasc Surg.* 1999;118(5):874–885.
148. Rein AJ, Preminger TJ, Perry SB, et al. Generalized arteriopathy in Williams syndrome: an intravascular ultrasound study. *J Am Coll Cardiol.* 1993;21(7):1727–1730.
149. Zalzstein E, Moes CA, Musewe NN, Freedom RM. Spectrum of cardiovascular anomalies in Williams-Beuren syndrome. *Pediatr Cardiol.* 1991;12(4):219–223.
150. Ewart AK, Jin W, Atkinson D, et al. Supravalvular aortic stenosis associated with a deletion disrupting the elastin gene. *J Clin Invest.* 1994;93(3):1071–1077.
151. Thistlethwaite PA, Madani MM, Kriett JM, et al. Surgical management of congenital obstruction of the left main coronary artery with supravalvular aortic stenosis. *J Thorac Cardiovasc Surg.* 2000;120(6):1040–1046.
152. Subahi SA, Nouh MS, Allam AR, Akhtar MJ. Diagnosis of supravalvular aortic stenosis by transesophageal echocardiography. *Echocardiography.* 1997;14(4):399–402.
153. Roldán FJ, Vargas-Barrón J, Romero-Cárdenas A, et al. Three-dimensional reconstruction of heart defects associated with Williams-Beurer syndrome. *Echocardiography.* 2002;19(4):337–340.
154. Faletra FF, De Castro S, Pandian NG, et al. *Atlas of Real Time 3D Transesophageal Echocardiography.* New York, NY: Springer; 2010.
155. Wessels MW, Berger RM, Frohn-Mulder IME, et al. Autosomal dominant inheritance of left ventricular outflow tract obstruction. *Am J Med Genet A.* 2005;134A(2):171–179.
156. Levine JC, Sanders SP, Colan SD, et al. The risk of having additional obstructive lesions in neonatal coarctation of the aorta. *Cardiol Young.* 2001;11(1):44–53.
157. Marx GR. "Repaired" aortic coarctation in adults: not a "simple" congenital heart defect. *J Am Coll Cardiol.* 2000;35(4):1003–1006.
158. Vukovic I, Lackovic V, Todorivic V, et al. Cytohistologic and immunohistochemical characteristics of the aortic intima and media in coarctation of the aorta of the adult type [in Serbian]. *Srp Arh Celok Lek.* 2004;132(suppl 1): 66–71.
159. Nihoyannopoulos P, Karas S, Sapsford RN, et al. Accuracy of two-dimensional echocardiography in the diagnosis of aortic arch obstruction. *J Am Coll Cardiol.* 1987;10(5):1072–1077.
160. Cyran SE. Coarctation of the aorta in the adolescent and adult: echocardiographic evaluation prior to and following surgical repair. *Echocardiography.* 1993;10(5):553–563.
161. Simpson IA, Sahn DJ, Valdes-Cruz LM, et al. Color Doppler flow mapping in patients with coarctation of the aorta: new observations and improved evaluation with color flow diameter and proximal acceleration as predictors of severity. *Circulation.* 1988;77(4):736–744.
162. Carvalho JS, Redington AN, Shinebourne EA, et al. Continuous wave Doppler echocardiography and coarctation of the aorta: gradients and flow patterns in the assessment of severity. *Br Heart J.* 1990;64(2):133–137.
163. Marx GR, Allen HD. Accuracy and pitfalls of Doppler evaluation of the pressure gradient in aortic coarctation. *J Am Coll Cardiol.* 1986;7(6):1379–1385.
164. Sugeng L, Cao QL, Delabays A, et al. Three-dimensional echocardiographic evaluation of aortic disorders with rotational multiplanar imaging: experimental and clinical studies. *J Am Soc Echocardiogr.* 1997;10(2):120–132.
165. Jiang L, Lee MY, Southern JD, et al. Quantitative three-dimensional reconstruction of aortic coarctation by intravascular ultrasonography. *J Am Soc Echocardiogr.* 2001;14(1):73–76.
166. Scohy TV, du Plessis F, McGhie J, et al. Rapid method for intraoperative assessment of aortic coarctation using three-dimensional echocardiography. *Eur J Echocardiogr.* 2009;10(8):922–925.

CHAPTER

10

THREE-DIMENSIONAL ECHOCARDIOGRAPHY OF COMPLEX OUTFLOW TRACT ANOMALIES

David A. Roberson, MD; Vivian Wei Cui, MD

ABSTRACT

Complex outflow tract anomalies are due to abnormal formation of one or several of the cardiac segment components and features including the ventricular septum, subarterial conus, ventriculoarterial connections, semilunar valves, and great vessel spatial relationships. They compromise a very broad collection of diagnoses, including anomalies such as tetralogy of Fallot, complete transposition of the great arteries, double-outlet right ventricle, interrupted aortic arch complex, and others. The value of three-dimensional echocardiography for imaging these anomalies is its ability to demonstrate the complex spatial relationships of all of the involved structures and to provide unique views of surfaces, in particular the ventricular septum and semilunar valves, which are not possible by two-dimensional echocardiography. In this chapter, we describe useful methods and views to demonstrate these features.

INTRODUCTION

Complex outflow tract anomalies, also known as conotruncal malformations, compromise a collection of defects that include abnormalities of some or all the following cardiac components: ventricular septum, subarterial conus, semilunar valves, ventriculoarterial connections, and great vessel relationships.[1,2] In this chapter, we illustrate a collection of representative three-dimensional (3D) echocardiograms of complex outflow tract anomalies acquired using the transthoracic and transesophageal modalities including live 3D, 3D zoom, and full-volume 3D.

We approach this topic in a segmental fashion[3–5] from most proximal to more distal structures, connections, and relationships. The important features that require analysis for each of the respective cardiac segments are discussed in detail in each specific section. Likewise, the best views and 3D modes for anatomic analysis from both transthoracic and transesophageal approaches are discussed in each section.

ANALYSIS OF THE VENTRICULAR SEPTUM

General considerations

Complex outflow tract defects often include a ventricular septal defect (VSD).[6–9] Although any type of VSD is possible, and all types of VSDs are encountered among the broad collection of complex outflow tract anomalies, the most common types associated with outflow tract anomalies are malalignment-type VSDs (see Figs. 10-1–10-8) and outlet VSDs (see Fig. 10-12). The echocardiographer must determine whether or not a VSD is present and, if so, determine the type, size, shape, and location of the defect.

Malalignment-type VSDs are due to deviation of the conal septum in either an anterior or a posterior direction relative to the muscular trabecular septum. Anterior deviation of the conal septum in the presence of normally related great vessels results in tetralogy of Fallot or double-outlet right ventricle (RV) with subaortic VSD. When the great arteries are transposed, anterior conal septal deviation results in double-outlet RV with subpulmonary VSD, also known as the Taussig–Bing anomaly. A malaligned VSD with posterior conal septal deviation and normally related great vessels results in subaortic stenosis and interrupted aortic arch complex or coarctation of the aorta. Posterior conal deviation is also present in complete transposition (discordant ventriculoarterial connection) with posterior malalignment VSD and left ventricular outflow tract obstruction.

The size of the VSD is important to define because it has a major impact on clinical decision making. For example, a restrictive VSD with a small left to right shunt may not need treatment unless other cardiac defects are present that require surgery. Larger defects or cases having surgery to repair associated anomalies will most often have VSD patch closure performed. In some cases of complex outflow tract anomalies such as double-outlet RV and interrupted aortic arch complex, the VSD may be the only functional egress from the left ventricle. If the VSD is restrictive, it will require enlargement in order to baffle the left ventricle output in an unobstructed fashion to the functional systemic semilunar valve through the VSD.

En face 3D views of the ventricular septum from either the right or the left ventricle side are ideal for demonstrating VSD size and shape. The shape of a VSD is usually oval or crescentic. Therefore, the size of the VSD is often underestimated by two-dimensional (2D) echocardiography if one relies only on the apical

Figure 10-1

Transthoracic subcostal full-volume mode acquisition with cropping from left to right demonstrates a sagittal view of tetralogy of Fallot with anterior deviation of the conus and a large malaligned VSD (*) with aortic override. AoV, aortic valve; C, conus; MV, mitral valve; PV, pulmonary valve; TV, tricuspid valve; VS, ventricular septum. Note the 3D orientation icon in the figure.

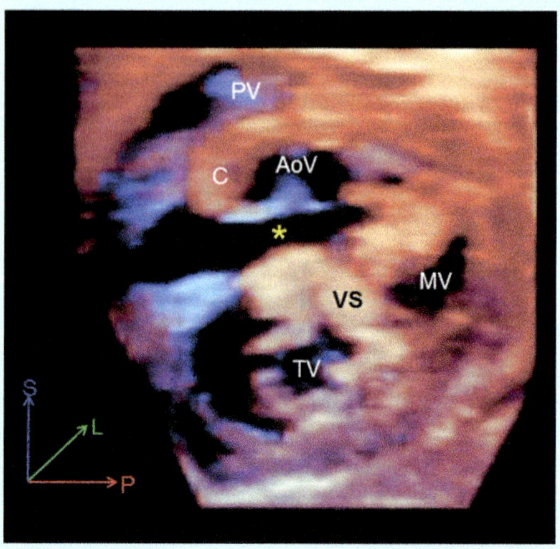

Figure 10-2

Transthoracic subcostal full-volume mode acquisition with cropping from left to right demonstrates a sagittal view of pulmonary atresia and VSD (*) with anterior deviation of the conus and a large malaligned VSD with aortic override. Ao, aorta; C, conus; MV, mitral valve; RVOT, right ventricular outflow tract; TV, tricuspid valve; VS, ventricular septum.

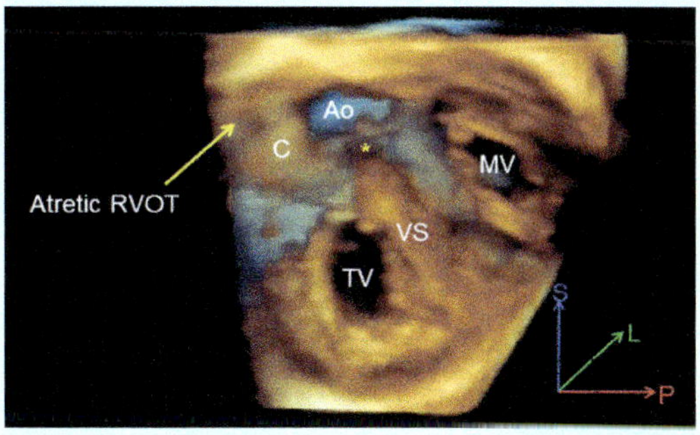

Figure 10-3

Subcostal live 3D mode view of double-outlet right ventricle with subaortic ventricular septal defect. The superior conus (C) portion of the septum is malaligned anteriorly with respect to the muscular trabecular septum (VS). The aorta overrides the VSD (*) and septum. The mitral and aortic valves are continuous (arrow), i.e., no conus is present between them. Ao, aorta; DORV, double-outlet right ventricle; LA, left atrium; LV, left ventricle; PA, pulmonary artery; VS, ventricular septum.

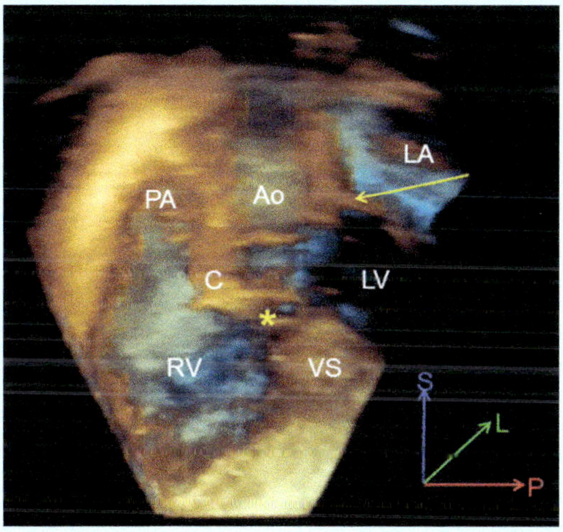

four-chamber view or the coronal view. In most cases, as evidenced by 3D ventricular septal en face views, the superior/basal to inferior/apical dimension as seen by apical 2D echo is often the smallest axis, whereas the anterior to posterior dimension, which is best seen in 3D en face views, is most commonly the longer axis of the defect. An additional interesting finding by 3D echo is the significant change in size of some VSDs over the cardiac cycle. In some cases, the area of the VSD orifice changes by more than 50% from diastole to

Figure 10-4

Midesophageal long-axis live 3D view of double-outlet RV (DORV) with mitral atresia. The conus separates the aortic valve from the right ventricular outflow tract. AoV, aortic valve; C, conus; LA, left atrium; RVOT, right ventricular outflow tract.

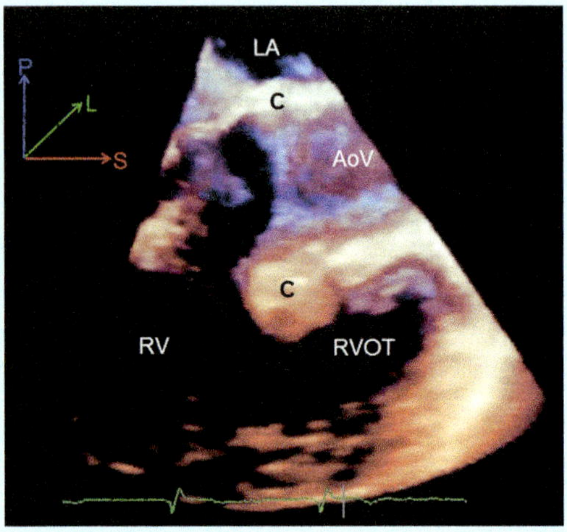

Figure 10-5

Midesophageal cropped 3D full-volume short- and long-axis views from a case of double-outlet RV (DORV) with anterior malposition of the aorta and pulmonary valve stenosis. Ao, aorta; AoV, aortic valve; C, conus; PA, pulmonary artery; PV, pulmonary valve.

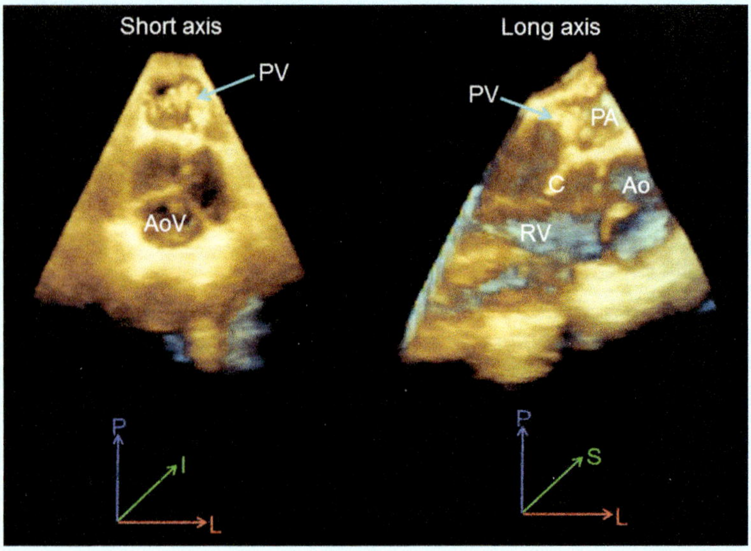

systole. Therefore, defects that are of borderline size at end diastole may become significantly narrow as systole proceeds. This may prove to be an important consideration in deciding whether VSD enlargement is required to achieve successful surgical repair.

The location of a VSD correlates with the particular diagnostic type of VSD, but it is also important to determine its anatomic spatial relationship to the semilunar valves. The relationship of a VSD to the systemic

Figure 10-6

Subcostal live 3D view of open common atrioventricular valve (AVV) and subpulmonic stenosis in a case of right dominant atrioventricular septal defect (AVSD) and double-outlet RV (DORV). AoV, aortic valve.

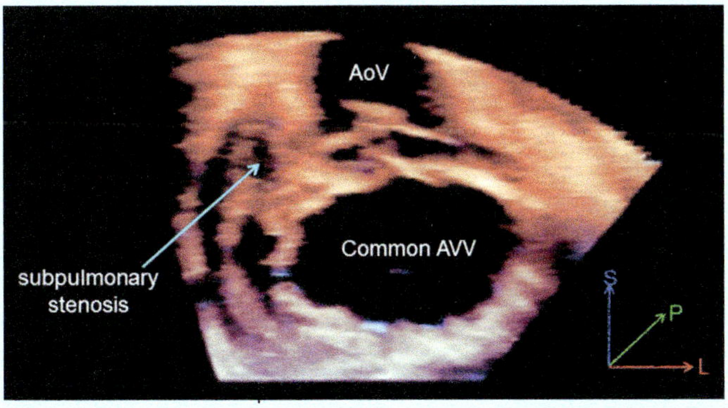

Figure 10-7

Subcostal 3D full-volume acquisition with frontal plane cropping (left image) demonstrates double-orifice RV (DORV) with subaortic VSD (*), subaortic stenosis, and hypoplastic aortic valve. The narrow subaortic outflow tract (1) is separated from the larger subpulmonary outflow tract (2) by the conus (C). Transverse view at the base shows the hypoplastic aorta and the large pulmonary valve. Ao, aorta; C, conus; PA, pulmonary artery; PV, pulmonary valve; RA, right atrium.

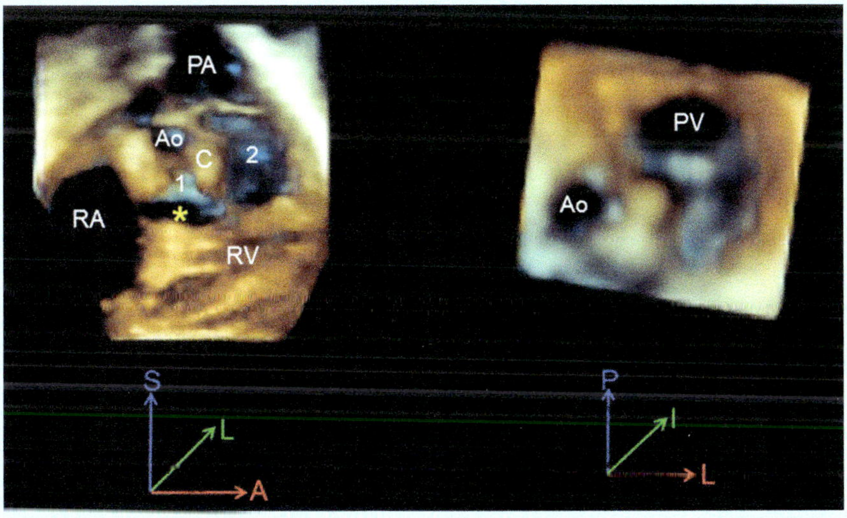

semilunar valve is particularly important because the goal of surgical correction is to connect the morphologic left ventricle to the systemic semilunar valve in an unobstructed fashion. Also, the approach to surgical closure of a VSD is sometimes best from a trans-semilunar valve approach in outlet-type defects, for example, a transpulmonary valve repair of a doubly committed subarterial (supracristal) VSD is usually the preferred approach. Therefore, VSD position must be clearly defined for complete anatomic analysis and appropriate surgical planning.

Figure 10-8

Transthoracic 3D views of interrupted aortic arch type B with malaligned VSD and subaortic stenosis. On the left is a 3D full-volume subcostal view cropped from anterior to posterior, which demonstrates malalignment of the muscular ventricular septum and outlet conal septum (C) with a VSD (*). The arrow points to the narrow subaortic area. There is also persistent subaortic conus (C). On the left is a suprasternal notch live 3D view of the type B interruption of the aorta. The right innominate artery (1) and the left carotid artery (2) arise from the aorta. The left subclavian artery arises from the descending aorta near the patent ductus arteriosus. Ao, aorta; IV, innominate vein; LA, left atrium; LSCA, left subclavian artery; MPA, main pulmonary artery; MV, mitral valve; PDA, patent ductus arteriosus; TV, tricuspid valve; VS, ventricular septum.

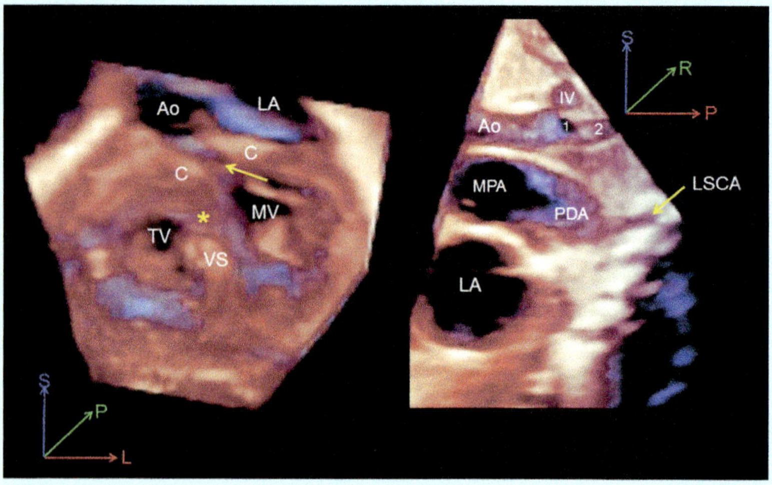

3D echocardiographic analysis of VSDs

In this and other sections, the reader should be cognizant of the fact that the comments regarding the performance of the 3D echocardiographic examination apply only in general terms. Each particular case may have its own unique characteristics that require modification of some of these recommended echocardiographic views.

Transthoracic 3D echo. The most useful views for the 3D echo examination of VSDs are acquired from apical and subcostal coronal four-chamber images using the 3D full-volume mode with postacquisition cropping to obtain en face views from both right- and left-sided perspectives. Apical long-axis views using live 3D mode with the image sector parallel to the ventricular septum can also be used to obtain en face views by using the trackball to electronically rotate the image 90° clockwise for the right side en face view versus 90° counterclockwise for the left side en face view.

Transesophageal 3D echo. As one might predict, transesophageal views that are analogous to transthoracic views are used to demonstrate the 3D features of VSDs. Views employed include midesophagus four-chamber and transgastric four-chamber acquisitions using 3D full-volume mode with en face cropping from the right and left sides, respectively. Longitudinal views of the ventricular septum and outflow tracts using full-volume and live 3D modes are also useful. The 3D zoom mode, which provides precropped live 3D views, albeit at slower volume rates, is more useful with transesophageal echocardiography (TEE) because the patients tend to be larger and the heart rate slower than in the smaller children. The fairly large size of the currently available 3D TEE transducer makes it unsuitable for patients with body weight < 20 kg.

ANALYSIS OF THE CONUS AND SUBARTERIAL OUTFLOW TRACTS

General considerations

Conus is defined as the portion of myocardium located between an atrioventricular valve and a semilunar valve. In the normal heart at birth, conus is present in the RV, resulting in a discontinuity between the tricuspid and pulmonary valves. In contrast, the normal left ventricle at birth lacks conus, thereby resulting in mitral to aortic valve continuity. Abnormalities of the conus are common in complex outflow tract anomalies, and in some types they are the primary etiologic anatomic defect, for example, anterior conal septal deviation in tetralogy of Fallot.

Malalignment of the conus in an anterior direction toward the RV is associated with anomalies such as tetralogy of Fallot[10–13] (see Fig. 10-1), pulmonary atresia with VSD (see Fig. 10-2), and double-outlet RV[14–19] (see Figs. 10-3–10-7). Posterior malalignment of the conus often results in subaortic stenosis, which is usually associated with more distal left obstructive abnormalities (see Fig. 10-8) including aortic valve stenosis, aortic coarctation, and interrupted aortic arch.[20–22]

Abnormal persistence of conus between the mitral valve and the aortic valve occurs in anomalies such as tunnel-type subaortic stenosis and double-outlet RV. Bilateral deficiency of the conus is present in some of the very rare cases with double-outlet left ventricle. Hypertrophy of the conus, hypertrophy of other portions of the myocardium, anomalous muscle bundles, presence of accessory fibrous tissue, and abnormal atrioventricular valve malattachments may also cause obstruction at the outflow tract level. Combinations of one or several of these features may be present and, if so, they are often associated with obstruction at more distal sites. Specific surgical procedures have been developed to deal with multilevel outflow obstruction. Figures 10-8 and 10-9 demonstrate multilevel left-sided obstructions. Two of the more common types of surgical repair for multilevel outflow obstruction, namely, the Damus–Kaye–Stansel procedure (see Fig. 10-10) and the Konno procedure (see Fig. 10-11), are also illustrated.

Figure 10-9

Transesophageal 3D full-volume view from the midesophagus, showing multilevel left-sided obstructions. The ventricular septum is very hypertrophied, resulting in midcavity narrowing. There is a discrete subaortic membrane. There is a small, thick, and doming aortic valve. LA, left atrium; LV, left ventricle; VS, ventricular septum.

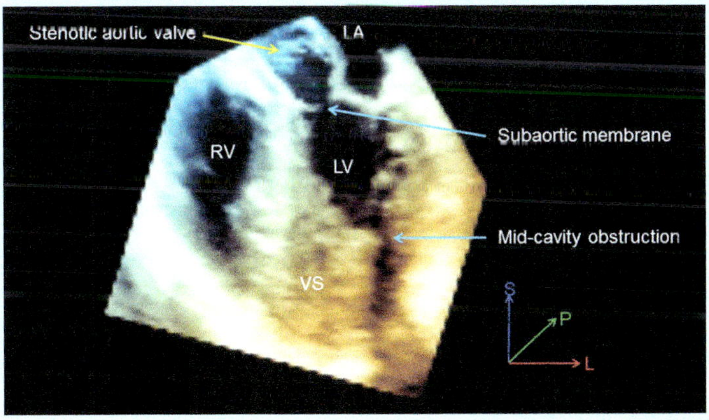

Figure 10-10

Transthoracic subcostal 3D full-volume with left to right cropping of a Damus–Kaye–Stansel (DKS) surgical aortopulmonary artery connection performed in a case of univentricular heart with subaortic stenosis. Ao, aorta; PA, pulmonary artery.

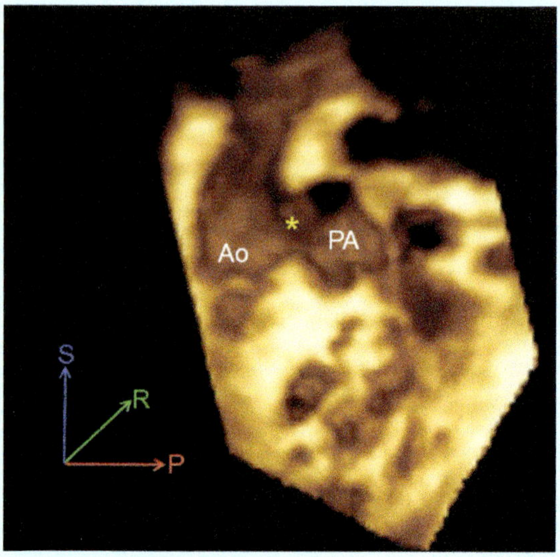

Figure 10-11

View of Konno procedure performed for subaortic stenosis and hypoplastic aortic valve. The VSD patch and prosthetic aortic valve are seen from the midesophagus long-axis view (left) and short-axis view (right) from the upper esophagus. AoV, aortic valve; LA, left atrium; LV, left ventricle; O, orifice; RVOT, right ventricular outflow tract; VS, ventricular septum.

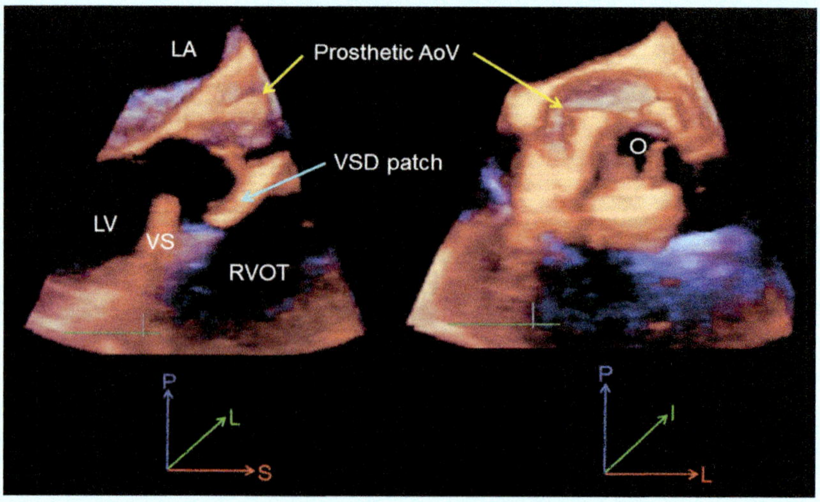

Figure 10-12

Transthoracic 3D full-volume subcostal (left) and apical (right) views with anterior to posterior cropping in a case with truncus arteriosus (T) type 1. On the left, the aortopulmonary connection (*) is seen. On the right, the outlet VSD (X) and truncal valve override is seen. Ao, aorta; LV, left ventricle; MPA, main pulmonary artery; RA, right atrium; VS, ventricular septum.

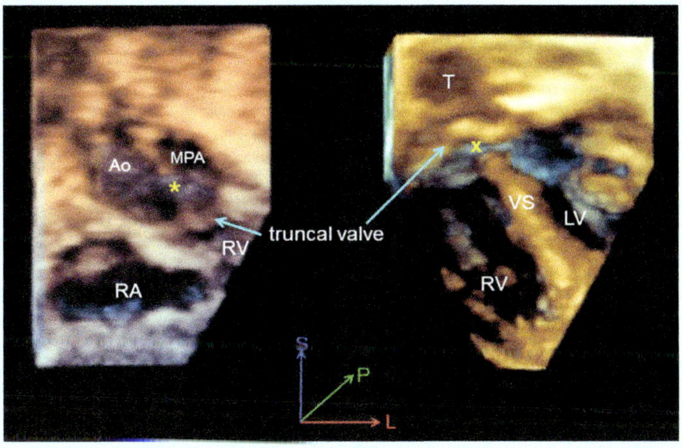

3D echocardiographic analysis of the conus

Transthoracic 3D echo. Analysis of the right ventricular outflow tract is in general best performed from the parasternal short-axis and subcostal sagittal views. Analysis of the left ventricular outflow tract is usually best performed from the parasternal long-axis view and subcostal coronal views. 3D full-volume acquisitions provide a large sample volume and are therefore quite useful to demonstrate the primary anomaly and surrounding structures of interest. As previously noted, however, stitch artifact can be a serious limitation of full-volume 3D in some cases. Live 3D is often best in small infants, especially from the subcostal transducer position, which allows the structures of interest to be situated in the far field where the 3D image sector is the widest and thickest. Full-volume 3D remains limited in some neonates and smaller children due to the stitch artifact caused by their relatively fast heart rates and lack of breath-holding ability.

Transesophageal 3D echo. The view of the right ventricular outflow tract obtained from the midesophagus with the transducer array at 45°–60° rotation often provides a high-quality view of right ventricular outlet structures. The left ventricular outflow tract is best seen at the same level with a transducer array orientation of 90°–110°. Transgastric views equivalent to the subcostal sagittal views of RV can be obtained from a transgastric right ventricular outflow tract view at 0°–20° transducer array rotation with the transducer not quite as deep as the left ventricular outflow tract view position. Insertion of the transesophageal transducer to a slightly greater depth reveals the left ventricular outflow tract transgastric view, which is analogous to the subcostal coronal surface echo views. At this position, rotation of the transducer array to approximately 60° will result in another sagittal view of the right ventricular outflow tract as well as the tricuspid valve inlet into the RV. In general, live 3D mode is used in those with a faster heart rate and 3D full-volume with postacquisition cropping is used for those with a slower hear rate.

ANALYSIS OF SEMILUNAR VALVES

General considerations

3D echo analysis of semilunar valves must include the determination of the number of semilunar valves present. If only a single semilunar valve is present it must be determined whether it is due to the presence of truncus arteriosus[23–27] versus atresia of one of the semilunar valves (see Figs. 10-2 and 10-9). Important features to analyze include the assessment of valve annulus size, the number of leaflets and commissures, leaflet mobility, and valve orifice size. The intrinsic anatomic features such as thickening, dehiscence, sites of insufficiency, coaptation failure, and perforations must be defined. Views of the stenotic pulmonary valve are presented in Figures 10-1 and 10-5. Views of the common types of bicuspid aortic valve and an example of the unicuspid aortic valve are presented in Figures 10-13 and 10-14, respectively.

3D echocardiographic analysis of semilunar valves

Transthoracic 3D echo. The parasternal short-axis and subcostal sagittal views are the best views to demonstrate the anatomy of the pulmonary valve. The parasternal short-axis, parasternal long-axis, and apical long-axis left ventricular outflow tract views are the best to demonstrate the aortic valve. Live 3D is usually the best mode because fast volume rates are needed and the leaflets do not have great depth. Therefore, the relatively narrow sector of live 3D mode is usually sufficient.

Transesophageal 3D echo. The pulmonary valve views from the esophagus are at the midesophagus with 60° transducer array rotation into the right ventricular outflow tract view and at the upper esophagus basal short-axis right ventricular outflow tract and pulmonary valve views with a transducer array orientation of 0°–20°. The pulmonary valve views from the transgastric position include the right ventricular outflow tract and pulmonary valve sagittal view from either the 0° array orientation more shallow position or the 60° array

Figure 10-13

Live 3D TEE images from the upper esophagus, showing unicuspid aortic valve in the open position during systole (left) and in the closed position during diastole (right). I, inferior; L, left; P, posterior.

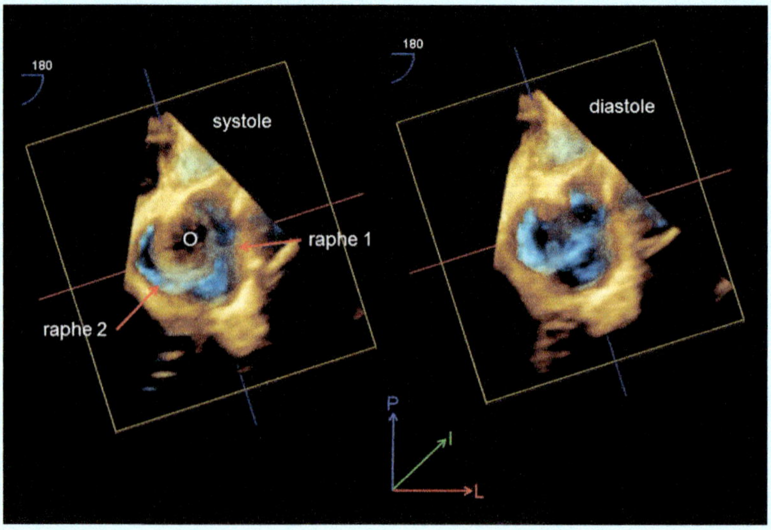

Figure 10-14

Live 3D TEE images from the upper esophagus showing normal aortic valve (top), bicuspid aortic valve with fused left to right commissure (left), and bicuspid aortic valve with fused right to noncoronary commissure (right). AoV, aortic valve; I, inferior; L-R, left to right; P, posterior; R-N, right to noncoronary.

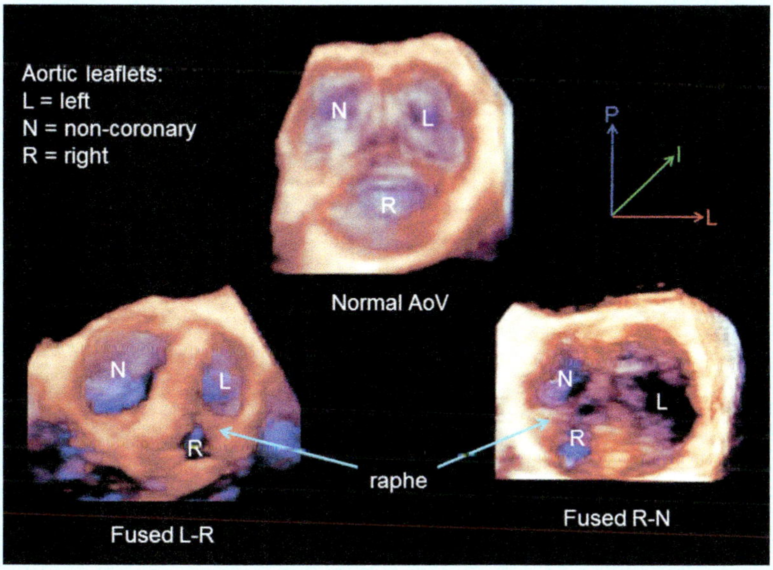

orientation slightly deeper position. The aortic valve is best seen from the upper esophagus basal short-axis view using live 3D with the array at 30°–60°. Excellent cross-sectional views of the aortic valve are obtained in this position (see Figs. 10-13 and 10-14). The long-axis view of the aortic valve is obtained at the midesophagus level with 90°–110° array rotation.

VENTRICULOARTERIAL CONNECTIONS AND SPATIAL RELATIONSHIPS OF GREAT VESSELS

General considerations

Over the years, several methods for describing ventriculoarterial connections and spatial relationships have been published[28–34] and applied quite effectively. In this chapter, we use a simple descriptive approach defining the connections as the ventricle to which the great artery (semilunar valve) connects. Connections are described as normal, overriding (see Figs. 10-1 and 10-2), double outlet (see Figs. 10-3–10-7), or discordant. Examples of discordant ventriculoarterial connections include both congenitally corrected transposition (see Fig. 10-15) and complete transposition (see Figs. 10-16–10-18). The relationships are described according to the anatomic position in 3D space of the aorta valve relative to the pulmonary valve in simple directional terminology: anterior versus posterior, superior versus inferior, and right versus left. The relative spatial positions of great vessels (see Fig. 10-19) and whether or not they cross one another in the normal arrangement or have a parallel relationship, as seen in transpositions of various types, should also be defined. See the bottom image of Figure 10-18 for an example of complete transposition with parallel great vessels.

Figure 10-15

Levo-transposition of the great arteries (L-TGA) four-chamber (left) and four-valve (right) views acquired in 3D full-volume mode at the midesophagus level. AoV, aortic valve; LA, left atrium; LAA, left atrial appendage; LV, left ventricle; MV, mitral valve; PV, pulmonary valve; RA, right atrium.

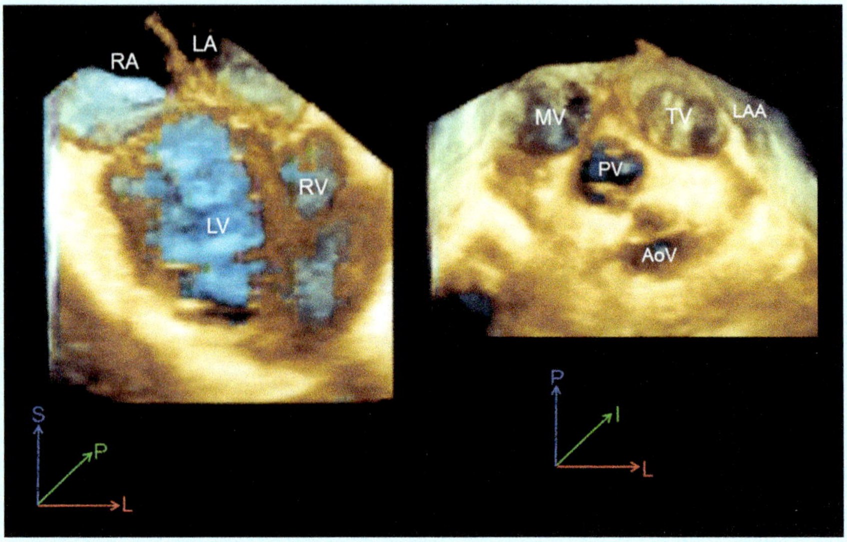

Figure 10-16

Views of complete transposition with VSD acquired from the subcostal position in 3D full-volume mode including a right side en face view (left), frontal view (center), and left side en face view (right). Ao, aorta; LA, left atrium; LV, left ventricle; PA, pulmonary artery; VS, ventricular septum.

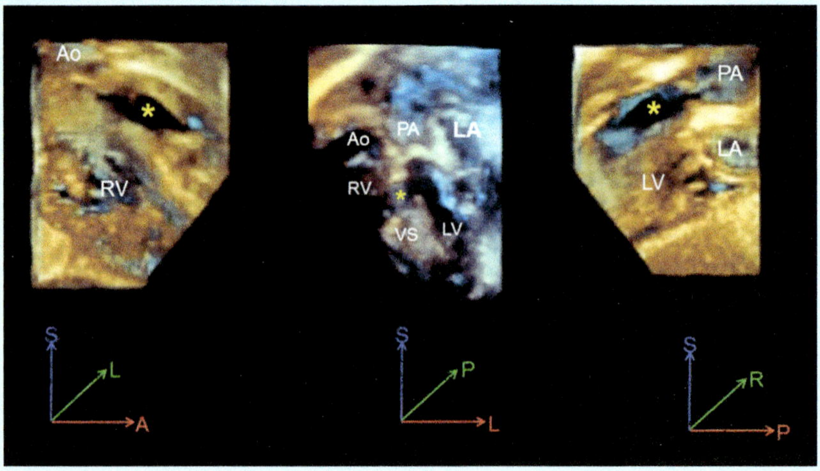

Figure 10-17

Transesophageal live 3D long-axis views of complete transposition after the Mustard procedure. The anatomies of the systemic venous baffle (SVB) and the pulmonary venous baffle (PVB) are demonstrated. TV, tricuspid valve.

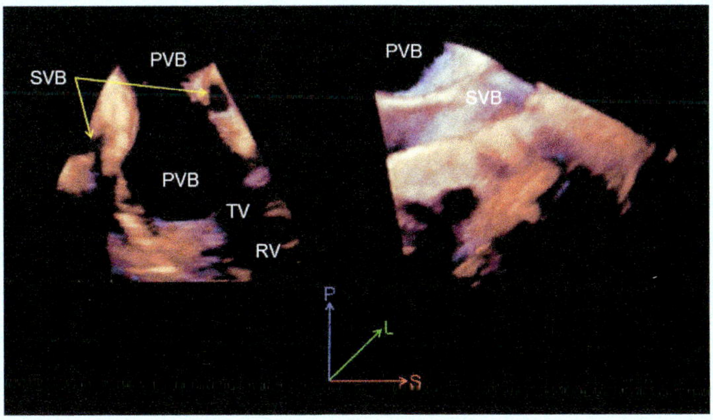

Figure 10-18

Transesophageal 3D full-volume echocardiograms of complete transposition after the Mustard procedure. The top two images were acquired at the midesophagus level and cropped from anterior to posterior. The bottom figure is a sagittal view acquired at the transgastric level and cropped from left to right. Ao, aorta; L, left; LV, left ventricle; P, posterior; PA, pulmonary artery; PVB, pulmonary vein baffle; R, right; S, superior; SVB, systemic vein baffle; TGA, transposition of the great arteries.

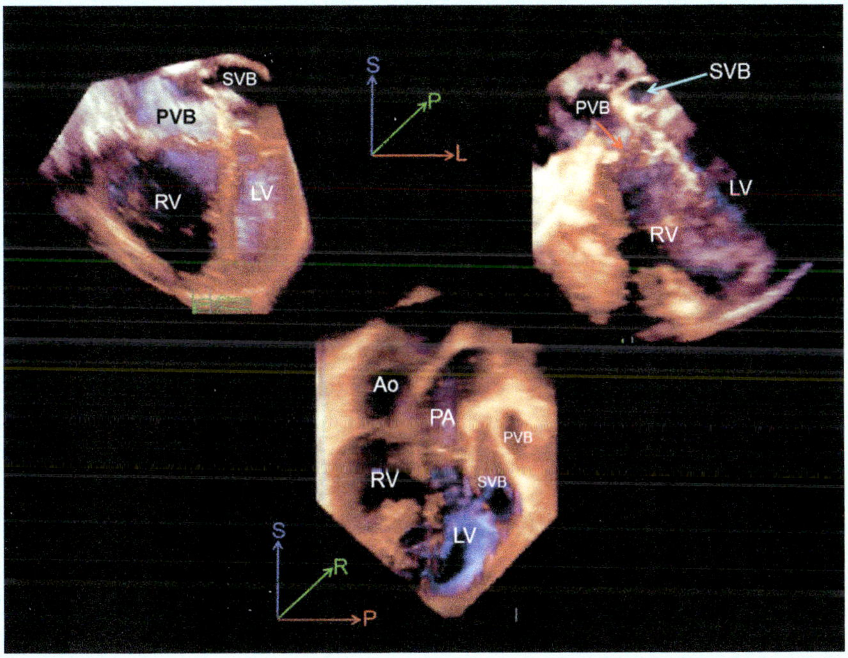

Figure 10-19

Views of the base of the heart in cases with transposed anterior aorta obtained using 3D TEE full-volume acquisition from the midesophagus. On the top, the aorta is directly anterior to the pulmonary valve (PV). On the bottom left, the aorta is rightward and anterior to the PV. On the bottom right, the aorta is leftward and anterior to the PV. Ao, aorta; AoV, aortic valve; AP, anterior to posterior; D-TGA, D-transposition of the great arteries; I, inferior; L, left; LAA, left atrial appendage; L-TGA, L-transposition of the great arteries; MV, mitral valve; P, posterior; PA, pulmonary artery; PVB, pulmonary vein baffle; SVB, systemic vein baffle; TV, tricuspid valve.

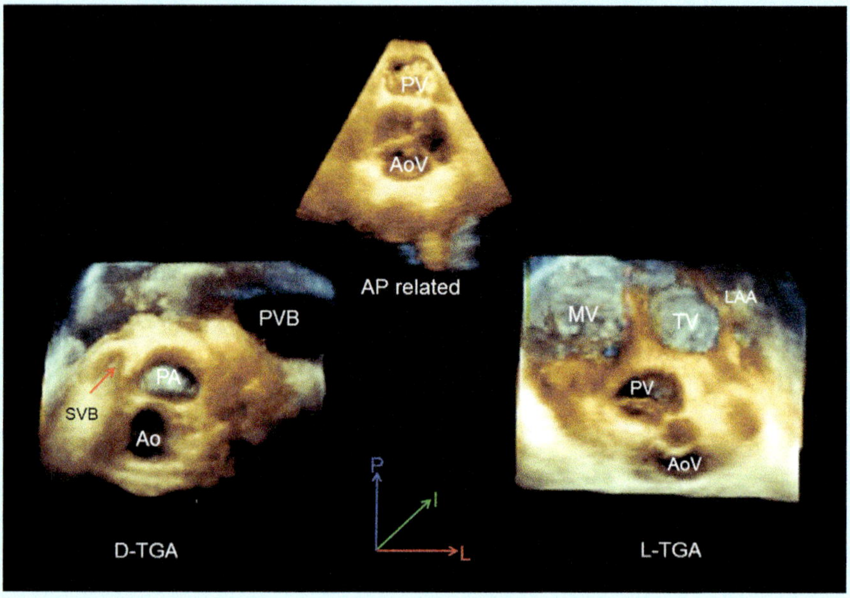

3D echocardiographic analysis of ventriculoarterial connections and relationships

Transthoracic 3D echo. Ventriculoarterial connections and spatial relationships of great vessels are often seen best from parasternal long- and short-axis, subcostal sagittal, and subcostal coronal views. 3D full-volume acquisitions with anterior to posterior cropping viewed from anterior and superior to inferior cropping viewed from superior are typically the most useful methods to assess connections and relationships. Alternatively, in those with faster heart rates or rapid respirations live 3D mode may be used.

Transesophageal 3D echo. A very useful view that is unique to 3D transesophageal echo is the four-valve full-volume 3D view. It is obtained by acquiring a full-volume four-chamber view at the midesophagus level with 0°–20° array orientation and cropping a small amount from anatomic superior to inferior (in the blue plane), and tilting the image forward 90°. All four valves, when they are present, and the spatial relationships of the semilunar valves are demonstrated in this view (see Figs. 10-15). Additional views that demonstrate the connections and relationships include the transgastric sagittal view; midesophagus 60°–110° transducer array rotation, which shows the respective right and left ventriculoarterial connections; and basal short-axis view at the superior esophagus.

CONCLUSION

Both transthoracic and transesophageal 3D echocardiographies provide unique and useful views of the component anatomic features of complex outflow tract anomalies. Great progress has clearly been made with transducer and software technology. However, a few limitations persist. To resolve them, faster volume rates, one-beat acquisition, and further development of rapid quantitative methods are required.

REFERENCES

1. Hagler DJ, Tajik AJ, Seward JB, et al. Wide-angle two-dimensional echocardiographic profiles of conotruncal abnormalities. *May Clin Proc.* 1980;55:73–82.
2. Sanders SP, Bierman FZ, William RG. Conotruncal malformations: diagnosis in infancy using subxiphoid 2-dimensional echocardiography. *Am J Cardiol.* 1982;50:1361–1367.
3. Anderson RH, Becker AE, Freedom PM, et al. Sequential segmental analysis of congenital heart disease. *Pediatr Cardiol.* 1984;5:281–287.
4. Freedom RM, Culham JAG, Moes CAF. The application of segmental nomenclature. In: Dew MTN, ed. *Angiography of Congenital Heart Disease.* New York: Macmillan Publishing Co.; 1984:17–45.
5. Anderson RH, Ho SY. Sequential Segmental analysis–description and categorization for the millennium. *Cardiol Young.* 1997;7:98–116.
6. Bierman FZ, Fellows K, Williams RG. Prospective identification of ventricular septal defects in infancy using subxiphoid two-dimensional echocardiography. *Circulation.* 1980;62:807–817.
7. Sutherland GR, Godman MJ, Smallhorn JF, et al. Ventricular septal defects. Two dimensional echocardiographic and morphologic correlations. *Br Heart J.* 1982;47:316–328.
8. Smallhorn J, Anderson RH, Macartney FJ. Morphological characteristics of ventricular septal defects associated with coarctation of the aorta by cross-sectional echocardiography. *Br. Heart J.* 1983;49:485–494.
9. Schmidt KG, Cassidy SC, Silverman NH, Stanger P. Doubly-committed subarterial ventricular septal defects: Echocardiographic features and surgical implications. *J Am Coll Cardiol.* 1988;12:1538–1546.
10. Van Praagh R, Van Praagh S, Nebesar RA, et al. Tetralogy of Fallot: underdevelopment of the pulmonary infundibulum and its sequelae. *Am J Cardiol.* 1970;26:25–33.
11. Anderson RH, Allwork SP, Ho SY, et al. Surgical anatomy of tetralogy of Fallot. *J Thorac Cardiovasc Surg.* 1981;81:887–896.
12. Silverman NH. Tetralogy of Fallot and related lesions. In: Pine JW, ed. *Pediatric Echocardiography.* Baltimore: Williams & Wilkins; 1993:195–214.
13. Bharati S, Lev M. Tetralogy of Fallot. In: Lincoln AB, ed. *The Pathology of Congenital Heart Disease.* Armonk NY: Futura Publishing Co; 1996:67–134.
14. Lev M, Bharati S, Meng CC, et al. A concept of double outlet right ventricle. *J Thorac Cardiovasc Surg.* 1972;64:271–281.
15. Lev M, Bharati S. Double outlet right ventricle. Association with other cardiovascular anomalies. *Arch Pathol.* 1973;95:117–122.
16. Sridaromont S, Ritter DG, Feldt RH, et al. Double-outlet right ventricle. Anatomic and angiocardiographic correlations. *Mayo Clin Proc.* 1978;53:555–577.
17. Hagler DJ, Tajik AJ, Seward JB, et al. Double-outlet right ventricle: Wide-angle two-dimensional echocardiographic observations. *Circulation.* 1981;63:419–428.
18. Macartney FJ, Rigby ML, Anderson RH, et al. Double outlet right ventricle. Cross sectional echocardiographic findings, their anatomical explanation, and surgical relevance. *Br Heart J.* 1984;52:164–177
19. Roberson DA, Silverman NH. Malaligned outlet septum with subpulmonary ventricular septal defect and abnormal ventriculoarterial connection: A morphologic spectrum defined echocardiographically. *J Am Coll.* 1990;16:459–468.
20. Smallhorn JF, Anderson RH, Macartney FJ. Cross-sectional echocardiographic recognition of interruption of aortic arch between left carotid and subclavian arteries. *Br Heart J.* 1982;48:229–235.
21. Smallhorn JF, Anderson RH, Macartney FJ. Morphological characterisation of ventricular septal defects associated with coarctation of aorta by cross-sectional echocardiography. *Br Heart J.* 1983;49:485–494.
22. Bharati S, Lev M. Absence of transverse arch (interrupted aortic arch) with ventricular septal defect. In: Lincoln AB, ed. *The Pathology of Congenital Heart Disease.* Armonk NY: Futura Publishing Co; 1996:1361–1370.

23. Collett RW, Edwards JE. Persistent truncus arteriosus: a classification according to anatomic types. *Surg Clin North Am.* 1949;29:1245–1270.
24. Van Praagh R, Van Praagh S. The anatomy of common aorticopulmonary trunk (truncus arteriosus communis) and its embryologic implications: a study of 57 necropsy cases. *Am J Cardiol.* 1965;16:406–425.
25. Bharati S, McAllister HA Jr, Rosenquist GC, et al. The surgical anatomy of truncus arteriosus communis. *J Thorac Cardiovasc Surg.* 1974;67:501–510.
26. Houston AB, Gregory NL, Murtagh E, Goleman EN. Two-dimensional echocardiography in infants with persistent truncus arteriosus. *Br Heart J.* 1981;46:492–497.
27. Smallhorn JF, Anderson RH, Macartney FJ. Two-dimensional echocardiographic assessment of communications between ascending aorta and pulmonary trunk or individual pulmonary arteries. *Br Heart J.* 1982;47:563–572.
28. Silverman NH, Payot M, Stanger P, Rudolph AM. The echocardiographic profile of patients after Mustard's operation. *Circulation.* 1978;58:1083–1093.
29. Bierman FZ, Williams RG. Prospective diagnosis of d-transposition of the great arteries in neonates by subxyphoid, two-dimensional echocardiography. *Circulation.* 1979;60:1496–1502.
30. Anderson RH, Tynan M. Complete transposition. The significance of describing separately connections, arterial relationships and infundibular morphology. *Int J Cardiol.* 1984;5:19–20.
31. Anderson RA, Henry GW, Becker AE. Morphologic aspects of complete transposition. *Cardiol Young.* 1991;1:41–53.
32. Silverman NH. Ventriculoarterial discordance (transposition of the great arteries). In: Pine JW, ed. *Pediatric Echocardiography.* Baltimore: Williams & Wilkins;1993:245–278.
33. Van Pragh R. What is congenitally corrected transposition? *N Engl J Med.* 1970;282:1097–1098.
34. Freedom RM, Dyck JD. Congenitally corrected transposition of the great arteries. In: Blow JB, ed. *Moss and Adams 5th edition Heart Disease in Infants, Children and Adolescents.* Baltimore Maryland: Williams & Wilkins; 1995:1222–1245.

CHAPTER

11

THREE-DIMENSIONAL ECHOCARDIOGRAPHY OF THE UNIVENTRICULAR HEART

David A. Roberson, MD; Vivian Wei Cui, MD

ABSTRACT

This chapter describes a three-dimensional echocardiographic (3DE) approach to the analysis of univentricular hearts. Transthoracic and transesophageal images from the available 3DE imaging modalities are presented. Illustrative cases include tricuspid atresia, double-inlet left ventricle, unbalanced atrioventricular septal defect, and others. 3DE examples of atrioventricular valve annular override, atrioventricular leaflet straddling, views of the Fontan, and some 3D quantitative methods are also included.

INTRODUCTION

Univentricular heart, also known as single ventricle, common ventricle, and univentricular atrioventricular connection, includes a broad and complex variety of diagnoses with the common feature of having the atrioventricular valve or valves connected exclusively or predominantly to one ventricle.[1–4] Through the years, concepts, definitions, and nomenclature of these anomalies have been debated.[5–8] Notwithstanding this debate, the treatment of univentricular hearts and similar lesions typically consists of a final stage palliation through a Fontan procedure. This chapter avoids engaging in these debates and focuses on the three-dimensional echocardiographic (3DE) analysis of these defects. We do not catalogue and illustrate the myriad of morphologic possibilities but rather provide illustrative 3DE cases to demonstrate the concepts, key anatomic features, and capabilities of 3DE in the imaging of univentricular hearts.

The value of 3DE in the imaging of these anomalies is its ability to demonstrate complex anatomy and spatial relationships of the atrioventricular junction, atrioventricular valves, and complex ventricular morphology. Imaging of valve leaflet surfaces, chordal attachments, and the relationships of these to the atrioventricular connections and septal defects is greatly enhanced. Also, 3D means of quantifying left ventricular volume, ejection fraction, and synchrony, as well as measuring right ventricular volume and ejection fraction, all of which are free geometric assumptions, are now available and in clinical use.

3DE is useful in analyzing the important features of anomalies within this category, including tricuspid atresia,[9–11] mitral atresia with double-outlet right ventricle, double-inlet left ventricle,[12–14] unbalanced atrioventricular septal defect,[15] (Figs. 11-1–11-8), atrioventricular valve straddle, atrioventricular valve annulus override,[16–18] and criss-cross atrioventricular connections[19,20] (Figs. 11-9–11-13). The final common palliative treatment for these patients is usually the Fontan procedure (Figs. 11-14–11-16).

The five currently available 3DE imaging modes include X plane, live 3D, 3D zoom, full-volume 3D, and 3D color modes, each of which has strengths and limitations. These modalities are discussed in detail in Chapter 6.

We use a systematic segmental approach from the proximal to the distal anatomic structures as a framework to demonstrate the capabilities of 3DE in analyzing these anomalies. Both transthoracic and transesophageal images are included. Readers should note that a careful and complete, organized segmental approach examination of these complex defects is required. This chapter focuses on the 3DE assessment of the atrioventricular junction and the important anatomy related to univentricular heart anatomy, physiology, and palliation.

ATRIAL SEPTUM

General considerations

Chapter 6 is devoted to atrial septal defect (ASD); therefore the discussion of ASD in this chapter is brief in order to avoid redundancy. A specific type of ASD is present in univentricular hearts. It is important to determine the type and size of the ASD because unobstructed interatrial blood flow is essential in order

Figure 11-1

Tricuspid atresia acquired from the transthoracic apical position using 3D X-plane mode demonstrating simultaneous biplane live 2D images. Upper left, left ventricular (LV) long-axis view; upper right, four-chamber view. The bottom row figures were acquired with transesophageal echocardiogaphy (TEE) using full-volume 3D acquisition and cropped in the frontal plane. Lower left, LV longitudinal view with the transducer array at 100°; lower right, four-chamber view with the transducer array at 0°. The site of tricuspid valve atresia is marked at the X. A pigtail catheter is present in the LV. Ao, aorta; LA, left atrium; RA, right atrium; RV, right ventricle.

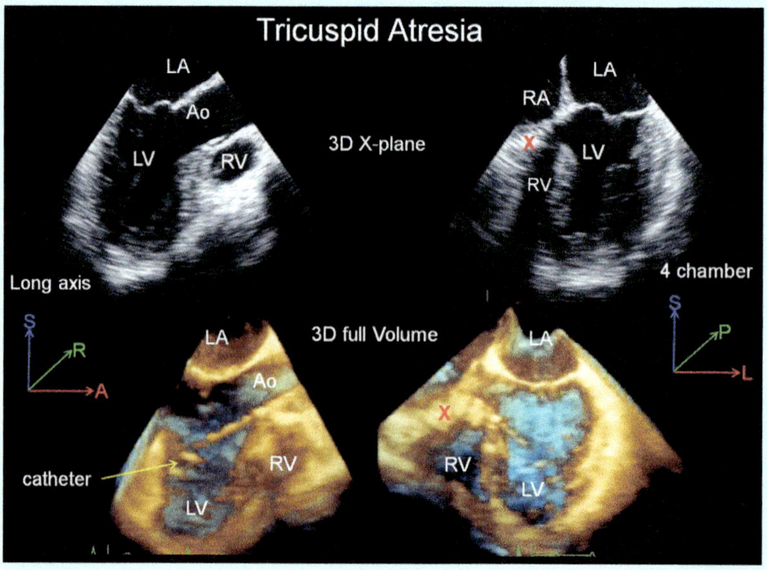

Figure 11-2

Tricuspid valve hypoplasia, dextrocardia, inlet ventricular septal defect (VSD), and cor triatriatum (cor t.) as seen from various 3D transesophageal echocardiography (TEE) modes. *A*, From a full-volume, four-chamber 3D view with frontal cropping. *B*, 3D zoom mode acquisition showing the cor triatriatum orifice. *C*, X-plane color Doppler flow map showing simultaneous biplane orthogonal views of turbulent flow through the obstructive orifice. cor t., cor triatriatum obstructive membrane; LAd, distal left atrial chamber; LAp, proximal left atrial chamber; LV, left ventricle; RA, right atrium; RV, right ventricle; TV, tricuspid valve.

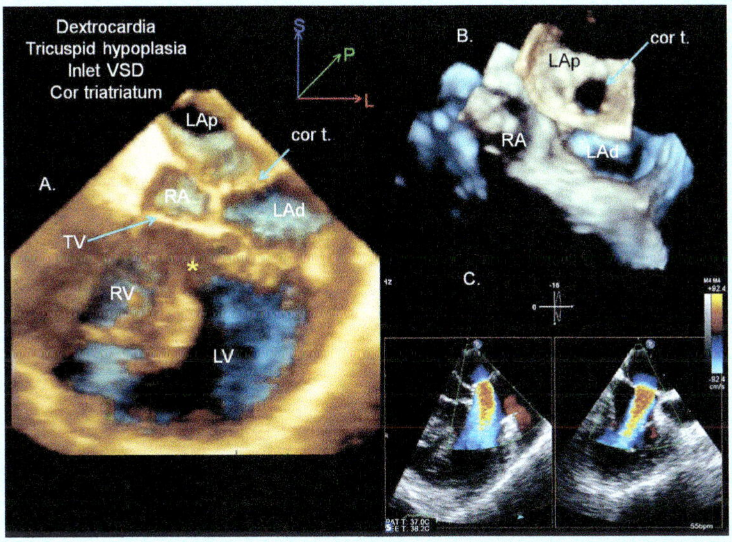

Figure 11-3

Double-inlet left ventricle image acquired with full-volume 3D transthoracic echocardiography. Left, Apical view with frontal cropping of the right (1) and left (2) atrioventricular valves connecting to the left ventricle. Right, Subcostal sagittal view with cropping from apex toward the base demonstrating the right (1) and left (2) atrioventricular valves, the pulmonary valve (PV), and the subaortic outlet chamber (OC). LA, left atrium; LV, left ventricle; RA, right atrium.

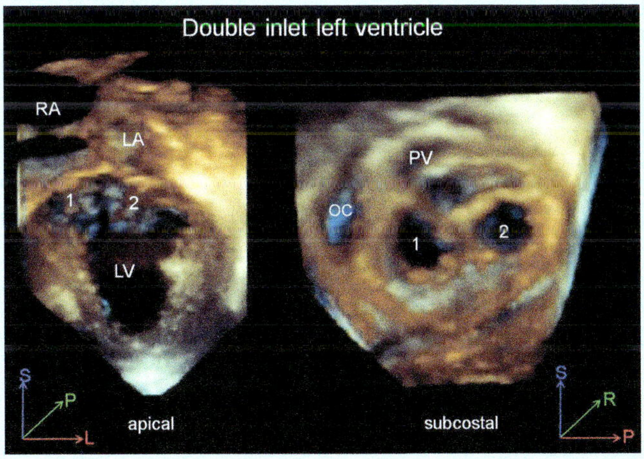

Figure 11-4

Double-inlet left ventricle (LV) transthoracic views acquired in full-volume 3D mode. Left, Apical view of the two atrioventricular (AV) valves opening into the left ventricle. Top right, Cross-section of the AV junction viewed from the atrium showing the open right (1) and left (2) AV valves. Bottom right, From the same cross-section frame now viewed from the LV apex. It shows both AV valves opening into the LV. LA, left atrium; RA, right atrium.

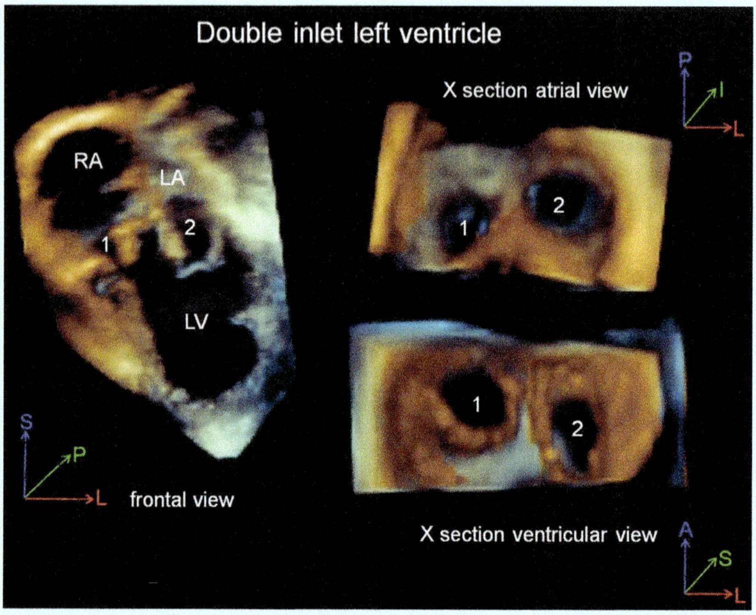

Figure 11-5

Double-inlet left ventricle (LV) after septation procedure as seen from a transesophageal four-chamber, full-volume 3D acquisition with frontal cropping. LA, left atrium; RA, right atrium; RV, right ventricle.

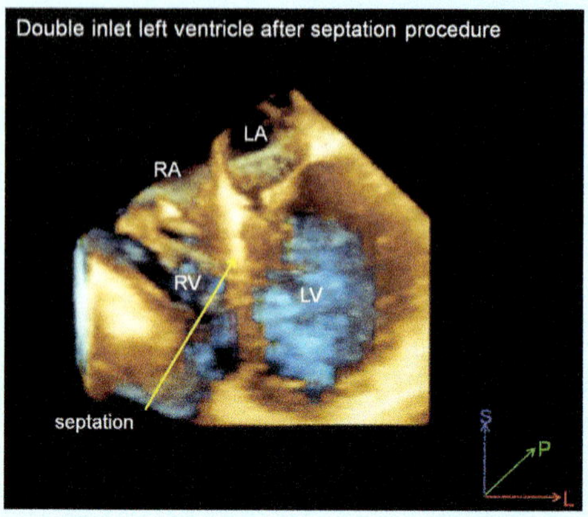

to prevent systemic venous obstruction in cases of tricuspid atresia or significant tricuspid stenosis, or alternatively to avoid pulmonary venous obstruction in mitral atresia or significant mitral stenosis. The secundum type of ASD may reduce in relative or absolute size over time. Therefore, baseline and ongoing assessment for unobstructed patency of the interatrial communication is required in some univentricular hearts. Primum ASD, a component of atrioventricular septal defect, is present in the unbalanced type of atrioventricular septal defect, this being one of the common types of univentricular heart. However, primum ASD seldom causes interatrial obstruction and does not spontaneously reduce in size.

A rarely encountered abnormality of malalignment between the atrial septum and ventricular septum can be detected using four-chamber views. In our experience, this malalignment is often the harbinger of abnormalities of the atrioventricular junction, in particular atrioventricular valve straddle and atrioventricular valve override, which result in significant hypoplasia of one of the ventricles.

Figure 11-6

Unbalanced atrioventricular septal defect. Left, Right dominant unbalanced atrioventricular (AV) septal defect, common atrium (CA), and right atrial isomerism. A thin band of tissue extends across the common atrium. The atrioventricular valve is committed entirely to the right ventricle. The left ventricle is essentially absent. This patient also had a double-outlet right ventricle (RV) (not demonstrated in this frame). This figure is from a 3D transesophageal full-volume acquisition with frontal plane cropping. Right, Left dominant atrioventricular septal defect with hypoplastic right ventricle. This is a live 3D mode transthoracic acquisition with the transducer in the subcostal position. The common atrioventricular valve is closed in this early systolic frame. An atrial septal defect (*) and ventricular septal defect (+) are present. LA, left atrium; LV, left ventricle; RA, right atrium; VS, ventricular septum.

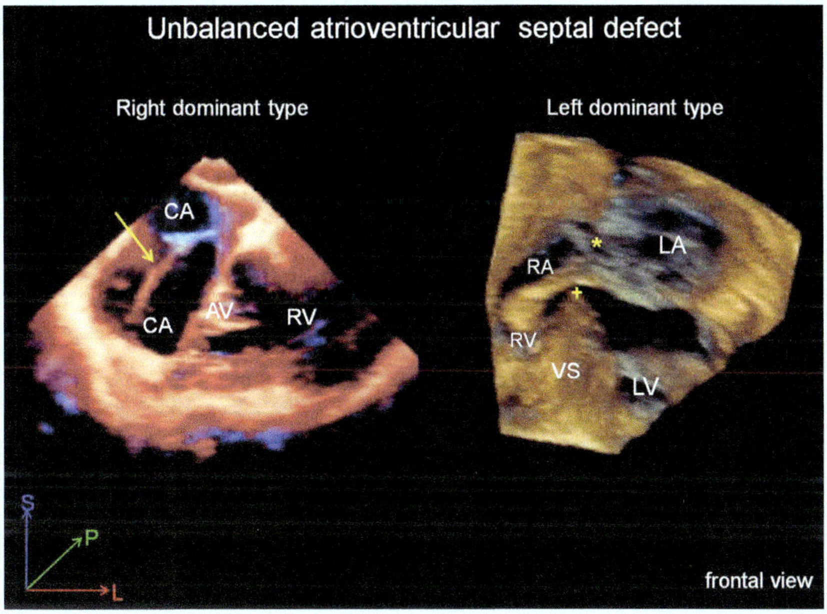

3DE analysis

Transthoracic full-volume 3D data sets should be obtained from the apical and subcostal four-chamber views and may be cropped laterally from both sides to yield en face views of the atrial septal anatomy. Cropping from anterior to posterior in the frontal plane is also useful to demonstrate the ASD type, location, and size. If the heart rate is not too fast, 3D zoom mode is similarly useful to obtain en face views of the ASD. Transthoracic live 3D mode, with its faster frame rate and no stitch artifact, is useful in smaller children with faster heart rates and limited breath-holding ability.

Transesophageal 3DE analysis of the atrial septum is best performed using the 3D zoom en face views, midesophagus four-chamber view acquired with full-volume 3D, and live 3D deep transgastric views. Detailed methods of these are described and illustrated in Chapter 6.

ATRIOVENTRICULAR JUNCTION

General considerations

Abnormalities of the atrioventricular junction resulting in absence or limited direct blood flow into, and limited development of, the ventricle from which blood flow has been diverted are the key feature of univentricular hearts. Detailed assessment of whether the atrioventricular valve is atretic, stenotic, or

Figure 11-7

An example of mitral atresia with a large atrial septal defect after atrial septostomy, small muscular ventricular septal defect (VSD), and hypoplastic left ventricle (LV). The acquisition is a full-volume 3D transesophageal echocardiogram from the four-chamber view at the midesophagus level. Double-outlet right ventricle (RV) was also present but is not visualized in this frame. LA, left atrium; MV, mitral valve; RA, right atrium; TV, tricuspid valve.

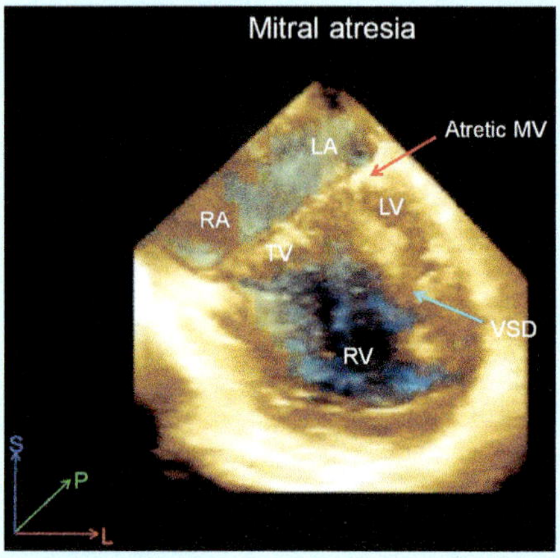

Figure 11-8

Parachute mitral valve deformity demonstrated by live 3D transesophageal echocardiogram acquired from the midesophagus with counterclockwise transducer rotation. This patient had double-inlet left ventricle (LV) with severe stenosis of the left-sided parachute mitral valve. LA, left atrium; PM, papillary muscle.

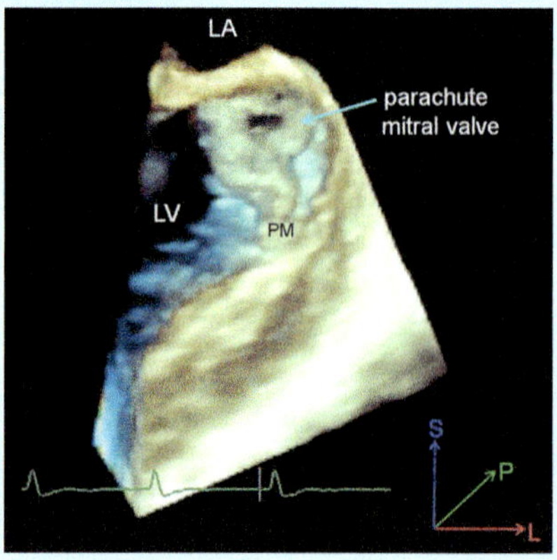

fully patent is required. The valves must be identified as tricuspid, mitral, or common-atrioventricular-valve type. It must also be determined whether there is normal atrioventricular valve alignment and attachment, as opposed to abnormal annular override, straddling, or both.

Atresia is defined as the congenital absence of the opening of a valve. This chapter is concerned with atresia of the tricuspid or mitral valve. Atrioventricular valve atresia (Figs. 11-1 and 11-7) may be of a muscular type in which there is complete or virtually complete absence of any apparent valve tissue. In its place is a muscular floor of the respective atrium in which a small dimple is found at the site where the valve failed to develop. Alternatively and less commonly, malformed fused leaflets and chordae that lack any perforation may be present.

Stenosis is defined as the presence of a congenital narrowing of an atrioventricular valve. It is caused by annular hypoplasia, shortened valve chordae, fused chordae, fused leaflets, hypoplastic leaflets, papillary muscle malposition, or absence of a papillary muscle. Any single feature or combination of these features may be present in a given case. In the case of the parachute mitral valve (Fig. 11-8) form of mitral valve stenosis, most or all of these abnormalities are present. Figure 11-2 shows a case of tricuspid valve annular hypoplasia causing stenosis in association with other complex defects.

Atrioventricular valve annulus override (Figs. 11-9–11-11) refers to the abnormal arrangement in which the atrioventricular junction is malaligned such that the atrioventricular valve annulus is shifted toward the contralateral side, thereby becoming positioned directly above a ventricular septal defect in such a manner as to partially override, and therefore empty into, both ventricles. Normally, the atrioventricular valve annulus is positioned directly and exclusively above its respective ventricle only: the tricuspid valve to the morphologic right ventricle and the mitral valve to the morphologic left ventricle.

Many valves with annular override also have the feature of straddling. Straddling of the tensor apparatus of an atrioventricular valve is the abnormal situation in which valve leaflets and chordae are malformed and abnormally attached such that they traverse a ventricular septal defect to insert within the contralateral ventricle to malpositioned papillary muscles. Straddling may be present with or without annular override (Figs. 11-10 and 11-12). It commonly results in hypoplasia of the ventricle opposite to the direction of straddling. For example, with straddling of the tricuspid valve attachments through an

Figure 11-9

Right dominant atrioventricular septal defect as seen from the cardiac base looking toward the apex. Note that the left side of the atrioventricular (AV) valve orifice is much smaller than the right side. The AV valve is closed in the systolic frame (left) and open in the diastolic frame (right). The secundum atrial septum is seen dividing the unbalanced atrioventricular orifice. LAVV, left atrioventricular valve; RAA, right atrial appendage; RAVV, right atrioventricular valve; S2, septum secundum.

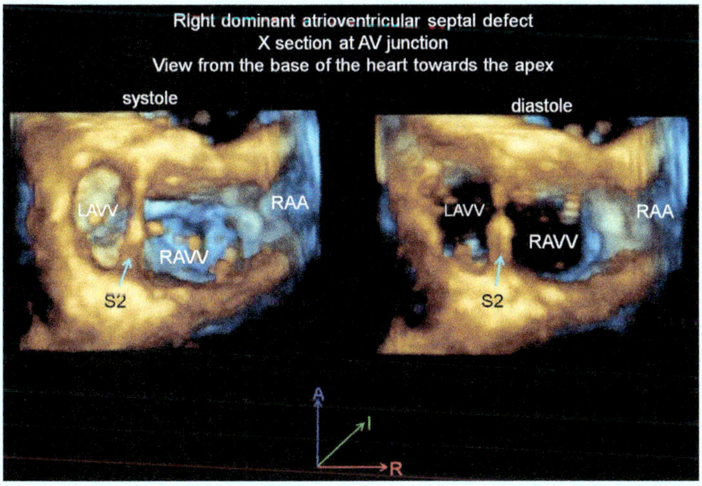

Figure 11-10

Overriding and straddling mitral valve, malaligned ventricular septal defect (*), and double-outlet right ventricle (RV). Left, Annular override of the mitral valve. The *yellow arrow* bisects the mitral annulus and points directly to the ventricular septum. Right, straddling of the mitral valve. The *blue arrow* points to chordal attachments of the mitral valve on the right side of the ventricular septum at the junction of the moderator band. The inlet ventricular septum (1) and outlet ventricular septum (2) are malaligned with respect to each other. LA, left atrium; LV, left ventricle; MB, moderator band; RA, right atrium.

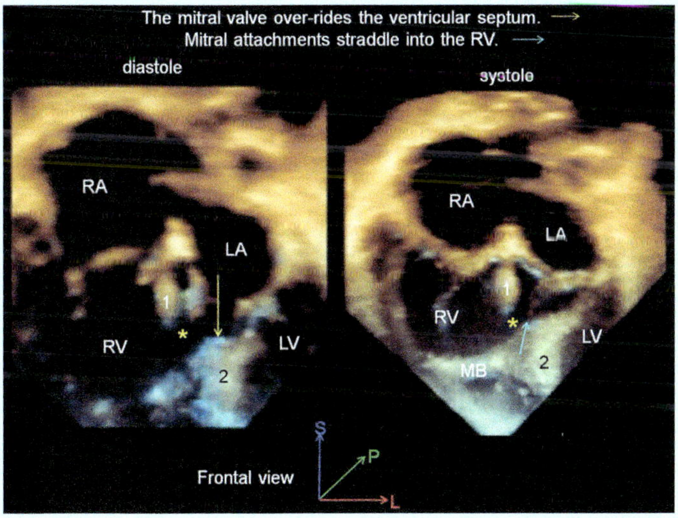

Figure 11-11

From the same patient as Figure 11-8, a cross-sectional view from the apex toward the base showing that the mitral valve (MV) orifice during diastole is positioned directly above the ventricular septum; therefore it is overriding. LV, left ventricle; LVOT, left ventricular outflow tract; RV, right ventricle; TV, tricuspid valve.

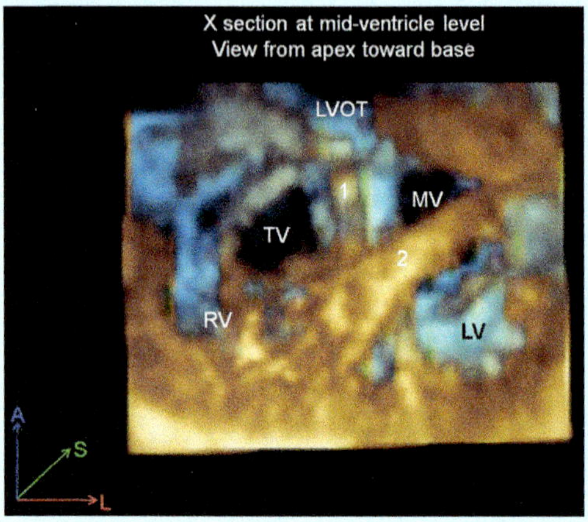

Figure 11-12

Straddling of tricuspid valve (TV) chordae through a large ventricular septal defect (*) to insert into the left ventricle (LV). Live 3D acquisition from a transthoracic subcostal coronal transducer position. RA, right atrium; RV, right ventricle; VS, ventricular septum.

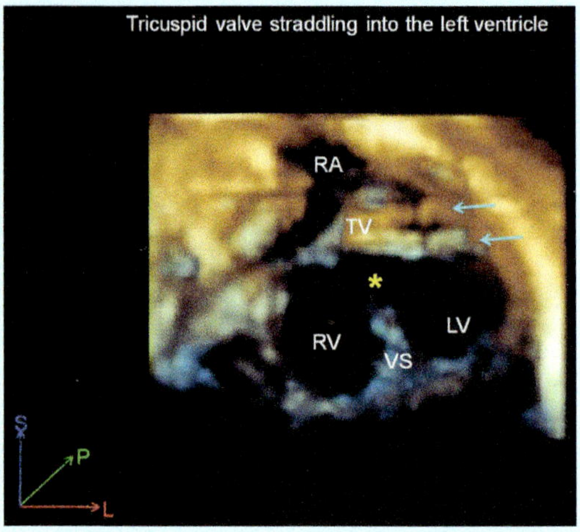

inlet ventricular septal defect to attach within the left ventricle, one would predict the presence of right ventricular hypoplasia. Most commonly the tricuspid valve straddles through ventricular septal defects located within the inlet portion, whereas the mitral valve typically straddles through ventricular septal defects located in the outlet portion of the ventricular septum. Mitral valves that straddle are often cleft.

Abnormal ventricular septal attachments of the mitral valve chordae are another important and common abnormality of the tension apparatus of the mitral valve. This chordal malattachment is present in atrioventricular septal defect and other defects. Occasionally these malattachments are extensive and associated not only with left ventricular outflow tract obstruction but also with multilevel left-sided obstruction resulting in important left ventricular hypoplasia, thereby directing some of these cases to the single-ventricle palliation therapy tract.

3DE analysis

Transthoracic full-volume 3D acquisitions from the apical four-chamber and subcostal coronal transducer positions with frontal plane anterior to posterior cropping are used to demonstrate the features of valve anatomy, patency, annular override, and straddling. In smaller patients with faster heart rate and respiratory rate, live 3D sweeps in the apical and subcostal positions may be substituted or added.

Cross-sectional views of the atrioventricular junction are obtained by additional cropping of the full-volume 3D set acquired in the apical position. Cropping is performed in the vertical plane from both the base and the apex toward the atrioventricular junction. The image is rotated 90° forward in the frontal plane to view it from the base. Alternatively it may be rotated 90° backward to view the atrioventricular junction from the apex. Figures 11-4 and 11-7 are examples of such a view of the cross-section of the atrioventricular junction as seen from the base of the heart, and Figures 11-4 and 11-9 illustrate this cropping scheme as seen from the apex. This cross-sectional view of the atrioventricular junction allows determination of tricuspid versus mitral versus common-atrioventricular-valve type; reveals the presence of annular override; and allows visualization of valve straddling.

Figure 11-13

Criss-cross heart with atrioventricular discordance and small right ventricle (RV). This full-volume 3D transthoracic acquisition is from a subcostal position and cropped from anterior to posterior in the frontal plane. Note that the anatomic axis of the tricuspid valve (TV) (left panel, *yellow arrow*) is perpendicular to the anatomic axis of the mitral valve (MV) (right panel, *blue arrow*). LA, left atrium; LV, left ventricle; PA, pulmonary artery; RA, right atrium; VS, ventricular septum.

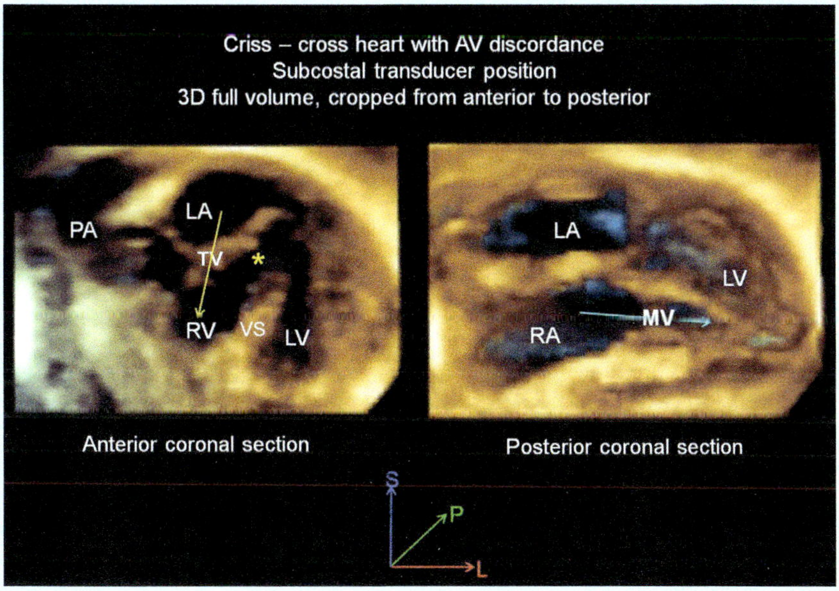

Transesophageal 3DE of the atrioventricular junction morphology also makes use of full-volume 3D acquisition from the four-chamber view with subsequent frontal plane anterior to posterior cropping. Base to apex cropping to obtain cross-sectional views analogous to that used with transthoracic 3DE is used as well. 3D zoom mode is similarly used to demonstrate the cross-section of the atrioventricular junction, albeit at a slow frame rate.

ANALYSIS OF THE VENTRICLE

General considerations

The intrinsic defining features of a normal morphologic right ventricle are the presence of a moderator band; a tricuspid atrioventricular valve; more apical position of the leaflets of the tricuspid valve relative to the mitral valve; a septal band; prominent apical trabeculations; and subarterial conus separating the tricuspid valve from the semilunar valve. The intrinsic defining features of a normal morphologic left ventricle are the presence of smooth septal surface; a mitral valve; absence of septal attachments of atrioventricular valve chordae; more basal positioned AV valve leaflets relative to the tricuspid valve; fine apical trabeculations; and atrioventricular to semilunar valve continuity. In complex malformed hearts, some of these features may be absent or extremely difficult to demonstrate. The cardiac position, relative spatial relationships of the right versus left ventricle, and the respective contribution of each ventricle to cardiac apex formation must be defined as well. All of these features are well defined on 3DE; however, space limitations prohibit illustrating all of them here. 3DE is ideal for measuring right and left ventricular volume and ejection fraction, as discussed below.

3DE analysis

Transthoracic full-volume 3D acquisitions from the four-chamber view, apical long-axis view, and subcostal sagittal and coronal views are used to assess ventricular qualitative and quantitative anatomy. In patients with fast heart rates or limited respiratory gating, live 3D mode sweeps from the same positions can be used to analyze the qualitative anatomy; however, this mode is not suitable for 3D volumetric quantitation because the entirety of the ventricle cannot usually be captured in one acquisition, owing to the relative thinness of the live 3D sector size as compared with the large full-volume 3D mode.

Transesophageal full-volume 3D images are acquired from the four-chamber views and left ventricular long-axis views at the midesophagus level. Deep transgastric views that are equivalent to the transthoracic subcostal views are quite effective for additional views of both ventricles but especially the right ventricle. These views are the equivalent of subcostal coronal views obtained from transthoracic echocardiography. Full-volume acquisitions are used for quantitative analysis. We prefer the real-time, live modalities of 3D zoom mode and live 3D mode for qualitative analysis of anatomy during transesophageal echocardiography.

ANALYSIS OF THE VENTRICULAR OUTFLOW TRACT

General considerations

Unobstructed outflow tract patency is important because obstruction beneath the systemic semilunar valve is particularly detrimental to single-ventricle function. Often with univentricular hearts, the systemic semilunar valve and its immediate subvalvular region are positioned in the substernal position; therefore, examination of this region is challenging in a number of patients who have typically had sternotomies. Also fairly commonly, such as in tricuspid atresia with transposition and also with double-inlet left ventricle with rudimentary subaortic right ventricular outflow chamber, a muscular ventricular septal defect serves as the potentially or actually obstructed outlet from the functional systemic ventricle to the native systemic semilunar valve. The nature of this muscular ventricular septal defect, also called *bulboventricular foramen*, is to undergo spontaneous narrowing with time. Abnormal conal septal deviation and hypertrophy may also cause narrowing of the systemic ventricular outflow tract. Additional causes of obstruction in this region are anomalous muscle bundles, proliferation of fibrous tissue, and occasional malattachment of atrioventricular valve chordae into the outflow tract.

3DE analysis

Transthoracic short-axis serial tomographic views from apical and basal perspectives are often quite useful and are best obtained from an apical full-volume acquisition. Subsequently, they can be cropped from base toward apex and vice versa with the top/base of the 3D data set tilted 90° forward to view the base, or the bottom/apex tilted 90° forward to view from the apex. This technique is analogous to that described above to demonstrate the atrioventricular junction in cross-section. Variable apical, long-axis, and subcostal views demonstrating side and en face views of the outflow tract should also be obtained.

Transesophageal deep transgastric views using live 3D are quite useful because of favorable alignment with the long axis of both outflow tracts. The midesophagus views with the transducer array orientation at 90° to 120° are favorable for the left ventricular outflow tract and 60° to 80° is usually best for the right ventricular outflow tract. Full-volume 3D mode acquisitions are often useful as well and are cropped in similar fashion to the transthoracic acquisitions.

PALLIATIVE PROCEDURES FOR THE UNIVENTRICULAR HEART

Most patients with univentricular hearts survive through the completion of Fontan procedure palliation. In our practice, we have far more univentricular heart patients, both children and adults, in the post-Fontan stage than in the pre-Fontan stage. Therefore, one must become familiar with the 3DE appearance of the palliative procedures.

Glenn procedure

General considerations. The classic Glenn procedure involves connection of the superior vena cava to the right pulmonary artery and ligating the connection of the right pulmonary artery to the main pulmonary artery. Today, the more commonly used version of the superior vena cava to right pulmonary artery anastomosis is the bidirectional Glenn, in which the connection of the right pulmonary artery to the main pulmonary artery is maintained. In the instances in which a persistent left superior vena cava is present, it is anastomosed to the left pulmonary artery, resulting in the bilateral bidirectional Glenn. Finally, occasional cases have maintenance of a small amount of restrictive antegrade flow across the pulmonary valve into the pulmonary artery along with the bidirectional Glenn, resulting in a pulsatile bidirectional Glenn.

3DE analysis. The best views of cavopulmonary connections are obtained from the suprasternal or subclavicular transthoracic positions and from the superior transesophageal position with clockwise rotation of the transducer. Live 3D is used to demonstrate superior vena cava size and patency of the anastomosis. Full-volume 3D color Doppler flow is used to demonstrate low-velocity laminar antegrade flow with respiratory variation from the cava into the pulmonary artery. Flow reversal may sometimes be seen in the presence of pulsatile Glenn or significant systemic to pulmonary arterial collateral flow.

Fontan procedure

General considerations. The total cavopulmonary connection or Fontan procedure in its classic original variation consists of a right atrial appendage to pulmonary artery connection (Fig. 11-14). This version results in a large venous capacitance subpulmonary structure that causes significant flow energy loss. It was therefore replaced by the lateral tunnel type of Fontan in which the lateral aspect of the Fontan is prosthetic patch or

Figure 11-14

Classic Fontan from an adult patient with tricuspid atresia. This transesophageal echocardiographic basal short-axis image was acquired in 3D zoom mode at the upper esophagus. The large atrial portion of the Fontan wraps around the anterior aspect of the heart. AoV, aortic valve; IVC, inferior vena cava; LA, left atrium; PA, pulmonary artery.

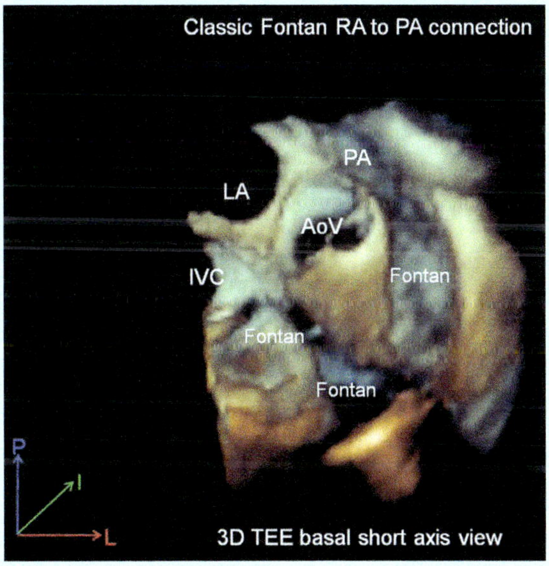

pericardium and the medial aspect is atrial tissue (Fig. 11-15). The latest version is the extracardiac Fontan, in which the inferior vena cava to pulmonary artery connection is a prosthetic tube graft and the superior cavopulmonary connection is a bidirectional Glenn (Fig. 11-16). Minor variations of these basic types are used by some.

Figure 11-15

Lateral tunnel Fontan for tricuspid atresia as seen from transesophageal 3D images. Left, Cross-section seen from the base of the heart, acquired in 3D zoom mode. Right, long-axis view of the left ventricle (LV) acquired in full-volume 3D mode and cropped in the frontal plane. This view is suitable for 3D quantitation of LV volume, function, and synchrony. AMV = anterior mitral valve leaflet; Ao, aorta; LA, left atrium; LAA, left atrial appendage; PMV, posterior mitral valve leaflet.

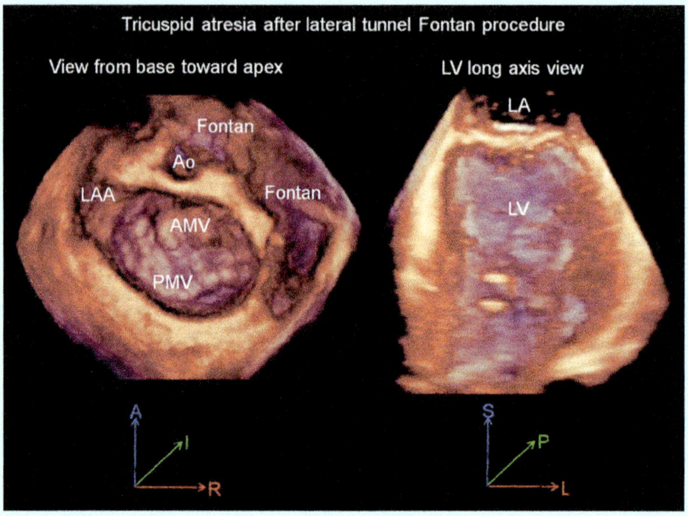

Figure 11-16

Three sections of extracardiac Fontan as seen on live 3D transesophageal echocardiography. Bottom, From a transgastric position at 0° array orientation with rightward twist of the transducer. Middle, From the midesophagus with 90° array orientation. Upper, From the upper esophagus, array 0°, with rightward twist of the transducer. IVC, inferior vena cava; LPA, left pulmonary artery; PA, pulmonary artery; RPA, right pulmonary artery.

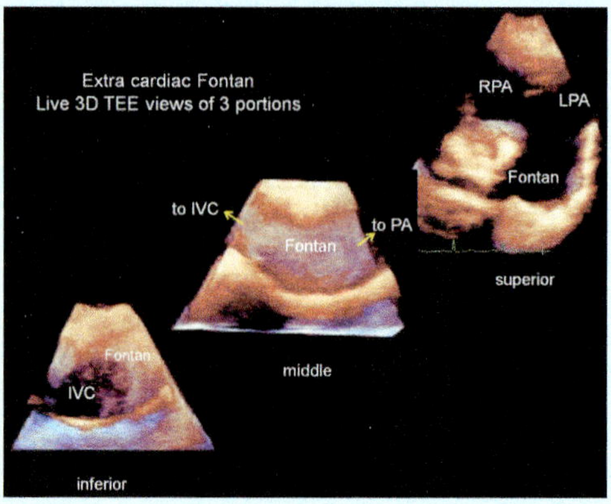

3DE analysis. The Fontan is often challenging to image in older patients using transthoracic echocardiography. The subcostal transducer position is usually the best for transthoracic imaging of the inferior vena cava, hepatic veins, and inferior Fontan. The superior Fontan to pulmonary artery connection is often the most difficult region to visualize in larger patients. It may be seen best from modified high parasternal views.

Using the transesophageal approach, image quality is usually significantly better. The transgastric view is best for visualization of the inferior vena cava, hepatic veins, and proximal Fontan. The middle to upper esophagus longitudinal view with a transducer array orientation of 90° to 110° using 3D zoom or live 3D is frequently the most useful for the middle of the Fontan. A high transesophageal position with 0° array orientation and rightward rotation using live 3D is best to visualize the Fontan conduit to pulmonary artery connection (Fig. 11-14). Slow antegrade flow patterns with respiratory variability and abnormal right to left shunts can be seen using X-plane color Doppler and live 3D color Doppler methods.

3D QUANTITATIVE VOLUMETRIC TECHNIQUES

Left ventricular volumetric measurements that are free of geometric shape assumptions are now in clinical use. With the advanced Philips QLAB 3DQ software (Amsterdam, Netherlands), ventricular volume, ejection fraction, stroke volume, and synchrony can be rapidly measured from full-volume 3D data sets in rapid semiautomated fashion (Fig. 11-17). Similarly right ventricular volume, ejection fraction, and stroke volume can be measured using commercially available TomTec (Chicago, IL) 4DRV software.

Figure 11-17

Ventricular synchrony and function study using advanced dedicated 3D software. Image from a 13 year old with double-inlet left ventricle after septation procedure and biventricular pacing (bipace). Top left, pre bipace; top right, post bipace. Left lower table summarizes the changes in synchrony, volume, and ejection fraction (EF) before and after bipace; right lower panel is an example of volume and synchrony curves from a normal heart. The data show improvement but not normalization after bipace. EDV, end-diastolic volume; ESV, end-systolic volume; TMSV, time to minimal systolic volume.

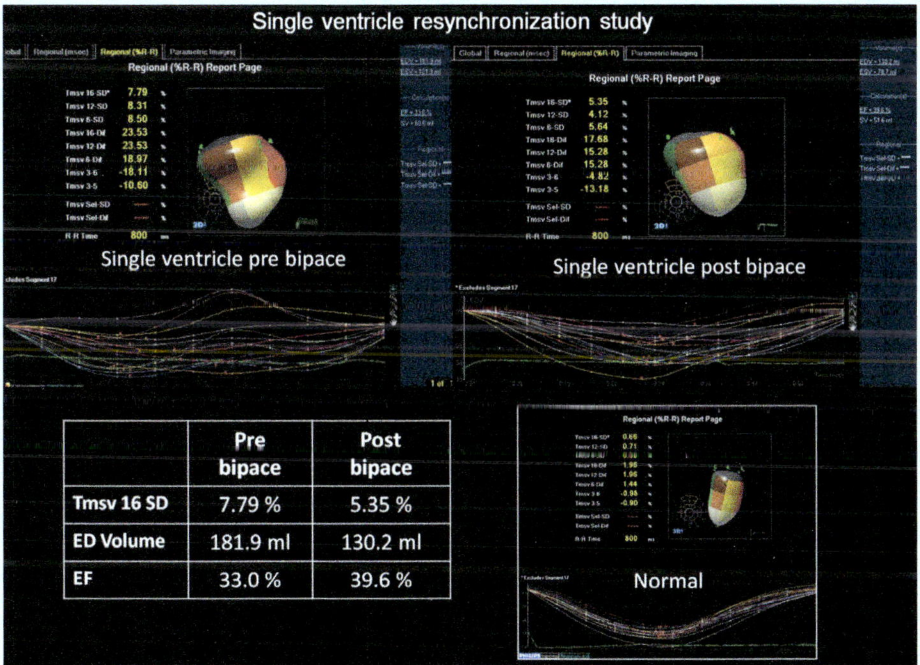

REFERENCES

1. Silverman NH. Univentricular atrioventricular connections (complex with one dominant ventricle – single ventricle). In: Silverman NH, ed. *Pediatric Echocardiography*. Baltimore, MD: Williams & Wilkins; 1993. pp. 279–302.
2. Huhta JC, Seward JB, Tajik AJ, et al. Two-dimensional echocardiographic spectrum of univentricular atrioventricular connection. *J Am Coll Cardiol*. 1985;5(1):149–157.
3. Rigby ML, Anderson RH, Gibson D, et al. Two-dimensional echocardiographic categorization of the univentricular heart, morphology, type and mode of atrioventricular connection. *Br Heart J*. 1981;46(6):603–612.
4. Sahn DJ, Harder JR, Freedom RM, et al. Cross-sectional diagnosis and classification of univentricular hearts: imaging studies of atrioventricular valves, septal structures and rudimentary outflow chambers. *Circulation*. 1982;66(5):1070–1077.
5. Anderson RH, Becker AE, Macartney FJ, et al. "Tricuspid atresia" a univentricular heart? *Pediatr Cardiol*. 1979;1:51–56.
6. Bharati S, Lev M. The concept of tricuspid atresia complex as distinct from that of the single ventricle complex. *Pediatr Cardiol*. 1979;1:57–62.
7. Van Praagh R, David I, Van Praagh S. What is a ventricle? The single-ventricle trap. *Pediatr Cardiol*. 1982;2(1):79–84.
8. Anderson RH, Macartney FJ, Tynan M, et al. Univentricular atrioventricular connection: the single ventricle trap unsprung. *Pediatr Cardiol*. 1983;4(4):273–280.
9. Van Praagh R, Ando M, Dungan WT. Anatomic types of tricuspid atresia: clinical and developmental implications. *Circulation*. 1971;44(suppl 2):111–115.
10. Bharati S. Tricuspid atresia. In: Bharati S, Lev M, eds. *The Pathology of Congenital Heart Disease*. Vol 1. Armonk, NY: Futura Publishing; 1996. pp. 403–420.
11. Weinberg PM. Anatomy of tricuspid atresia and its relevance to forms of surgical therapy. *Ann Thorac Surg*. 1980;29(4):306–314.
12. Van Praagh R, Ongley PA, Swan HJ. Anatomic types of single or common ventricle in man: morphologic and geometric aspects of 60 necropsied cases. *Am J Cardiol*. 1964;13:367–386.
13. Van Praagh R, Van Praagh S, Vlad P, Keith JD. Diagnosis of the anatomic types of single or common ventricle. *Am J Cardiol*. March, 1965;15:345–366.
14. Bharati S. Single ventricle with small outlet chamber. In: Bharati S, Lev M, eds. *The Pathology of Congenital Heart Disease*. Vol 2. Armonk, NY: Futura Publishing; 1996. pp. 1049–1114.
15. Smallhorn JF, De Tommasini G, Macartney FJ. Two-dimensional echocardiographic assessment of common atrioventricular valves in univentricular hearts. *Br Heart J*. 1981;46(1):30–34.
16. Smallhorn JF, Tommasini G, Macartney FJ. Detection and assessment of straddling and overriding atrioventricular valves in univentricular hearts. *Br Heart J*. 1981;46(3):254–262.
17. Milo S, Ho SY, Macartney FJ, et al. Straddling and overriding atrioventricular valves: morphology and classification. *Am J Cardiol*. 1979;44(6):1122–1134.
18. Bharati S. Straddling and displaced atrioventricular orifices and valves. In: Bharati S, Lev M, eds. *The Pathology of Congenital Heart Disease*. Vol 2. Armonk, NY: Futura Publishing; 1996. pp. 1115–1148.
19. Anderson RH, Shinebourne EA, Gerlis LM. Criss-cross atrioventricular relationships producing paradoxical atrioventricular concordance or discordance. Their significance to nomenclature of congenital heart disease. *Circulation*. 1974;50(1):176–180.
20. Marino B, Sanders SP, Pasquini L, et al. Two-dimensional echocardiographic anatomy in crisscross heart. Am J Cardiol. 1986;58(3):325–333.

CHAPTER 12

THREE-DIMENSIONAL ECHOCARDIOGRAPHIC ASSESSMENT OF THE MITRAL VALVE

Jeffrey F. Smallhorn, MBBS, FRACP, FRCP(C)

ABSTRACT

Assessment of abnormalities of the mitral valve is one of the current strengths of three-dimensional echocardiographic (3DE) imaging. The current imaging platform permits an accurate anatomical diagnosis and enhances two-dimensional echocardiographic data. It also enables the echocardiographer to speak the same language as the surgeon when describing and displaying the pathology. The application of 3D display and analysis has provided unique insights into the function of both the normal and the abnormal mitral valve, including congenital abnormalities such as isolated cleft of the anterior leaflet, straddling mitral valve, mitral valve dysplasia, double-orifice mitral valve, mitral valve prolapse, mitral valve in corrected transposition, and parachute mitral valve. 3DE also provides superior imaging of lesions associated with mitral valve stenosis, including supramitral valve stenosis and mitral valve stenosis secondary to leaflet thickening, chordal shortening, and fusion.

INTRODUCTION

The mitral valve has been extensively evaluated using three-dimensional echocardiography (3DE). Most investigations have been done in adults, with attention to rheumatic mitral valve stenosis, ischemic mitral valve regurgitation, and prolapse.[1–4] The function of the mitral annular shape has also been a topic of interest, as has the location of the papillary muscle in patients with ischemic regurgitation.[5–10] 3DE has improved our understanding of normal and abnormal mitral valve function and is currently used in clinical decision making. For years, echocardiographers strove to educate their surgical colleagues on two-dimensional echocardiographic (2DE) evaluation of the mitral valve; however, what the echocardiographer showed and what the surgeon saw were very different. When the mitral valve is demonstrated on 3DE, with the images displayed in a surgical view from the left atrium, our surgical colleagues instantaneously appreciate the pathology, often with more confidence than the echocardiographer. Moreover, 3DE morphological and functional assessment of the mitral valve is physiological, whereas surgical evaluation through inspection and saline testing is not.[11] This does not mean that we should abandon 2D assessment of the mitral valve but rather we should strive to determine the incremental value of 3DE.[2,3,11]

NORMAL MITRAL VALVE

The mitral valve functions as a unit, with all components acting in unison to maintain valve competency.[12] The valve annulus is saddle shaped to minimize leaflet stress, with two high and two low points (Figs. 12-1A and 12-1B),[9,13] an important concept that will be expanded in the section on "Mitral valve prolapse." The annulus changes shape throughout the cardiac cycle and is very heterogeneous,[8] unlike its tricuspid counterpart, which is homogeneous (Fig. 12-1A). Annular forces also vary such that during systole the left ventricular outflow

Figure 12-1A and B

A, Montage demonstrating the shape of the mitral annulus as seen from the left atrial view, as well as graphic examples of annular shape and a heterogeneous contraction pattern, as seen in the upper right panel. The lower left panel shows the 3D shape of annular coordinates, which is taken from the same normal population as shown in the upper right panel. The lower right panel is a cartoon from the same population demonstrating the numbering of the annular segments. *B*, Two images demonstrating the saddle shape of the tricuspid annulus in the left panel, as well as the bending angle in a pediatric population. The annulus bends along the line of the commissures between the anterior and posterior leaflets. Note that the bending of the annulus starts in later systole and continues through isovolumic relaxation and into diastole. A, anterior; AL, anterior leaflet; AO, aorta; AVC, aortic valve closure; AVO, aortic valve opening; DF, diastolic phase; EP, ejection phase; IC, isovolumic contraction; IR, isovolumic relaxation; LA, left atrium; MVC, mitral valve closure; MVO, mitral valve opening; P, posterior; TV, tricuspid valve.

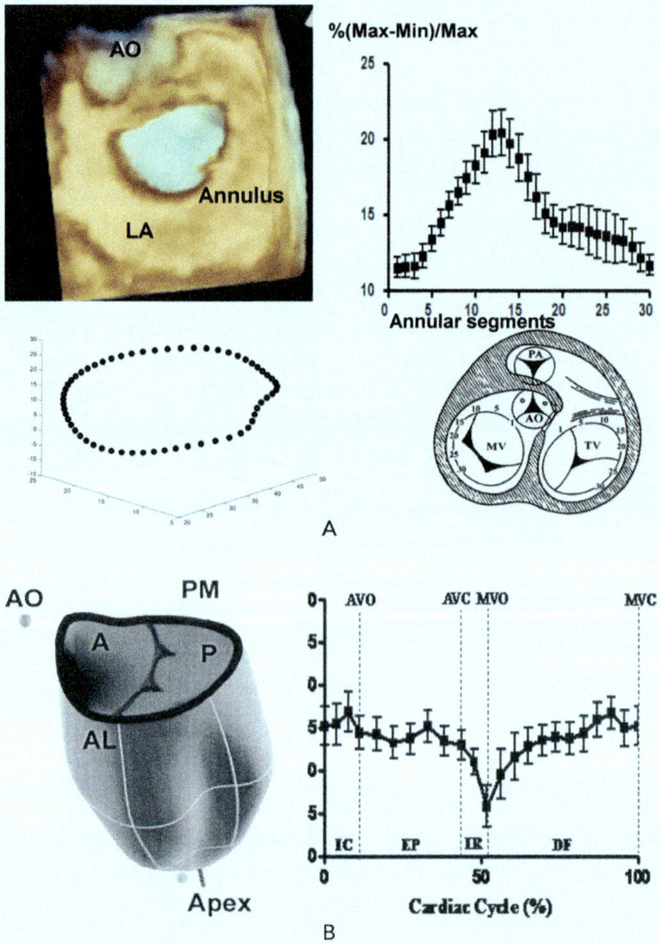

tract maintains maximum dimension to permit unimpeded flow to the aorta.[7,10] The normal mitral valve leaflets have an element of tethering and prolapse related to the insertion points of the chordae.[14] The leaflets roll over each other in such a way as to maintain maximum coaptation throughout systole. The anterior or aortic leaflet is smaller than its posterior or mural counterpart, with a curved zone of apposition between the two during systole (Fig. 12-2A).

Mitral valve chordae are multiple and complex (Fig. 12-2B).[12] Two main strut chordae insert onto the anterior leaflet, with the attachments running from the free margins onto the belly of the leaflet. These provide major support to the leaflet and are responsible for tethering in patients who have ischemic mitral valve regurgitation and secondary papillary muscle displacement. The free edges of the anterior leaflet are supported by rough zone chordae, which are smaller, multiple, and prevent leaflet prolapse. Medially and laterally, there are commissural chordae that are shared by both the anterior and posterior leaflets. The posterior leaflet has a series of scallops, which are supported by cleft chordae. The leaflets are supported by two papillary muscles that may have a single or multiple heads. The papillary muscles have a broad base of attachment and maintain a constant angle with the annulus throughout the cardiac cycle (Fig. 12-2C). This arrangement is important because it maintains minimal stress on the leaflets. All of the above findings can be appreciated on 3DE, and indeed it is this technique that has provided these unique insights into mitral valve function.

CONGENITAL MITRAL VALVE ABNORMALITIES

An understanding of the types of congenital abnormalities is important when embarking on an echocardiographic evaluation of the abnormal mitral valve.[15–18] The lesions divide generally into those that produce predominant stenosis or regurgitation, though there is overlap.

Isolated cleft of the anterior leaflet

Isolated cleft of the anterior leaflet results in mitral valve regurgitation, the severity of which is determined in part by the extent of the cleft.[19–22] In some cases, the cleft runs from the free edge of the leaflet to its base, whereas in others the extension is incomplete. The cleft differs from that seen in an atrioventricular septal defect in that it points toward the left ventricular outflow tract rather than the interventricular septum and right ventricle.[19] The exception is in hearts with abnormal ventriculoarterial connections, where it is often eccentric.[23,24] The papillary muscles are in the normal location in hearts with an isolated cleft, unlike in an atrioventricular septal defect, where the posterior-medial papillary muscle is rotated more laterally.[19] In most cases, the free edges of the cleft are unsupported; however, in some patients, there are accessory chordae supporting the leaflet, which usually results in valve competency. The accessory chordae may attach to the interventricular septum, whereas in other cases they cross the ventricular septum through a defect, resulting in mitral valve straddling. Although this lesion was first described after visualization on 3DE, the recent 3D technique permits a more complete evaluation of the extent of the cleft, as well as any associated chordal attachments. An isolated cleft can be reconstructed from either an apical four-chamber, full-volume data set or from a parasternal long-axis view. An apical rendered view from below provides optimal images for reasons mentioned in the section on "Normal Mitral Valve"; however, for our surgical colleagues, it can be displayed from above (Figs. 12-3A and 12-3B). From the parasternal long-axis view, an image cropped from above, such that the interventricular septum is removed, provides optimal visualization of the anterior mitral leaflet and a cleft. Neither of these two latter views is possible on 2DE, thus demonstrating the uniqueness of 3DE.

Straddling mitral valve

A straddling mitral valve is seen more frequently in hearts with an abnormality of the ventriculoarterial connection, in particular ventriculoarterial discordance, or double-outlet right ventricle. The degree of straddling is important, because the presence of balanced ventricles determines whether a biventricular or functionally single ventricle repair is undertaken.[25,26] The straddling mitral valve may insert into the crest of the interventricular septum, toward its base or in a more anterior location. In the former situation, a

Figure 12-2A, B and C

A, Two images showing the 3D features of the normal mitral valve as seen on transesophageal echocardiography. Note the broad anterior and smaller posterior or mural leaflet. Also observe the commissures, as seen in the right panel, as well as the scalloped nature of the mural leaflet, seen in the right panel in diastole. The left panel shows the peaks and valleys of the leaflet. The video clips show the same features, seen from above (*Fig. 12-2 movie 1*) and below (*Fig. 12-2 movie 2*). *B*, Chordal apparatus as seen on 3DE, as well as in a pathological specimen. Note the strut chords that tent the anterior leaflet toward the left ventricular cavity. The marginal chords can be seen on the coaptation zone of the leaflets. The video clip shows the 3DE features (*Fig. 12-2 movie 3*). *C*, 3DE appearance of the anterior and posterior papillary muscles of the mitral valve. Note the chords inserting into the anterior muscle and the broad base of the posterior papillary muscle. The video clips show the same features as the still images (*Fig. 12-2 movies 4 and 5*). ANT PM, anterior papillary muscle; AL, anterior leaflet; AO, aorta; LA, left atrium; LV, left ventricle; MC, marginal chords (or rough zone); ML, mural or posterior leaflet; POST PM, posterior papillary muscle; PM, papillary muscle; RZ, rough zone chords; SC, strut chords.

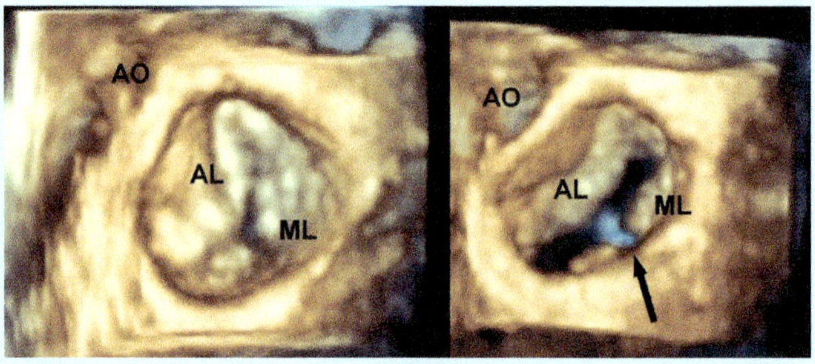

A

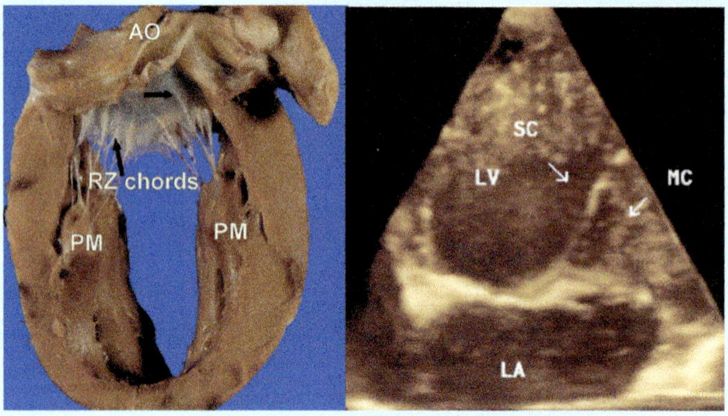

B

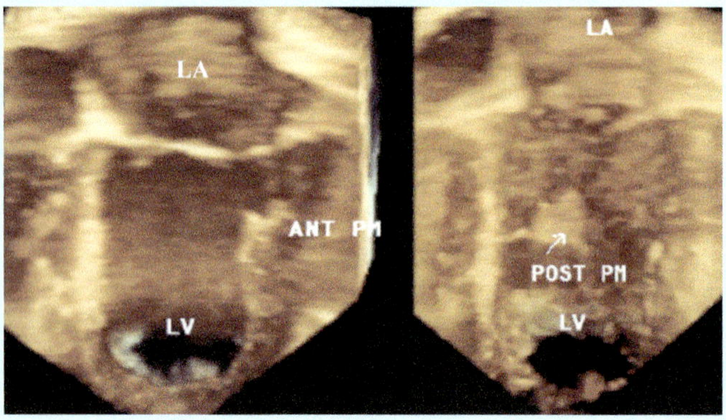

C

Figure 12-3A and B

A, Montage showing the 2D and 3D appearance of an isolated mitral cleft of the mitral valve (*black arrow* in left panel and *asterisk* in right panel). The *white arrow* shows the point of mitral aortic continuity. Note in the left panel that the 3D image shows the full extent of the cleft, whereas the right panel does not. The video clip (*Fig. 12-3 movie 1)* shows the same features in real time. The 2D color video clip (*Fig. 12-3 movie 2*) shows the regurgitation. *B*, An eccentric cleft as seen on 3DE, from the left ventricular (right panel) and left atrial (left panel) aspects. Note that the cleft does not point toward the left ventricular outflow tract. Note in the right panel that the papillary muscles are close together. This patient had an arterial switch operation for transposition of the great arteries. The video clips (*Fig. 12-3 movie 3*) and MV below (*Fig. 12-3 movie 4*) show the features in real time. AL, anterior leaflet; AO, aorta; ML, mural or posterior leaflet; MV, mitral valve; PM, papillary muscle.

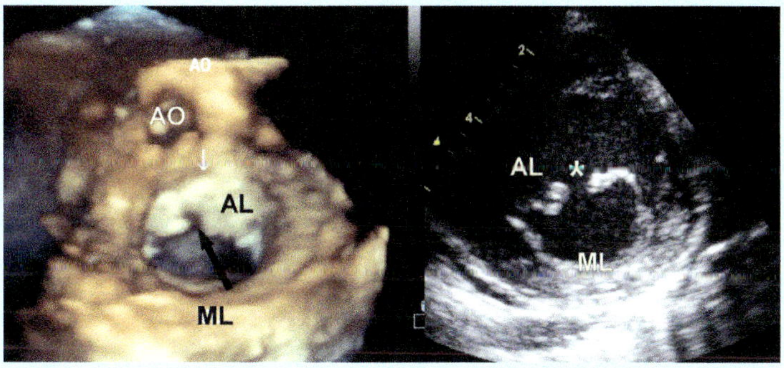

A

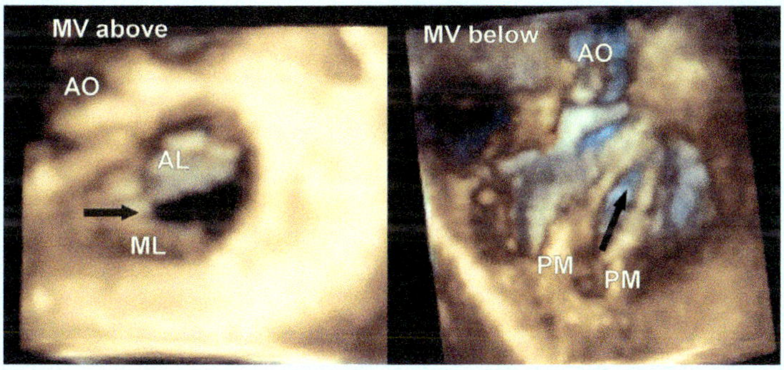

B

biventricular repair can be considered; however, in the latter case, two-single-ventricle palliation is usually the treatment of choice. Because it has higher frame rates, 2DE still provides superior detail when imaging fine chordal structures; however, it is inferior when attempting to determine the spatial relationship of these structures in a 3D space. Whether a ventricular septal defect can be closed depends on these relationships, and this is where 3DE is very valuable. Most importantly, it provides the surgeons with a mental image of what they will encounter and thus it may prevent unnecessary surgical exploration and improve preoperative planning. Because mitral valve chords always straddle through an anterior defect in the interventricular septum, they are best appreciated on 3DE from the parasternal location, as this provides optimal resolution and imaging in the axial plane. This is not to say that the mitral valve chords cannot be imaged from other locations, but this approach is optimal. The view that we have found most useful is that obtained when the anterior crop plane is adjusted, because the septal defect, chords, and any accessory papillary muscles are readily appreciated (Fig. 12-4).

Figure 12-4

2D and 3D appearance of a straddling mitral valve in the setting of transposition of the great arteries, and a ventricular septal defect, plus pulmonary outflow tract obstruction. Note that the mitral valve straddles through a large anterior muscular ventricular septal defect, with chords inserting into a papillary muscle that resides in the right ventricle. The video clips demonstrate the features far better than the still images. *Fig. 12-4 movies 1 and 2* are the same images as in the still Figure 12-4. *Fig. 12-4 movie 3* shows the unique features of the muscular ventricular septal defect as viewed from the right ventricular aspect, as well as the location of the abnormal mitral valve papillary muscle. Note the second perimembranous ventricular septal defect. IVS, interventricular septum. The *black arrow* points to the chords. LV, left ventricle; PM, perimembranous; RV, right ventricle; TV, tricuspid valve; VSD, ventricular septal defect.

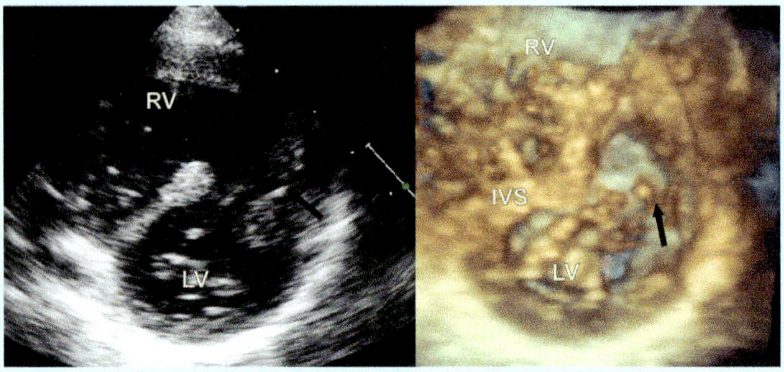

Mitral valve dysplasia

Mitral valve dysplasia usually results in mitral valve regurgitation or stenosis due to leaflet deficiency, tethering, and poor zones of coaptation.[27] The posterior mitral leaflet is usually more affected than its anterior counterpart. 2DE demonstrates leaflets that appear thickened and relatively immobile, often tethered with areas of poor coaptation. 3DE can demonstrate the same; however, the amount of tethering and the leaflet area can be determined.

Double-orifice mitral valve

Double-orifice mitral valve may be responsible for mitral valve regurgitation, although in other cases it is found incidentally during evaluation for an associated lesion.[28] The orifices may be equal sized or one may be much smaller. One or both orifices may be regurgitant, which is problematic when attempting repair, because if the regurgitant orifice is closed, the other may be too stenotic. In most cases, each orifice has its own support mechanism, unlike those seen in atrioventricular septal defect, where one may appear merely as a perforation in the leaflet. Double-orifice mitral valves have often been described by 2DE; however, evidence is scant as to the reliability of detecting them. 2DE falls short in diagnostic accuracy of the left atrioventricular valve in hearts with an atrioventricular septal defect, so the same may be true for its mitral counterpart. Whether 3DE is superior will be determined only from longitudinal studies. From an imaging standpoint, a full-volume data set acquired from the apical four-chamber or parasternal long-axis view should provide optimal imaging to aid in diagnosis of this lesion (Fig. 12-5).

Mitral valve prolapse

Mitral valve prolapse is rarely encountered in children except in those with abnormalities of elastic tissue, such as Marfan syndrome and Ehlers–Danlos syndrome. The incidence of mitral valve prolapse in the general population is about 2.4%, much lower than was previously thought.[29] The culprit for overdiagnosis was M-mode echocardiography and a poor understanding of the normal structure of the mitral annulus.

Figure 12-5A and B

A, Two- and three-dimensional features of a double-orifice mitral valve, labeled 1 and 2, in an otherwise normal heart. *Fig. 12-5 movie 1* shows the same features. *B*, Montage taken from a multiplanar reconstruction 3D data set in another patient with a double-orifice mitral valve (1 and 2). Note the smaller anterior orifice. *Fig. 12-5 movie 2* shows the same features. LA, left atrium; LV, left ventricle; LVOT, left ventricular outflow tract.

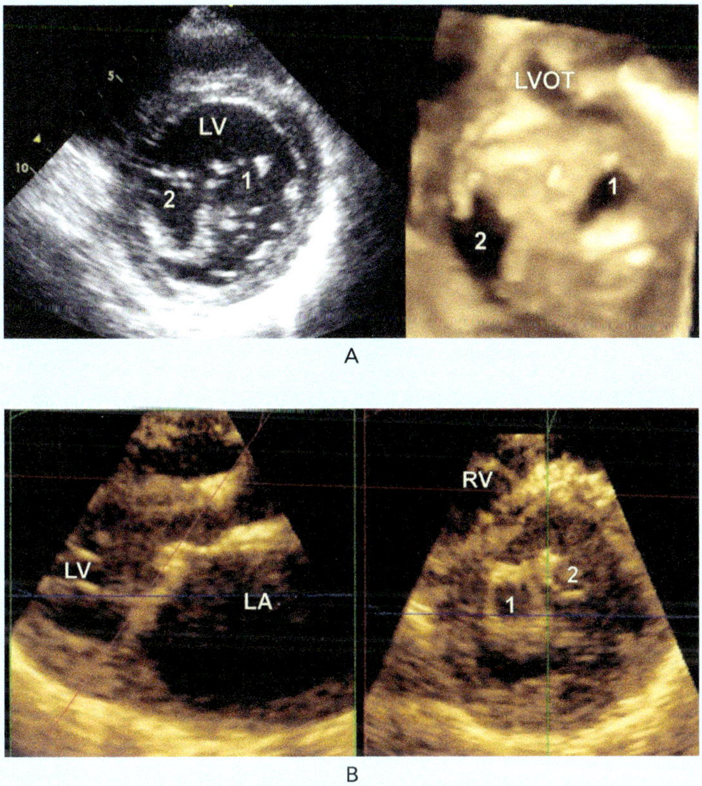

This overdiagnosis was corrected when the true shape of the mitral annulus was appreciated, most importantly by early work in 3DE showing that the mitral annulus is saddle shaped, with two high and two low points. Therefore, evaluation by 2DE in the parasternal long-axis view provided a more accurate assessment than was possible from the apical four-chamber view, as the former images the two high points of the annulus, whereas the latter mode images the two low points.[13] More advanced 3DE systems (in particular transesophageal 3DE) permit imaging of both the annulus and leaflets from multiple imaging planes, providing a very sensitive evaluation of localized prolapse.[30] This more sophisticated approach is important, particularly as the normal mitral valve has inbuilt prolapse and tethering, which is an intrinsic component of normal valve function.[14] Compared with 2DE, which requires multiple imaging planes to determine the precise location of mitral valve prolapse,[31] a 3D approach provides instantaneous accurate data that the surgeon readily understands (Fig. 12-6). Not only can this technique determine the location of the prolapse, but with quantitative packages the volume of prolapse can also be measured. Indeed, this has been one of the major steps forward in the evaluation of mitral valve prolapse. The other advantage of 3DE is that the imager is not limited to standard 2D planes; rather the valve can be imaged from multiple locations. Therefore, the current evidence is that 3DE provides better anatomic and functional data than its 2D counterpart.

Figure 12-6

Montage from a patient with mitral valve prolapse with associated leaflet dysplasia. The left panel shows the transesophageal echo appearance at 122°. Note in the right panel all of the leaflets can be seen with significant prolapse on A1 and A2. The middle panel was taken during diastole and shows the commissures and irregular nature of the anterior leaflet. AO, aorta; LV, left ventricle. Letters A1–A3 and P1–P3 represent the individual segments of the anterior and posterior leaflets. *Fig. 12-6 movies 1 and 2* show the real-time features of the prolapse.

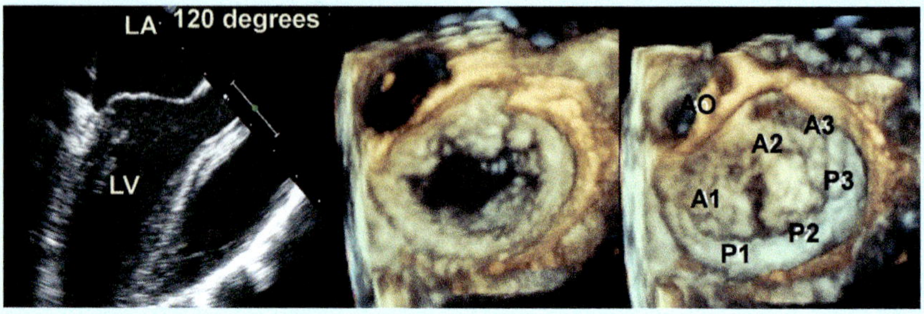

Mitral valve in corrected transposition

Mitral valve in corrected transposition is frequently abnormal and has a significant impact on decision making in treating patients in whom an anatomical repair of the heart is considered. The valve may have a cleft in the anterior leaflet, shortened chordae, or multiple leaflets (Fig. 12-7). Also, abnormal chordal attachments may obstruct the pulmonary outflow tract or straddle an anterior ventricular septal defect. 2DE provides some detail and can be helpful in the diagnosis of a cleft and straddling of chordal apparatus. Conversely, 3DE can provide greater detail in patients with multiple leaflets and commissural abnormalities. As well, vena contracta site and size are more readily defined on 3DE in patients with regurgitation. Imaging from the four-chamber view usually provides an optimal data set; however, the valve frequently lies at more of an angle to the transducer beam, resulting in less optimal imaging than with its tricuspid counterpart.

ASSESSMENT OF MITRAL VALVE REGURGITATION

Accurate quantification of mitral valve regurgitation has been the "holy grail" of echocardiographers, because it provides the key to determining whether a change in chamber size or function is merely secondary to an increased volume load or represents deterioration in pump function. Multiple 2D and Doppler techniques have been agreed upon by the American Society of Echocardiography[32]; however, they are often difficult to obtain and are based on geometrical assumptions. The eventual key to quantitative assessment will lie with 3D techniques.[33] What 3DE has demonstrated is that for many

Figure 12-7

Corrected transposition and a cleft in the morphological mitral valve, as indicated by the *black arrow*. The video clips (*Fig. 12-7 movies 1 and 2*) demonstrate the features. MLV, morphological left ventricle; MRV, morphological right ventricle.

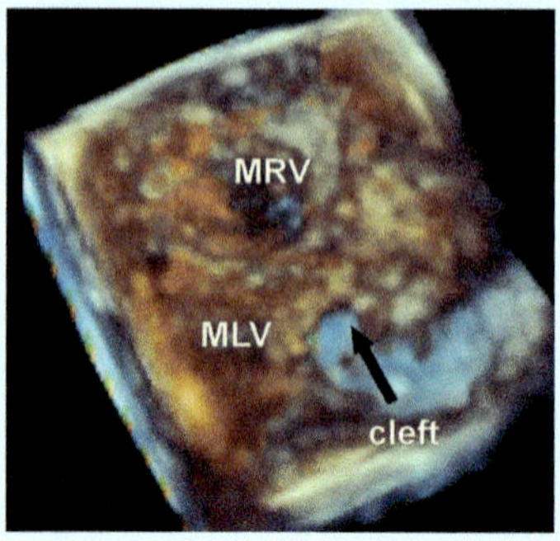

jets, the proximal isovelocity surface area is not a hemisphere, particularly when it is adjacent to a border.[34–36] Also, regurgitant jets are often multiple and irregularly shaped. The width of the 2D regurgitant jet, or vena contracta size, can be used as a semiquantitative measurement and indeed correlates well with that measured using 3D techniques.[37] Despite this correlation, studies using multivariate analysis have demonstrated that mechanisms of valve failure correlate better with 3D vena contracta size. 3D vena contracta size correlates well with volume regurgitation and can thus provide a semiquantitative method to assess severity of mitral valve regurgitation. If there are multiple jets of regurgitation, then they can be summated. The best approach to measuring vena contracta size is to obtain a data set from the apical four-chamber view, as the valve and its regurgitant jet are imaged in the axial plane, providing optimal resolution. Once the data set is acquired, it can be cropped from above and below, so that the vena contracta is sandwiched between the two planes, like the filling of an Oreo cookie (Fig. 12-8). The vena contracta area(s) can then be planimetered and then related to the size of the annulus. Although this method is only semiquantitative, it is a step in the right direction.

LESIONS ASSOCIATED WITH MITRAL VALVE STENOSIS

Supramitral valve stenosis

Supramitral valve stenosis rarely occurs in isolation and is usually associated with a more extensive abnormality of the mitral valve, with associated leaflet thickening and shortened chordae.[38] The lesion is situated just above the mitral annulus, which differentiates it from cor triatriatum, in which the membrane is located above the left atrial appendage. In supramitral stenosis, the ring may be complete or partial, which in part determines the severity of the obstruction. 2DE underestimates the extent of a supramitral membrane, just as it does in fibromuscular subaortic stenosis. With 3DE, the full extent of the ring is appreciated, particularly from a four-chamber full-volume data set (Fig. 12-9). Once again, this plane images the ring in the axial plane, providing superior resolution.

Figure 12-8

Vena contracta in a patient with mitral valve regurgitation. Note the regurgitant jet is located in the posterior aspect of the mitral valve. The video clips demonstrate the regurgitation in 3D. *Fig. 12-8 movie 1* is the same view as the still figure; *movie 2* shows the regurgitant jet at an angle; and *movie 3* shows the utility of 3DE with the jet being more posterior. AL, anterior leaflet; AO, aorta; LA, left atrium.

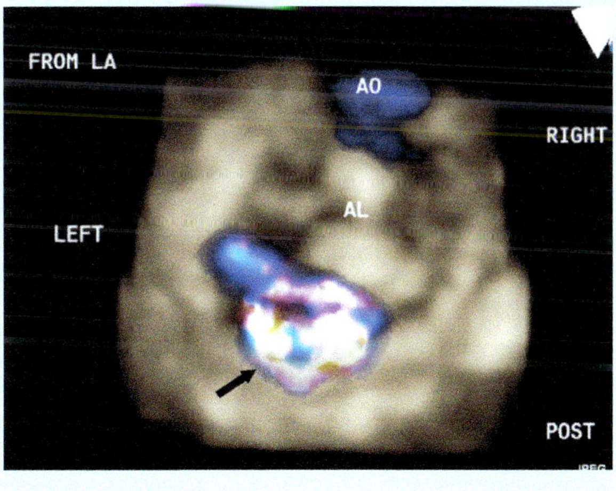

Mitral valve stenosis secondary to leaflet thickening, chordal shortening, and fusion

Mitral valve stenosis secondary to leaflet thickening, chordal shortening, and fusion is what is encountered most frequently. In this setting, the thickened leaflets are often attached to shortened chordae, such that it can be difficult to determine where the leaflet ends and the papillary muscle starts.[39] There may be a restrictive orifice at the tips of the leaflets; however, in many patients, slit-like eccentric orifices are seen along the length of the fused chordae (Fig. 12-10). The ultimate example of this is a mitral arcade with complete muscularization

Figure 12-9

Montage from a patient with mitral valve stenosis and an associated supramitral ring. The two images on the right show the 2D appearance, while the 3DE image shows the circumferential nature of the ring. The video clips show the 2D features (*Fig. 12-9 movie 1*) and 3D features (*Fig. 12-9 movie 2*). LA, left atrium; LV, left ventricle.

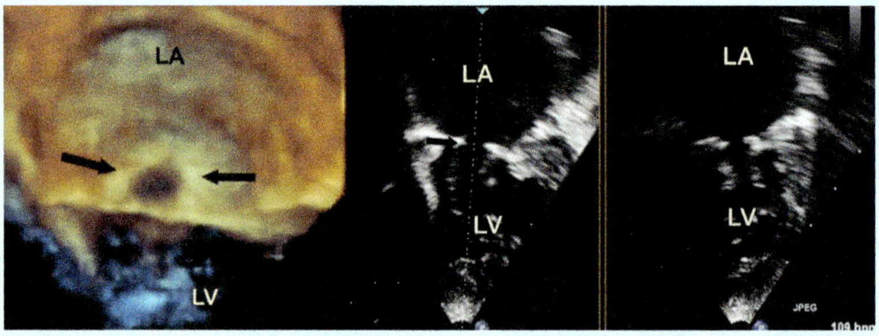

Figure 12-10

Two 3D images from a patient with mitral valve stenosis. The image on the left is seen from the front, with the interventricular septum removed, such that the chords and papillary muscles can be seen. The image on the right is seen from the left ventricular aspect and shows the papillary muscles and fused chords and leaflets. The video clips show the stenosis in real time. *Fig. 12-10 movie 1* shows the mitral valve with limited excursion, while *movie 2* shows the surgical view with a hypoplastic annulus. *Movie 3* shows the stenotic mitral valve from in front and is the same as the still image. *Movies 4* and *5* show the 2D features of the valve. *Movie 6* shows the obstruction starting at the valve level, in comparison with *movie 7*, in which the flow acceleration starts above the mitral annulus. AL, anterior leaflet; ANT PM, anterior papillary muscle; AO, aorta; LV, left ventricle; LVOT, left ventricular outflow tract; PM, papillary muscle; POST PM, posterior papillary muscle.

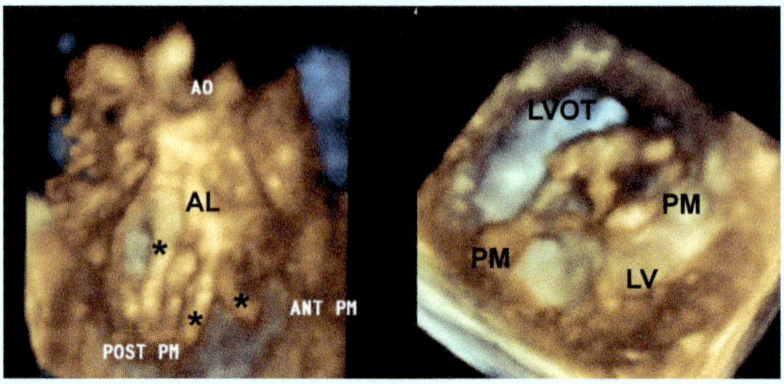

of the subvalve apparatus. 2DE can identify leaflet thickening and chordal shortening; however, the eccentric orifices and the complexity of the subvalve apparatus are best appreciated on 3DE (Figs. 12-11A and 12-11B). This technique can also provide quantitative data regarding the extent of tethering, which might be important to surgeons in the future.

Parachute mitral valve

Parachute mitral valve may result in stenosis, although in some instances it is an innocent bystander having no hemodynamic consequence. Although the classical parachute mitral valve consists of a solitary papillary muscle, in some patients there is one dominant muscle that provides most of the support to the leaflets, with a rudimentary smaller muscle that may or may not have chordal attachments. When the valve is stenotic, it is usually related to chordal shortening, fusion, and leaflet thickening. 2DE provides excellent delineation of a parachute mitral valve; however, its 3D counterpart is superior when imaging the leaflets and chordal apparatus.

Figure 12-11A and B

A, Images from a patient with a mitral arcade. Note the muscularized appearance of the subvalve apparatus in the right panel, and the thickened leaflets in the left panel. The video clip (*Fig. 12-11 movie 1*) shows the mitral arcade from the left ventricular view. AL, anterior leaflet; APM, anterior papillary muscle; LV, left ventricle; ML, mural leaflet; PPM, posterior papillary muscle. *B*, A multiplanar reconstruction (MPR) demonstrating the mitral arcade in a four-chamber view (upper left) and a two-chamber view (upper right), as well as the 3D image in the lower right panel, which shows the fused leaflets, chordae, and anterior papillary muscle. Image in the lower left shows the regurgitant jet in 3D, which is typical of this lesion. *Fig. 12-11 movie 2* shows the MPR images in real time, while *movie 3* shows the regurgitant jet. LA, left atrium; LV, left ventricle.

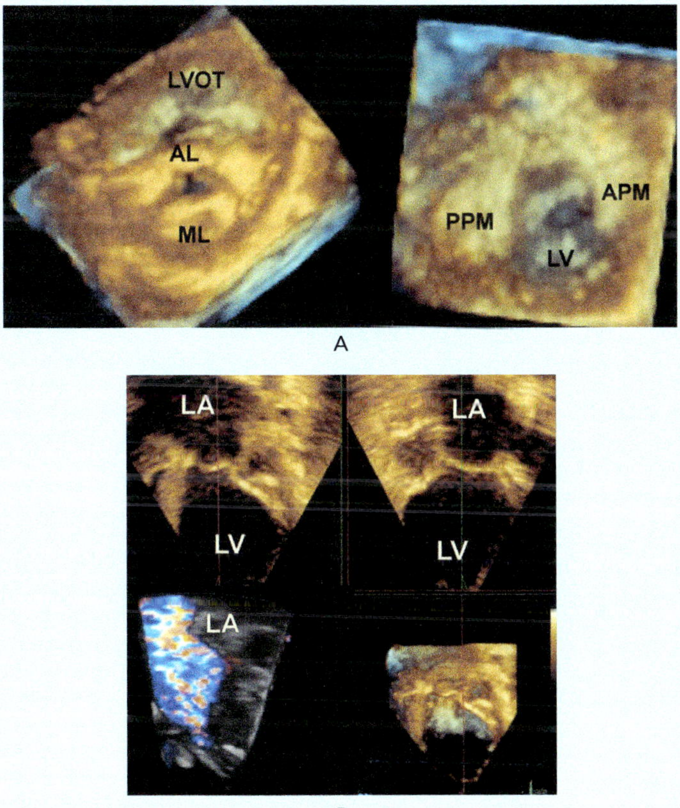

A

B

QUALITATIVE ASSESSMENT OF MITRAL VALVE STENOSIS

Color Doppler is a valuable modality in the qualitative assessment of mitral valve stenosis, particularly in helping locate the level of stenosis. It is unclear at this stage whether 3DE is superior to 2DE. From the four-chamber view, if the aliasing starts above the annulus, then this usually signifies associated supramitral valve stenosis (Fig. 12-10). Conversely, in some cases there is laminar flow at the annular level and down into the orifice, with the turbulence starting midway or lower owing to a fibrous ridge that is attached to the leaflets, protruding into the lumen of the valve. Also, by both techniques, the eccentric nature of the orifices can be appreciated, with jets of color emanating from the sides of the valve leaflets.

QUANTITATIVE ASSESSMENT OF MITRAL STENOSIS

In children, the most reliable technique for quantitative assessment of mitral stenosis thus far has been calculation of the mean gradient by continuous-wave Doppler.[40] Pressure half-time calculation is less useful owing to the higher heart rates in children, although this technique can be used in older adolescents with slower heart rates.[41] In the older age group, pressure half-time and valve area correlate well. Although pediatric echocardiographers use mean gradient assessment, this approach is highly dependent on cardiac output, which limits its value in clinical practice. Also, if there is associated mitral valve regurgitation, the mean gradient overestimates the severity of stenosis.

3DE has contributed to a reliable assessment of mitral orifice area in patients with rheumatic heart disease, in whom the restrictive orifice can be imaged in the axial plane from an apical four-chamber full-volume data set. For several reasons, similar data are not available in patients with congenital mitral valve stenosis. First, congenital mitral valve stenosis is a rare lesion, particularly in isolation. Second, it is unusual to have accurate hemodynamic correlations as to the severity, as most pediatric patients do not undergo hemodynamic evaluation. Finally, the lesion is anatomically different from its acquired counterpart, because the mechanism of stenosis is usually fusion of the chordae, such that there are often multiple orifices that are eccentric. Although this anatomical detail is important, it limits the ability to measure orifice area and obtain quantitative data.

REFERENCES

1. García-Orta R, Moreno E, Vidal M, et al. Three-dimensional versus two-dimensional transesophageal echocardiography in mitral valve repair. *J Am Soc Echocardiogr*. 2007;20(1):4–12.
2. Patel V, Hsiung MC, Nanda NC, et al. Usefulness of live/real time three-dimensional transthoracic echocardiography in the identification of individual segment/scallop prolapse of the mitral valve. *Echocardiography*. 2006;23(6):513–518.
3. Pepi M, Tamborini G, Maltagliati A, et al. Head-to head comparison of two-and three-dimensional transthoracic and transesophageal echocardiography in the localization of mitral valve. *J Am Coll Cardiol*. 2006;48(12):2524–2530.
4. Müller S, Müller L, Laufer G, et al. Comparison of three-dimensional imaging to transesophageal echocardiography for preoperative evaluation in mitral valve prolapse. *Am J Cardiol*. 2006;98(2):243–248.
5. Carlhäll C, Wigström L, Heiberg E, et al. Contribution of mitral annular excursion and shape dynamics to total left ventricular volume change. *Am J Physiol Heart Circ Physiol*. 2004;287(4):H1836–H1841.
6. Kwan J, Qin JX, Popović ZB, et al. Geometric changes of mitral annulus assessed by real-time 3-dimensional echocardiography: becoming enlarged and less nonplanar in the anteroposterior direction during systole in proportion to global left ventricular systolic function. *J Am Soc Echocardiogr*. 2004;17(11):1179–1184.
7. Lansac E, Lim KH, Shomura Y, et al. Dynamic balance of the aortomitral junction. *J Thorac Cardiovasc Surg*. 2002;123(5):911–918.
8. Nii M, Roman KS, Macgowan CK, Smallhorn JF. Insight into normal mitral and tricuspid annular dynamics in pediatrics: a real-time three-dimensional echocardiographic study. *J Am Soc Echocardiogr*. 2005;18(8):805–814.
9. Salgo IS, Gorman JH 3rd, Gorman RC, et al. Effect of annular shape on leaflet curvature in reducing mitral leaflet stress. *Circulation*. 2002;106(6):711–717.
10. Veronesi F, Corsi C, Sugeng L, et al. A study of functional anatomy of aortic-mitral valve coupling using 3D matrix transesophageal echocardiography. *Circ Cardiovasc Imaging*. 2009;2(1):24–31.

11. Takehashi K, Mackie AS, Rebeyka IM, et al. Two-dimensional versus transthoracic real-time three-dimensional echocardiography in the evaluation of the mechanisms and sites of atrioventricular valve regurgitation in a congenital heart disease population. *J Am Soc Echocardiogr.* 2010;23(7):726–734.
12. Lam JH, Ranganathan N, Wigle ED, Silver MD. Morphology of the human mitral valve. I. Chordae tendineae: a new classification. *Circulation.* 1970;41(3):449–458.
13. Levine RA, Triulzi MO, Harrigan P, Weyman AE. The relationship of mitral annular shape to the diagnosis of mitral valve prolapse. *Circulation.* 1987;75(4):756–767.
14. Watanabe N, Ogasawara Y, Yamaura Y, et al. Quantification of mitral valve tenting in ischemic mitral valve regurgitation by transthoracic real-time three-dimensional echocardiography. *J Am Coll Cardiol.* 2005; 45(5):763–769.
15. Ruckman RN, Van Praagh R. Anatomic types of congenital mitral stenosis: report of 49 autopsy cases with consideration of diagnosis and surgical implications. *Am J Cardiol.* 1978;42(4):592–601.
16. Asante-Korang A, O'Leary PO, Anderson RH. Anatomy and echo of the normal and abnormal mitral valve. *Cardiol Young.* 2006;16(suppl 3):27–34.
17. Carpentier A, Branchini B, Cour JC, et al. Congenital malformations of the mitral valve in children. Pathology and surgical treatment. *J Thorac Cardiovasc Surg.* 1976;72(6):854–866.
18. Daliento L, Thiene G, Chirillo F, et al. Congenital mitral valve malformations: clinical and morphological aspects [in Italian]. *G Ital Cardiol.* 1991;21(11):1205–1216.
19. Kohl T, Silverman N. Comparison of cleft and papillary muscle position in cleft mitral valve and atrioventricular septal defect. *Am J Cardiol.* 1996;77(2):164–169.
20. Sigfússon G, Ettedgui JA, Silverman NH, Anderson RH. Is a cleft in the anterior leaflet of an otherwise normal mitral valve an atrioventricular canal malformation. *J Am Coll Cardiol.* 1995;26(2):508–515.
21. Smallhorn JF, De Leval M, Stark J, et al. Isolated anterior mitral cleft. Two dimensional echocardiographic assessment and differentiation from "clefts" associated with atrioventricular septal defect. *Br Heart J.* 1982;48(2):109–116.
22. Fraisse A, Massih TA, Kreitmann B, et al. Characteristics of cleft mitral valve. *J Am Coll Cardiol.* 2003;42(11):1988–1993.
23. Wenink ACG, Gittenberger-de Groot AC, Brom AG. Developmental considerations of mitral valve anomalies. *Int J Cardiol.* 1986;11(1):85–98.
24. Otero Coto E, Quero Jimenez M, Deverall PB, Bain H. Anomalous mitral 'cleft' with abnormal ventriculo-arterial connection: anatomical findings and surgical implications. *Pediatr Cardiol.* 1984;5(1):1–6.
25. Aeba R, Katogi T, Takeuchi S, Kawada S. Surgical management of the straddling mitral valve in the biventricular heart. *Ann Thorac Surg.* 2000;69(1):130–134.
26. Serraf A, Nakamura T, Lacour-Gayet F, et al. Surgical approaches for double-outlet right ventricle or transposition of the great arteries with straddling atrioventricular valves. *J Thorac Cardiovasc Surg.* 1996;111(3):527–535.
27. Kalangos A, Oberhansli I, Baldovinos A, et al. Hypoplasia of the posterior leaflet as a rare cause of congenital mitral insufficiency. *J Card Surg.* 1997;12(5):339–342.
28. Anwar AM, McGhie JS, Meijboom FJ, Ten Cate FJ. Double orifice mitral valve by real-time three-dimensional echocardiography. *Eur J Echocardiogr.* 2008;9(5):731–732.
29. Freed LA, Levy D, Levine RA, et al. Prevalence and clinical outcome of mitral-valve prolapse. *N Engl J Med.* 1999;341(1):1–7.
30. Sugeng L, Shernan SK, Salgo IS, et al. Live three-dimensional transesophageal echocardiography: initial experience using a full-sampled matrix array probe. *J Am Coll Cardiol.* 2008;52(6):446–449.
31. Agricols E, Oppizzi M, De Bonis M, et al. American Society of Echocardiography. Multiplane transesophageal echocardiography performed according to the guidelines of the American Society of Echocardiography in patients with mitral valve prolapse, flail, and endocarditis: diagnostic accuracy in the identification of mitral regurgitant defects by correlation with surgical findings. *J Am Soc Echocardiogr.* 2003;16(1):61–66.
32. Zoghbi WA, Enriquez-Sarano M, Foster E, et al. American Society of Echocardiography. Recommendations for evaluation of the severity of native valvar regurgitation with two dimensional and Doppler echocardiography. *J Am Soc Echocardiogr.* 2003;16(7):777–802.
33. Sugeng L, Weinert BS, Lang RM. Real time 3-dimensional color Doppler flow of mitral and tricuspid valve regurgitation: feasibility and initial quantitative comparison with 2-dimensional methods. *J Am Soc Echocardiogr.* 2007;20(9):1050–1057.
34. Little SH, Igo SR, Pirat B, et al. In vitro validation of real-time three-dimensional color Doppler echocardiography for direct measurement of proximal isovelocity surface area in mitral regurgitation. *Am J Cardiol.* 2007;99(10):1440–1447.
35. Yosefy C, Levine RA, Solis J, et al. Proximal flow convergence region as assessed by real-time 3-dimensional echocardiography: challenging the hemispheric assumption. *J Am Soc Echocardiogr.* 2007;20(4):389–396.

36. Chao K, Moises VA, Shandas R, et al. Influence of the Coanda effect on color Doppler jet area and color encoding. In vitro studies using color Doppler flow mapping. *Circulation*. 1992;85(1):333–341.
37. Buck T, Plicht P, Hurold P, et al. Broad-beam spectral Doppler sonification of the vena contracta using matrix-array technology : a new solution for semi-automated quantification of mitral regurgitant flow volume and orifice area. *J Am Coll Cardiol*. 2005;45(5):770–779.
38. Sullivan ID, Robinson PJ, de Leval M, am TP Jr. Membranous supravalvular mitral stenosis: a treatable form of congenital heart disease. *J Am Coll Cardiol*. 1986;8(1):159–164.
39. Collins-Nakai RL, Rosenthal A, Castaneda AR, et al. Congenital mitral stenosis. A review of 20 years' experience. *Circulation*. 1977;56(6):1039–1046.
40. Banerjee A, Kohl T, Silverman NH. Echocardiographic evaluation of congenital mitral valve anomalies in children. *Am J Cardiol*. 1995;76(17):1284–1291.
41. Hatle L, Brubakk A, Tromsdal A, Angelsen B. Noninvasive assessment of pressure drop in mitral stenosis by Doppler ultrasound. *Br Heart J*. 1978;40(2):131–140.

CHAPTER 13

THREE-DIMENSIONAL ECHOCARDIOGRAPHIC ASSESSMENT OF THE TRICUSPID VALVE

Jeffrey F. Smallhorn, MBBS, FRACP, FRCP(C)

ABSTRACT

Three-dimensional echocardiography has and is still opening our eyes to the normal and abnormal anatomy and function of the tricuspid valve. An improved understanding of the tricuspid valve is going to be essential as patients survive into adult years with both congenital and acquired abnormalities of the tricuspid valve. Already this technique is invaluable in planning both primary and secondary surgical procedures of the tricuspid valve.

INTRODUCTION

The tricuspid valve has been the poor cousin of the mitral valve with regards to a detailed understanding, morphological description, pathology, and noninvasive evaluation. Those involved in congenital heart disease have had a greater interest, particularly as it is problematic in those patients with hypoplastic left heart syndrome who are on a Norwood/Fontan track, patients with complete or congenitally corrected transposition, Ebsteins malformation, tricuspid valve dysplasia, and secondary abnormalities related to right ventricular dilatation or damage from prior surgery to the right ventricular outflow tract +/– closure of a ventricular septal defect.

NORMAL ANATOMY

As with the mitral valve an understanding of the normal anatomy is an important starting point. Unlike its mitral counterpart the tricuspid annulus is elliptical in shape, with lateral annular forces being greater than in an antero-posterior direction (Fig. 13-1). This data has been gleaned from three-dimensional echocardiographic (3DE) assessment of normal mitral and tricuspid function in a pediatric population where it is possible to acquire simultaneous mitral and tricuspid annular data. The tricuspid annulus is also completely surrounded by muscle, unlike the mitral valve which has an area of fibrous continuity between it and the aortic outflow tract. The annulus is also shaped like a saddle, with two high and two low points, which like the mitral valve are important to minimize leaflet stress (Fig. 13-1). As well the dynamic annular changes are relatively homogenous, unlike the normal mitral valve (Fig. 13-2). The greater lateral forces maintain the elliptical

Figure 13-1

This illustration shows the elliptical nature of the tricuspid annulus, which is maintained by increased lateral forces, as indicated by the black arrows. As well the right hand picture demonstrates the saddle shape of the tricuspid annulus. AO, aorta; PA, pulmonary artery; RVOT, right ventricular outflow tract; TV, tricuspid valve.

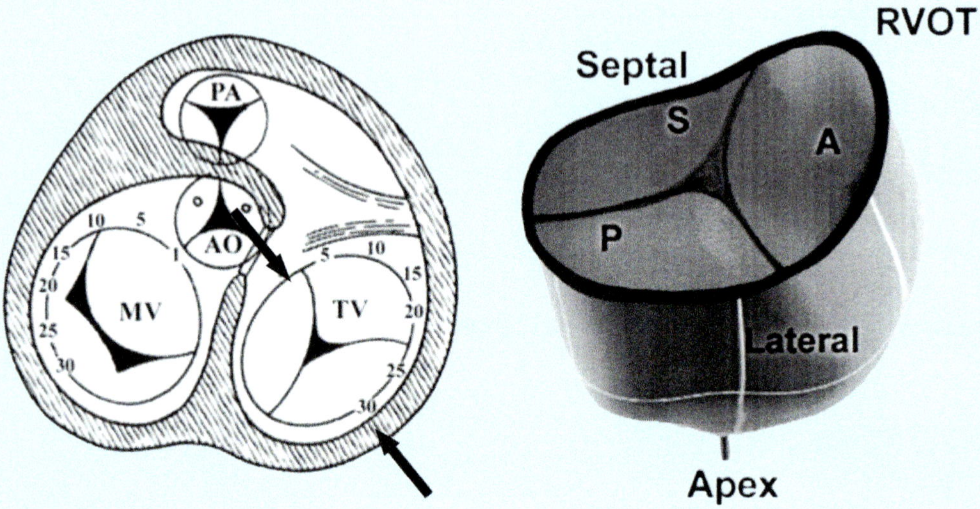

Figure 13-2

This graph represents the diameter change of each segment of the tricuspid valve in one cardiac cycle. Note the change is homogeneous.

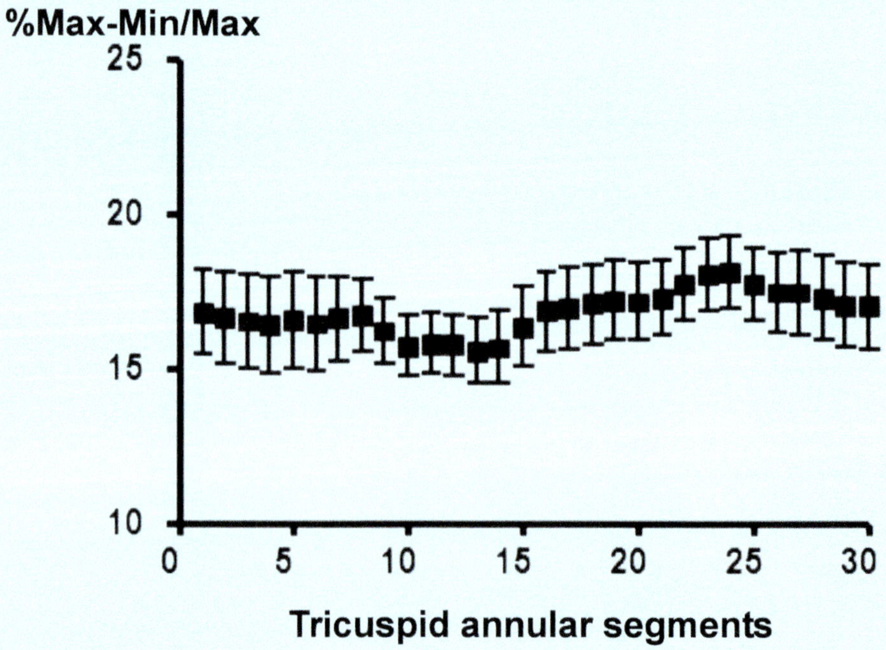

shape which is probably essential to maintain leaflet competency. The explanation for this may well be related to the fact that although the septal leaflet is very large it is supported by relatively short chordae that insert directly into the septum rather than by well-defined individual papillary muscles. The septal leaflet may also have a series of small clefts which may or may not be supported by chords. As a result the septal leaflet is relatively immobile when compared to the anterior and posterior leaflets of the tricuspid valve, or indeed both leaflets of the mitral valve. The anterior leaflet is supported by a large papillary muscle which usually inserts into the moderator band, again with some variability in insertion site (Fig. 13-3). This leaflet has further support in the vicinity of the anteroseptal commissure from the papillary muscle of the conus. The support of the posterior leaflet is less consistent, though there is usually a smaller more posteriorly situated muscle. There is also a variable commissure between the anterior and posterior leaflets, which may be well formed or almost completely fused (Fig. 13-3). The attachments to the anterior papillary muscle may also cross this commissure in some hearts.

What is evident is that unlike the mitral valve, its tricuspid counterpart has considerable anatomical variability, even in the normal heart. Understanding the nature of the leaflets provides part of the explanation as to why the annulus is elliptical in shape. The large size and relative immobility of the septal leaflet act as a door-jam against the more mobile anterior and posterior leaflets. If the annulus was more circular in shape, then this relationship would be less than ideal, resulting in poor leaflet coaptation and regurgitation. Indeed this is encountered clinically in volume and pressure loaded morphological right ventricles.

Figure 13-3

These two specimens demonstrate the pathology of the tricuspid valve. The image on the left is seen with the front of the right ventricle removed. Note the anterior leaflet is attached to a large papillary muscle that inserted into the moderator band. As well, the asterisk shows the papillary muscle of the conus, which supports the anteroseptal commissure. AL, anterior leaflet; AO, aorta; APM, anterior papillary muscle; MB, moderator band; PL, posterior leaflet; SL, septal leaflet.

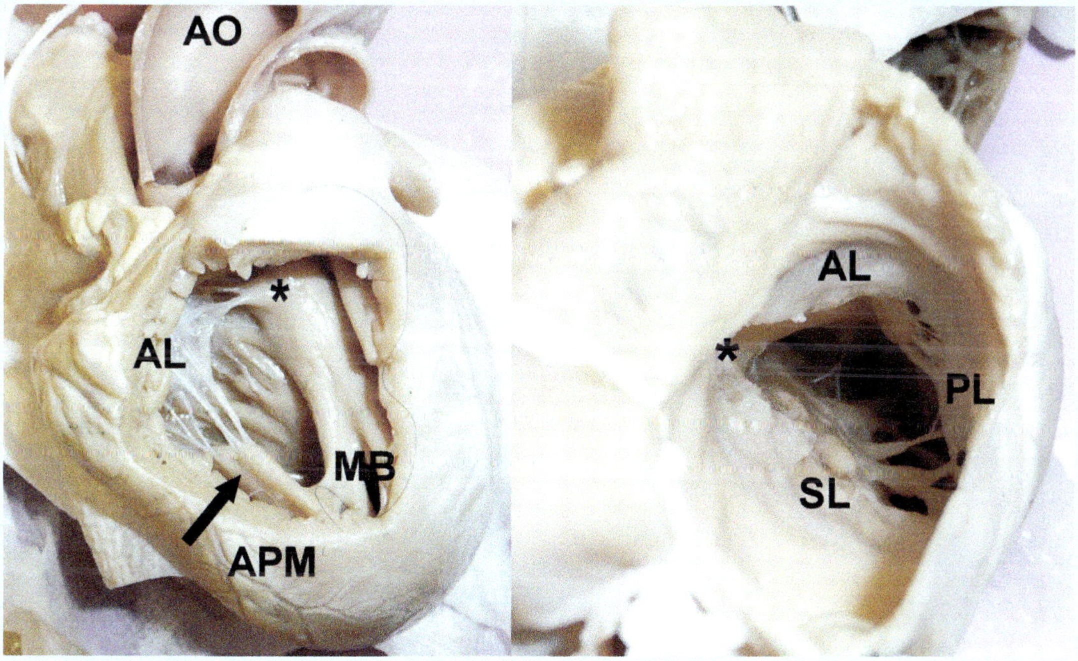

IMAGING THE TRICUSPID VALVE

Two-dimensional echocardiography (2DE) provides an incomplete assessment of the tricuspid valve, in particular an assessment of the commissures. It is difficult to determine where the anterior leaflet ends and the posterior starts as imaging the commissure between the two is a challenge. From the apical four chamber view with the transducer tilted toward the left ventricular outflow tract the anterior leaflet is seen, while from the same position, angling more posteriorly toward the coronary sinus the inferior leaflet is imaged. What is challenging is the area between the two, particularly as the size of the anterior and posterior leaflets can vary in the normal heart. As a result it is almost impossible to image the commissure between the two leaflets. Although it is possible to image the septal leaflet from a variety of views, identifying the various scallops in the leaflet, along with their chordal support apparatus, is a challenge.

Three-dimensional echocardiography overcomes most of these limitations, as the tricuspid valve can be imaged in its entirety.[1] For the mitral valve the transesophageal approach provides the optimal imaging approach in the adult and older child. This is related to the orientation of the mitral valve which lies almost at right angles to the transducer beam, such that the valve is imaged in an axial plane, resulting in optimal resolution. The tricuspid valve lies obliquely to the transesophageal beam, such that valve imaging suffers from the challenges of lateral resolution.[2] This is more of an issue if the three-dimensional zoom mode is used for image acquisition, as the frame rates are lower. Full volume breath held acquisitions can help, but still result in suboptimal imaging compared to the mitral valve. As a result of this limitation image acquisition from the four chamber view, particularly with the transducer in a slightly more midline location provides the optimal imaging plane. The exception to this is in functionally single ventricle hearts with a dominant morphological right ventricle, post Mustard or Senning procedure, or in hearts with corrected transposition. Once the full volume data set is acquired it is best to orient from one of two views. The enface view should be imaged in the surgical orientation with the location of the aortic root in the upper left hand quadrant (Fig. 13-4). It is also useful to image the valve from below, with the aorta being located in the upper right

Figure 13-4

These three-dimensional images demonstrate the tricuspid valve from above and below. The left hand image is from below and shows the commissures as well as the leaflets. Note it is possible to identify all three leaflets of the tricuspid valve. The video clips show the same features as the still images. AL, anterior leaflet; PL, posterior leaflet; SL, septal leaflet; TV, tricuspid valve.

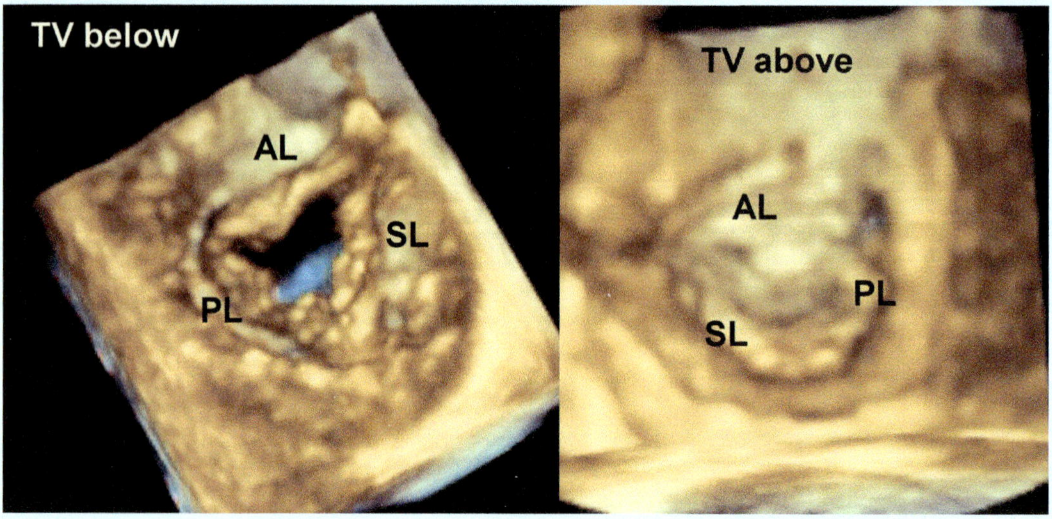

hand quadrant, when imaged by the echocardiographer (Fig. 13-4). As with the mitral valve, this provides optimal imaging of the commissures, as well as any clefts in the septal leaflet. It is also possible to image the attachment of the anterior leaflet to the papillary muscle of the conus (Figs. 13-3 and 13-4). The application of color Doppler helps determine the size and location of any regurgitant jets. As areas of dropout may occur at the hinge points with the tricuspid annulus, color Doppler is a valuable adjunct to confirm that these sites are not true defects in the leaflets (Fig. 13-5). Similarly in both normal and abnormal valves there are high points and low points, as leaflets are not flat (Fig. 13-4). In this setting the valleys usually appear darker and in many instances look like areas of dropout providing a challenge as to whether this is normal or represents a deficiency in the leaflet. Color Doppler is invaluable in this setting, as if there is no regurgitant jet at such a site then it just represents the normal morphology of that particular valve. Three-dimensional echocardiography is also more accurate in defining sites of regurgitation than either its two-dimensional counterpart, or saline testing at the time of surgical evaluation.[3] This is understandable as color Doppler provides a physiological evaluation, unlike saline testing.

Three-dimensional echocardiography also permits a more quantitative approach to the assessment of the tricuspid valve. By extracting the coordinates from the various components of the valve, dynamic annular geometry, leaflet motion, and papillary muscle location can be quantified.[4] Of interest using 3DE the papillary muscle angle in relationship to the annulus can be determined.[5,6] As well, these relationships can be

Figure 13-5

This montage is in the MPR mode and shows the tricuspid valve in both two- and three-dimensional formats. The lower left hand panel shows the color Doppler signal in three-dimensions, demonstrating that the regurgitant jet involves both the central part of the valve, as well as toward the anteroseptal commissure. The video clips show the tricuspid regurgitation in real-time. ANT, anterior leaflet; POST, posterior leaflet; RA, right atrium; RV, right ventricle; SEPT, septal leaflet.

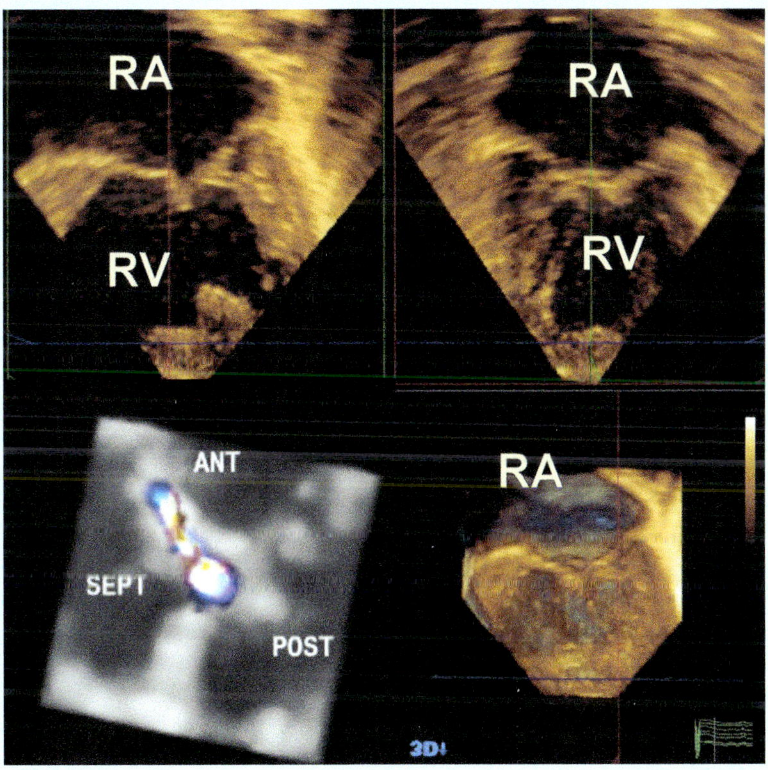

determined through the application of three-dimensional sonomicrometry crystals in animals.[7] This angle is approximately 90°, and is the same as has been measured using sonomicrometry crystals in an experimental animal model. An accurate knowledge of this relationship is important when attempting to understand mechanisms of valve failure.

ABNORMALITIES OF THE TRICUSPID VALVE

- *Tricuspid valve dysplasia*: can be seen in isolation, particularly in the fetal and neonatal periods, or can be associated with other congenital abnormalities, in particular pulmonary atresia and intact ventricular septum. The leaflets are usually thickened, deficient, and tethered, with areas of poor coaptation resulting in regurgitation (**Fig. 13-6**). The tethering is usually due to shortened chordae limiting the mobility of the anterior and posterior leaflets, such that they cannot abut against their septal counterpart. When imaged by 2DE the lack of mobility can be appreciated from the apical four chamber view, with the site of coaptation being below the level of the tricuspid annulus. In this setting the regurgitant jet usually appears to be in a central location. What is difficult to appreciate are abnormalities of the commissures, as well as the shape of the regurgitant jet. Three-dimensional echocardiography overcomes this limitation, as well providing optimal imaging of the commissures, particularly from the right ventricular aspect. Many of the regurgitant jets follow the lines of the commissures, so are quite irregular, limiting any quantitative approach by the PISA method (**Fig. 13-6A**). As well, although there is a good correlation between two- and three-dimensional echocardiographic vena contracta width and area, it is only the latter that correlates well with valve failure in a multivariate analysis.
- *Tricuspid valve prolapse*: has been a difficult entity to diagnose by 2DE, as there has been a poor understanding of annular shape with its high and low points, lack of correlative studies, and in general lack of interest. Those involved with congenital heart disease have been more interested, particularly in those hearts where the tricuspid valve is under systemic pressure. Even in this population defining prolapse has been difficult by two-dimensional imaging. As well, surgical definition of prolapse has been difficult, particularly as the valve is imaged in a nonphysiological mode. Indeed, in a correlative study both two- and three-dimensional techniques underestimated the presence of prolapse compared to surgical inspection.[3] This most likely relates to a lack of definition by the surgeons, rather than the echocardiographers. Primary congenital prolapse is unusual apart from patients with abnormalities of elastin. Acquired prolapse is more common, either secondary to surgical closure of a ventricular septal defect, balloon dilatation of pulmonary valve stenosis, or due to probable subendocardial ischemia and papillary muscle dysfunction. Three-dimensional echocardiographic quantitative methods can overcome this problem, and provide accurate quantitative information.[6] In the pediatric population the amount of "normal" tricuspid valve prolapse has been calculated, and can be used to compare those with valve failure where pathological prolapse is a mechanism of regurgitation.[3] The next logical step in the process is determining degrees of prolapse and how they can be factored into valve repair. For this to happen there has to be a close working relationship between surgeons, cardiologists, and engineers. Although a quantitative approach is ideal, valuable qualitative data can be gleaned from 3DE and factored into the decision-making process for valve repair. A data set acquired from the apical view usually provides all the necessary information. Enface views from above and below can be used, but are currently limited by viewing images on a flat screen. This limitation can be overcome by those centers that have the ability to image in three-dimensional cave, but this is still experimental, with difficulties in importing some of the data sets into such systems. Certainly this will be the imaging method of the future. This current limitation can be overcome by obtaining a full volume data set from the four chamber view and then imaging the three-dimensional data set from the side. By this approach it is possible to image the annulus and leaflets from multiple views, and determine the precise site of prolapse (**Fig. 13-7**).
- *Functional abnormalities of the tricuspid valve*: are being encountered more frequently. These are seen in hearts where there is secondary dilatation of the tricuspid valve annulus due to associated

Figure 13-6A and B

A, This monatage demonstrates the features of a dysplastic tricuspid valve as seen in the MPR mode. The bottom left hand panel is a view of the tricuspid valve from above and demonstrates the site of regurgitation. The video clip 3D VC above shows the anterior regurgitant jet, while the 2D video clip entitled 2D col compare reg shows the regurgitation using two-dimensional echo. The video clip 3D 4ch teth TV shows the tethered tricuspid valve leaflets in a 3D four chamber view. AL, anterior leaflet; PL, posterior leaflet; RA, right atrium; RV, right ventricle; SL, septal leaflet. *B*, This montage demonstrates a dysplastic tricuspid valve as seen from above (left hand panel) and below (right hand panel). The video clips entitled 3D TV above and 3D TV labels show the enface views of the tricuspid valve from above and below respectively. AL, anterior leaflet; AO, aorta; PL, posterior leaflet; SL, septal leaflet.

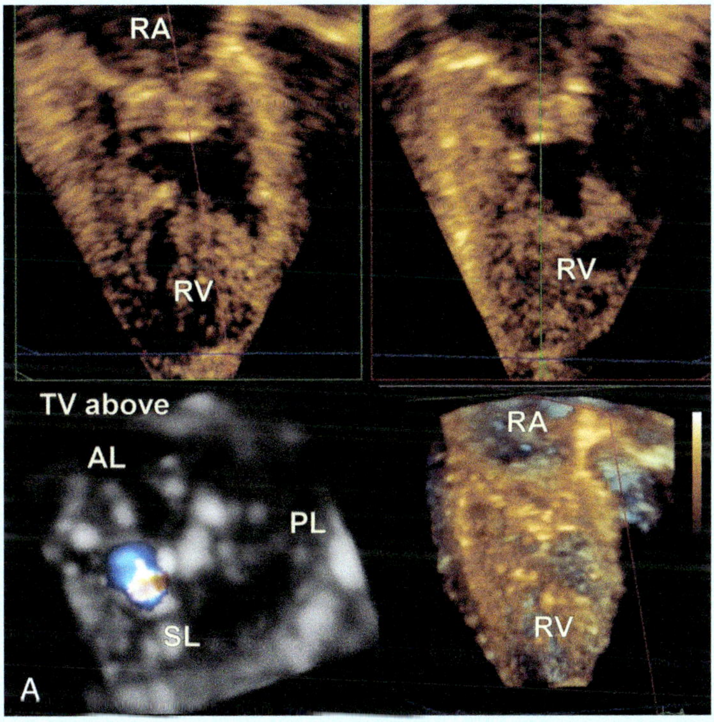

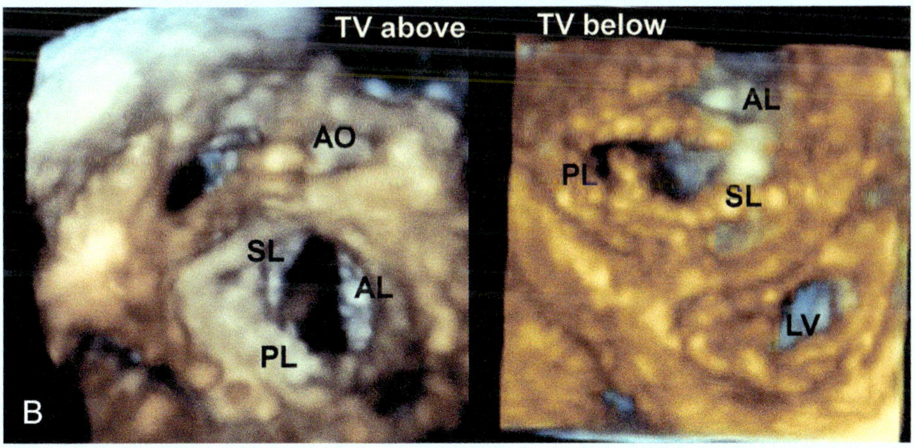

Figure 13-7

This montage is from a patient who underwent a Norwood/Sano procedure for hypoplastic left heart syndrome and subsequently developed tricuspid valve prolapse. The prolapse involves the anterior leaflet of the tricuspid valve and is seen in the left hand panel. The color Doppler signal shows the regurgitant jet, as seen from above. The video clips show the anterior prolapse of the tricuspid valve by two- and three-dimensional echo. ANT, anterior; POST, posterior; RA, right atrium; RV, right ventricle; SEPTAL, septal; TV, tricuspid valve.

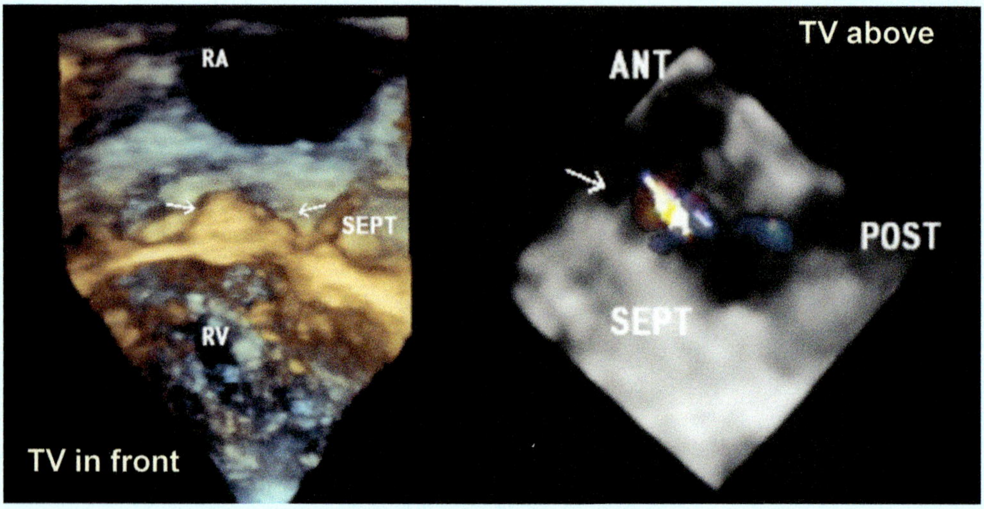

pulmonary valve regurgitation, pulmonary hypertension, or as a result of surgical damage at the time of ventricular septal defect repair,[8–10] The underlying pathology is often a combination of leaflet tethering and prolapse which are compounded by associated annular dilatation (**Fig. 13-8A** and **B**). In hearts with pulmonary hypertension leaflet tethering is often a mechanism responsible for tricuspid regurgitation, and is exacerbated by a more circular annulus due to the high right ventricular pressure. In those with a low pressure volume loaded right ventricle annular dilatation is usually the responsible mechanism for regurgitation, resulting in zones of poor coaptation along the areas of valve closure. In hearts where a ventricular septal defect has been previously closed leaflet damage in the vicinity of the anteroseptal commissure is often the mechanism responsible for the regurgitation, while in others it is due to surgical tethering of the septal leaflet. Our interventional colleagues are also responsible for some tricuspid valve trauma at the time of balloon dilatation of obstructive lesions of the right ventricular outflow tract. The most vulnerable component of the tricuspid valve is in the region of the anteroseptal commissure with avulsion of the papillary muscle of the conus resulting in tricuspid valve prolapsed in that region. 3DE is invaluable in helping to sort out the mechanisms of valve failure and determine the precise sites of regurgitation. The various imaging methods described in the previous sections can be applied to hearts with secondary tricuspid valve regurgitation. An improved understanding of the mechanisms of tricuspid valve failure through echocardiography[11] is beneficial in decision making with regards to repair versus replacement of the tricuspid valve.[12]

- *Ebsteins malformation of the tricuspid valve*: By definition this involves both leaflet displacement and dysplasia and is encountered in the fetus or newborn, which usually represents the more severe spectrum, to the older patient who presents with a murmur or supraventricular tachycardia. The septal leaflet is always displaced, with less variability in the posterior leaflet. The anterior leaflet is never displaced, however may have distal linear attachments to the anterior wall of the right ventricle,

Figure 13-8A and B

A, This three-dimensional image is from a postoperative case with a dilated poorly functioning right ventricle, with tethering of the tricuspid valve. The restriction of the valve is best appreciated in the real-time video clips entitled 3D front tethered and 3D TV below. The two-dimensional video clip entitled 2D 4c dil RV shows the features by two-dimensional echo. AL, anterior leaflet; PL, posterior leaflet; POT, pulmonary outflow tract; SL, septal leaflet. *B*, These images show the regurgitation of the tricuspid valve in the MPR mode, with the lower left hand image demonstrating the vena contracta in an enface view. The two video clips called 3D col MPR mode and 3D col TR above show the color Doppler imaging. ANT; anterior; POST, posterior; RA, right atrium; RV, right ventricle.

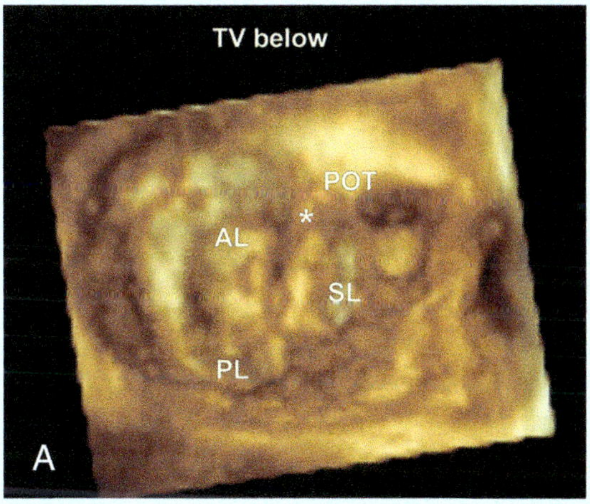

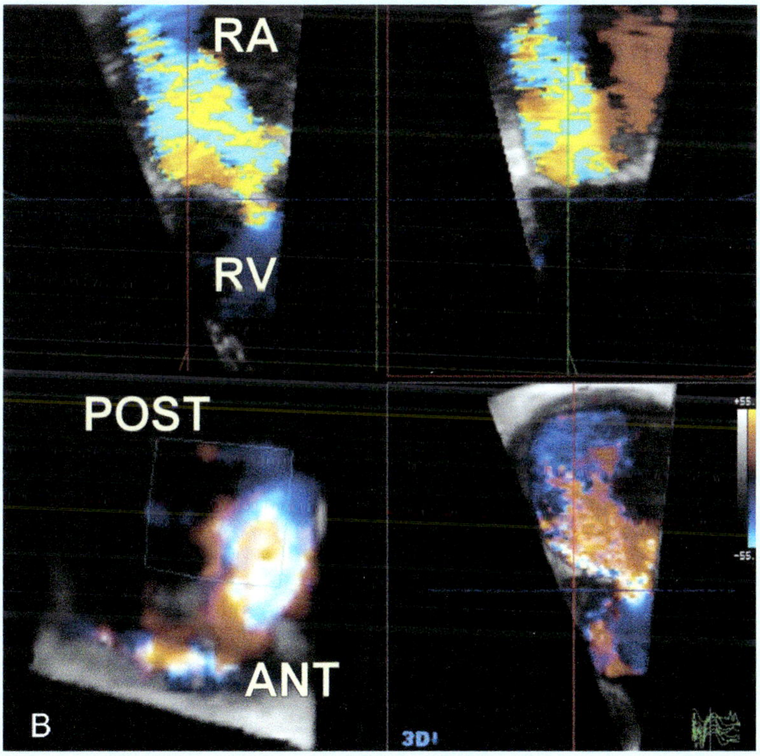

which in some cases result in obstruction to the right ventricular outflow tract (**Fig. 13-9**). As a result the true right ventricle may be much smaller than the atrialized component. As a result of the displacement the functional orifice of the tricuspid valve is oriented more toward the right ventricular outflow (**Fig. 13-9**). Associated tricuspid valve regurgitation is variable and tends to be more severe in those hearts with significant displacement and dysplasia (**Fig. 13-10**). The right atrium is frequently thin walled and patulous, resulting in significant cardiomegaly. Two-dimensional echocardiography has been the main mode of diagnosis in this lesion providing reliable and accurate data upon which most clinical decisions are made. Three-dimensional echocardiography can be challenged by this lesion, particularly in those hearts with very thin leaflets where considerable drop out occurs. As well, due to the abnormal orientation of the tricuspid valve it lies partly in the axial and lateral planes which impacts on image quality. In older patients the absolute size of the valve can limit the ability to image the whole valve in one full volume data set. Despite these limitations imaging the zones of leaflet coaptation as well as the true size and shape of the vena contracta in those with regurgitation is a valuable adjunct to two-dimensional imaging. The large sail like anterior leaflet can be imaged in the four chamber view, but as well its relationship to the right ventricular outflow tract is well appreciated in the subcostal view, with simultaneous imaging of the right ventricular outflow tract (**Fig. 13-11A**). It is also possible to obtain unique views of the tricuspid valve that can enhance our understanding of this lesion (**Fig. 13-11B**). As well it is possible with 3DE to determine the extent of the tricuspid regurgitation (**Fig. 13-11C**).

- *Tricuspid valve in corrected transposition*: is invariably dysplastic and occasionally displaced. The leaflets are frequently thickened with associated shortened chordae, resulting in leaflet tethering. When leaflet displacement is seen this often involves the posterior leaflet, unlike that seen in Ebsteins, where by definition it is always the septal leaflet (**Fig. 13-12A**). Tricuspid valve regurgitation is frequently encountered, if not at presentation later on as the child grows (**Fig. 13-12B**). The valve is under systemic

Figure 13-9

This montage is from a case with Ebsteins and significant distal linear attachments of the anterior leaflet. The keyhole orifice of the tricuspid valve is seen in the right hand picture, while the left hand one shows the distal linear attachments. The video clip entitled TV above 3D dist lin shows the same features as the still image. The video clip called atr RV 3D shows the true tricuspid annulus and the atrialized portion of the right ventricle. AO, aorta; TV, tricuspid valve; RV, right ventricle; RVOT, right ventricular outflow tract.

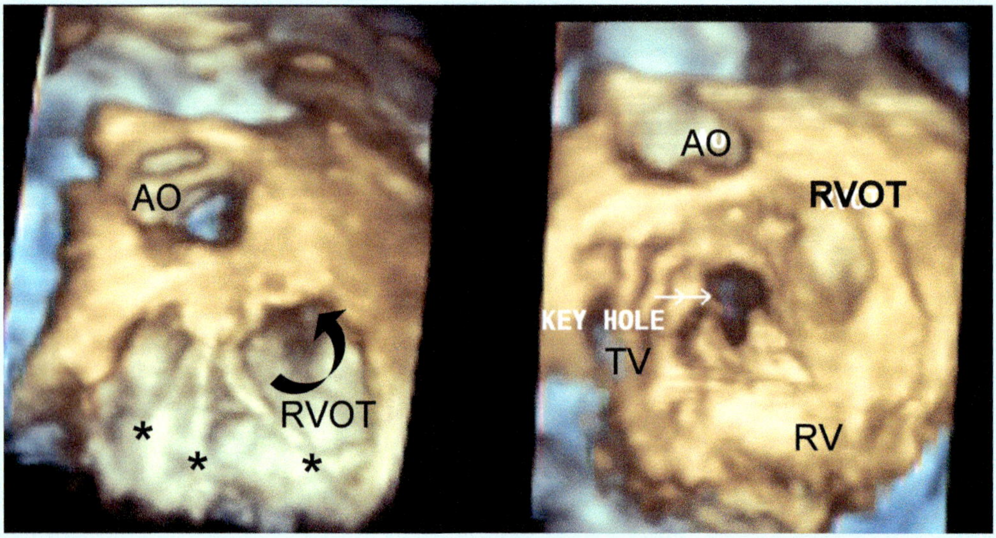

Figure 13-10A and B

A, The image on the left is a two-dimensional four chamber view of Ebsteins and significant tricuspid valve dysplasia. Note the thickened leaflets, a dilated right atrium, and septal leaflet displacement. The right hand image is a 3D image as seen from below demonstrating poor coaptation of the leaflets more posteriorly. The video clips called 2D 4ch and 2D 4ch reg show the dysplastic leaflets and the regurgitation. AL, anterior leaflet; PL, posterior leaflet; RA, right atrium; RV, right ventricle; SL, septal leaflet; TV, tricuspid valve. *B*, This is the same case as seen in Figure 13-10a, with a more anterior image in the left hand panel and more posterior in the right hand. Note the good coaptation anteriorly with a large gap between the leaflets posteriorly. The video clip called 3D TV below absent post leaf shows the same features. PL, posterior leaflet; RA, right atrium; RV, right ventricle; SL, septal leaflet.

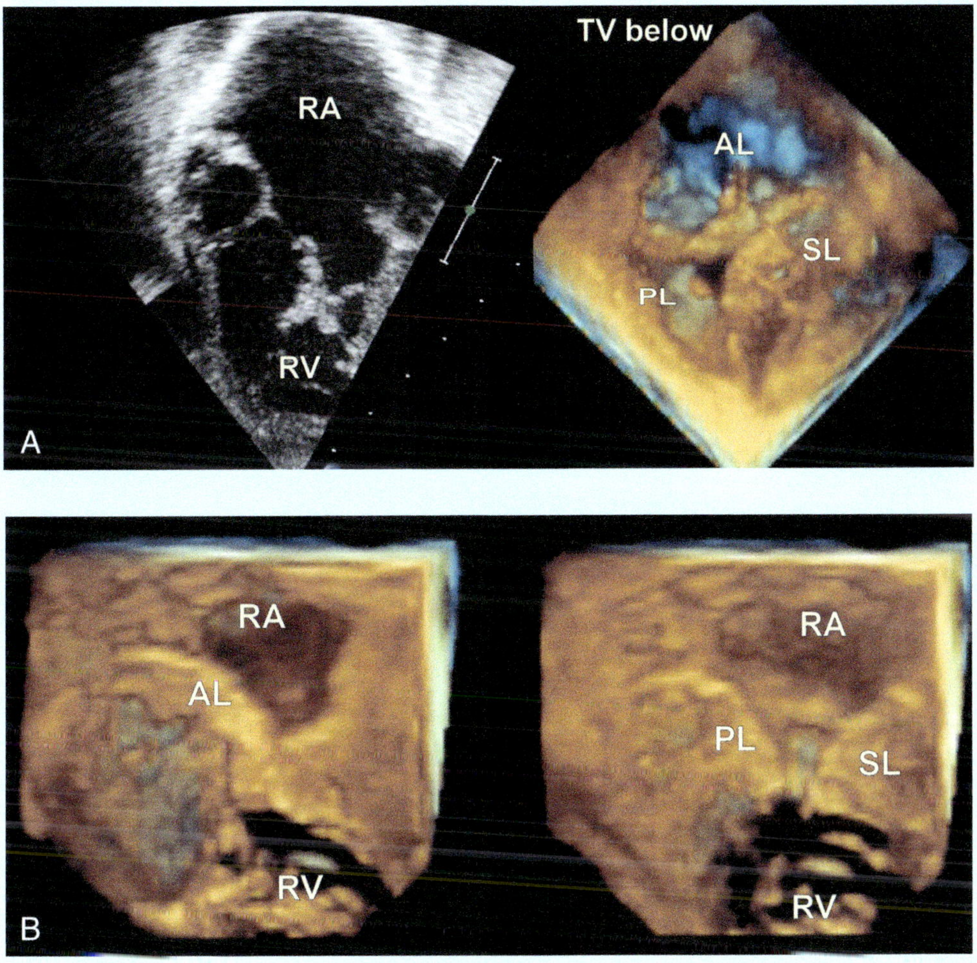

pressure, and a combination of a more circular annulus, in conjunction with leaflet dysplasia and chordal abnormalities, is responsible for the regurgitation. Regurgitation begets more regurgitation, as the dysplastic and tethered leaflets are unable to accommodate further annular dilatation, resulting in inadequate zones of apposition. Two-dimensional echocardiography can diagnose the lesion, however is surpassed by its three-dimensional counterpart when it comes to leaflet and commissural detail. Unlike the normal tricuspid valve which is not suited to imaging by a three-dimensional transesophageal approach, in corrected transposition the valve orientation is usually at right angles to the transducer beam in systole as a result of the more vertical orientation of the interventricular septum (**Fig. 13-13A–C**).

Figure 13-11A, B and C

A, This montage is from a patient with Ebsteins and a large sail like anterior leaflet, with minimal distal linear attachments. The left hand picture is the 3DE view of the anterior leaflet in a simulated right anterior oblique position. The right hand picture is the 2DE image of the anterior leaflet in the right anterior oblique view. The video clips called 3D RAO sail like ant leaf and RAO 2D show these features in real-time. The video clip called 4ch ant leaf TV shows the two-dimensional features in this case. AO, aorta; ALTV, anterior leaflet of tricuspid valve; PA, pulmonary artery; PLTV, posterior leaflet of the tricuspid valve; RA, right atrium; RV, right ventricle. *B*, This three-dimensional image is of the tricuspid valve Ebsteins as seen through the tricuspid orifice, being obtained from the subcostal view. Note the displaced septal leaflet with the larger anterior leaflet. The video clip called RAO view into TV orifice shows the same feature in real-time. AO, aorta; AL, anterior leaflet; PL, posterior leaflet; SL, septal leaflet. *C*, This montage shows the degree of tricuspid regurgitation. The right hand panel is in a four chamber view, while the left hand one images the vena contracta from below and shows that it is a small elliptical shaped jet. The video clips called 2D 4ch TR and 3D col TR 4ch show the regurgitation of the tricuspid valve. RA, right atrium; RV, right ventricle.

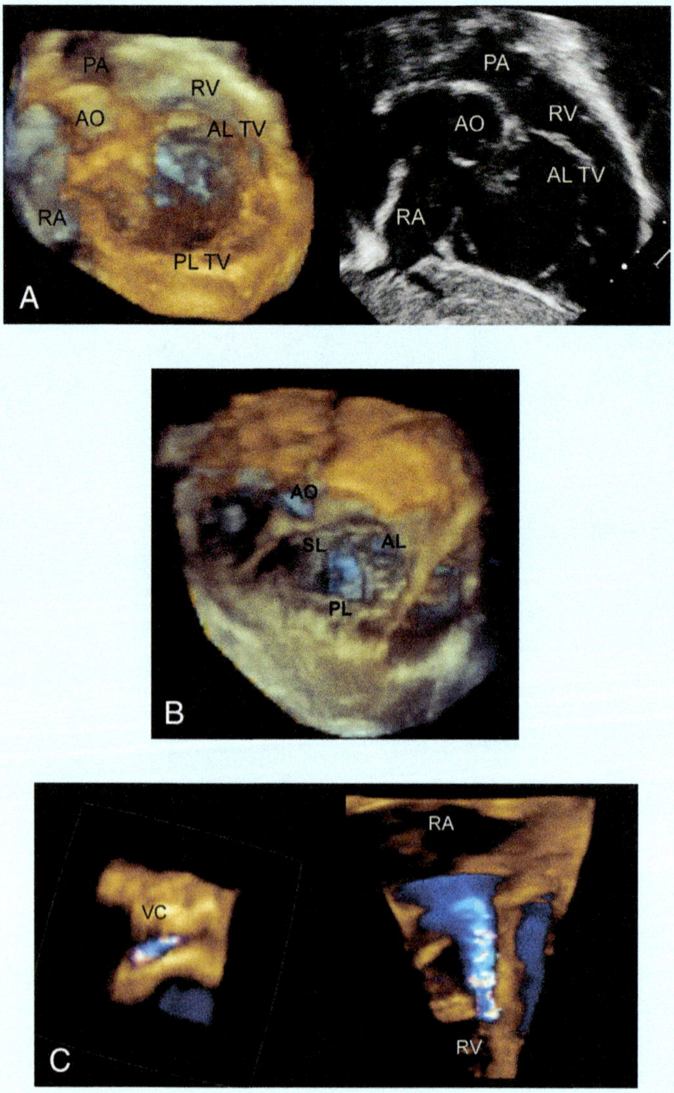

Figure 13-12A and B

A, These two images are from a case of corrected transposition with displacement and dysplasia of both the septal and posterior tricuspid valve leaflets. Note there is also associated mitral valve regurgitation. The video clips 2D 4ch TV1 and 2D 4ch TV col show the same features. LA, left atrium; LV, left ventricle; RA, right atrium; RV, right ventricle. *B*, This montage is from the same patient as Figure 13-12a. The left hand image is an enface view of the tricuspid valve which demonstrates the leaflets and the associated displacement and tethering. The right hand image is seen from below and shows the valve in systole with poor coaptation. The video clips 3D TV below 3 and 3D TR above show the three-dimensional features. AL, anterior leaflet; MLV, morphological left ventricle; MV, mitral valve; PL, posterior leaflet; SL, septal leaflet; TV, tricuspid valve.

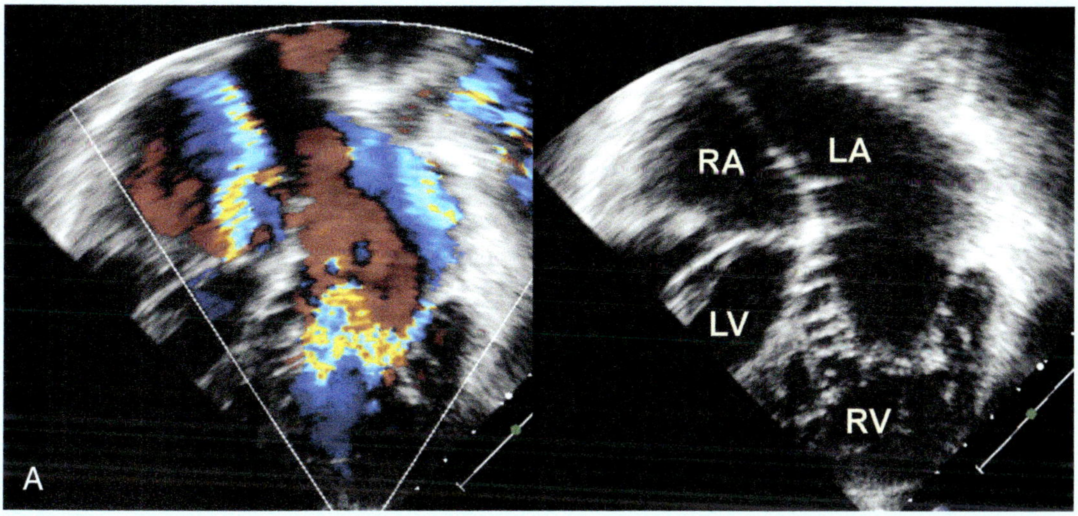

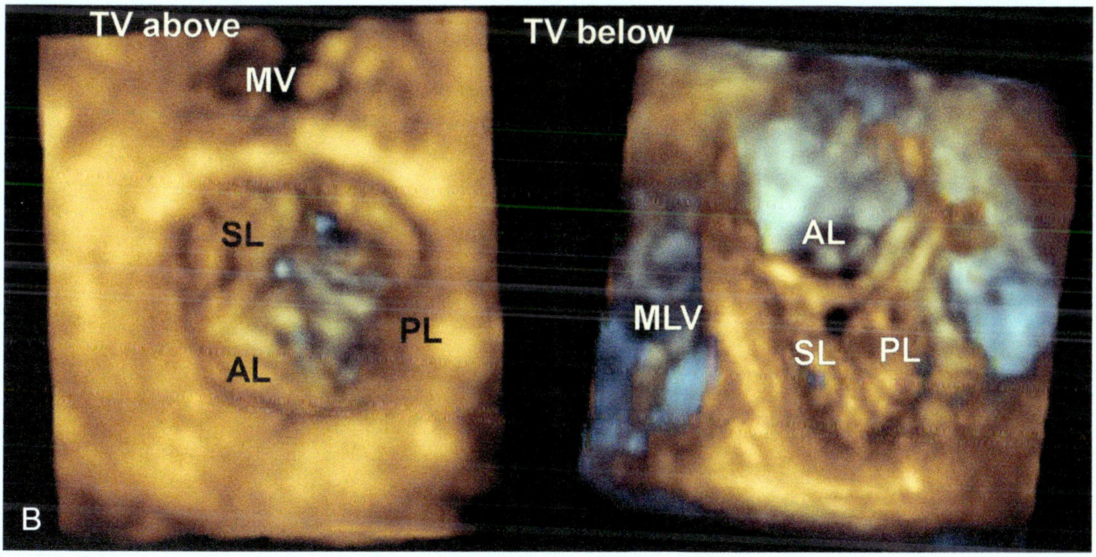

Figure 13-13A, B and C

A, This montage demonstrates the three-dimensional echo appearance of the tricuspid valve in corrected transposition by the transesophageal approach. The image on the right shows the commissures (asterisk), seen during diastole. The video clip 3D preop TV view 1 shows the valve in real-time from above. AL, anterior leaflet; PL, posterior leaflet; SL, septal leaflet. *B*, This MPR data set shows the more anterior aspect of the tricuspid valve in the upper left and right panel and the lower right panel. The lower left hand panel shows the tricuspid valve as seen from below. The video clip called 3D MPR ant cut TV shows the same features as in the still image. The video clip 3D preop TV below lower lev shows the tricuspid valve from below. ANT, anterior; LA, left atrium; PL, posterior leaflet; SL, septal leaflet. *C*, This MPR data set shows the site of the tricuspid regurgitation which is in the anterior aspect of the valve. The lower right hand picture is the three-dimensional enface view for orientation. The video clip called 3D col reg jet above 1 shows the site of the regurgitant jet from above. AL, anterior leaflet; LA, left atrium; POST, posteriror; PL, posterior leaflet; RV, right ventricle; SL, septal leaflet.

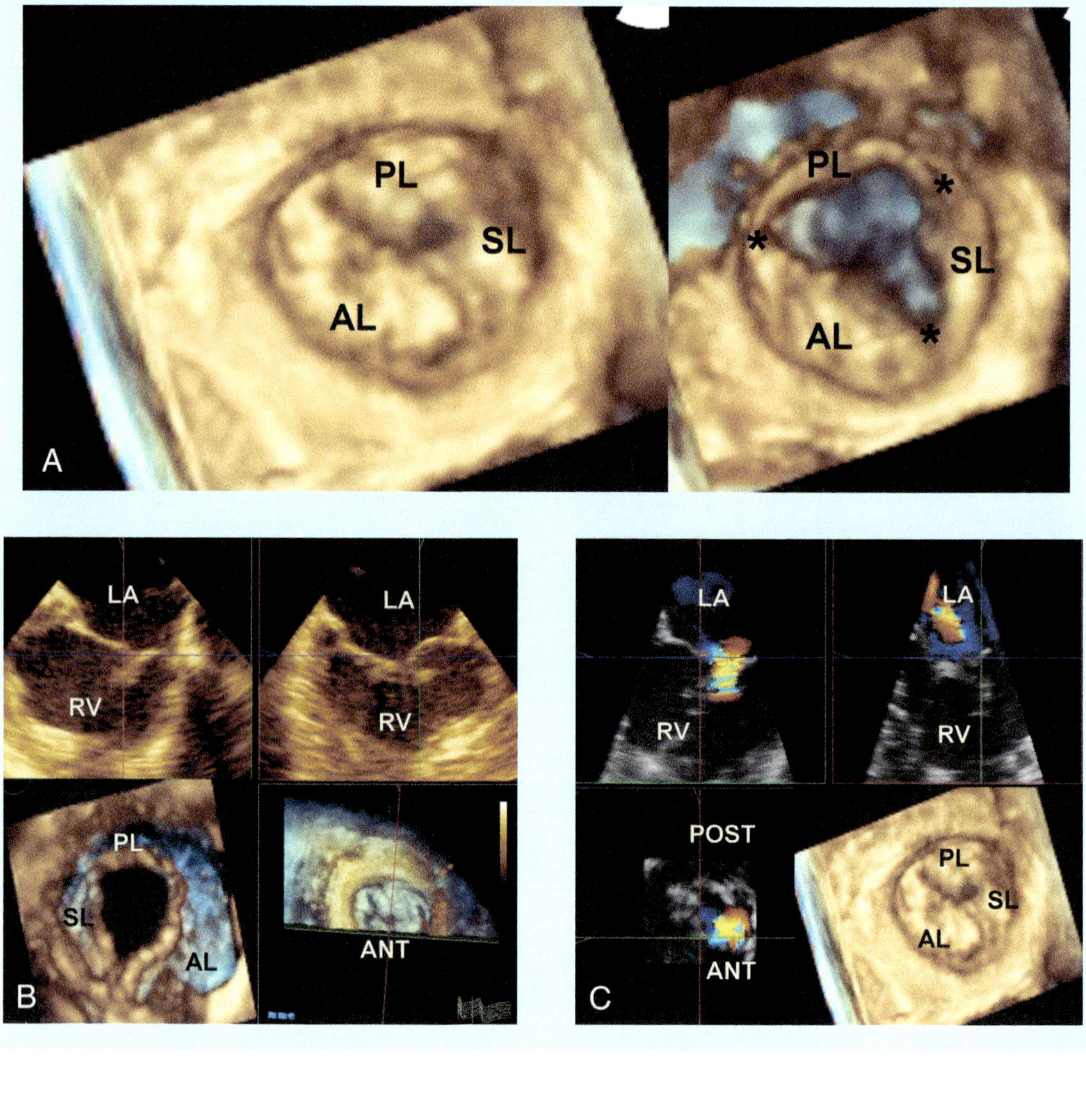

Figure 13-14A, B and C

A, Two-dimensional images of a straddling tricuspid valve. The left hand panel shows the septal leaflet straddling through a perimembranous ventricular septal defect into the left ventricle as indicated by the asterisk. The two video clips called 2D straddling TV SA and 2D subc stradd TV show these features in real-time. LA, left atrium; LV, left ventricle; RA, right atrium; RV, right ventricle. *B*, This three-dimensional long axis view shows the tricuspid valve straddling into the left ventricle. The leaflet inserts into a major papillary muscle in the left ventricle. The video clip calle 3D stradd TV above shows the same features as in the still. AO, aorta; LA, left atrium; MV, mitral valve; RV, right ventricle; TV, tricuspid valve; VSD, ventricular septal defect. *C*, These two images demonstrate the versatility of 3DE. The image on the left shows the right and left ventricle with part of the anterior wall removed such that the septal leaflet of the tricuspid valve is seen straddling the ventricular septal defect (asterisk). The image on the right is a similar short axis view as in *A*, but the added depth from three-dimensional echo provides greater definition of the tricuspid valve. The two video clips called 3D subc pap through VSD 1 and 3D subc stradd TV show the straddling tricuspid valve by three-dimensional echo. LV, left ventricle; MV, mitral valve; RV, right ventricle; S, interventricular septum; TV, tricuspid valve.

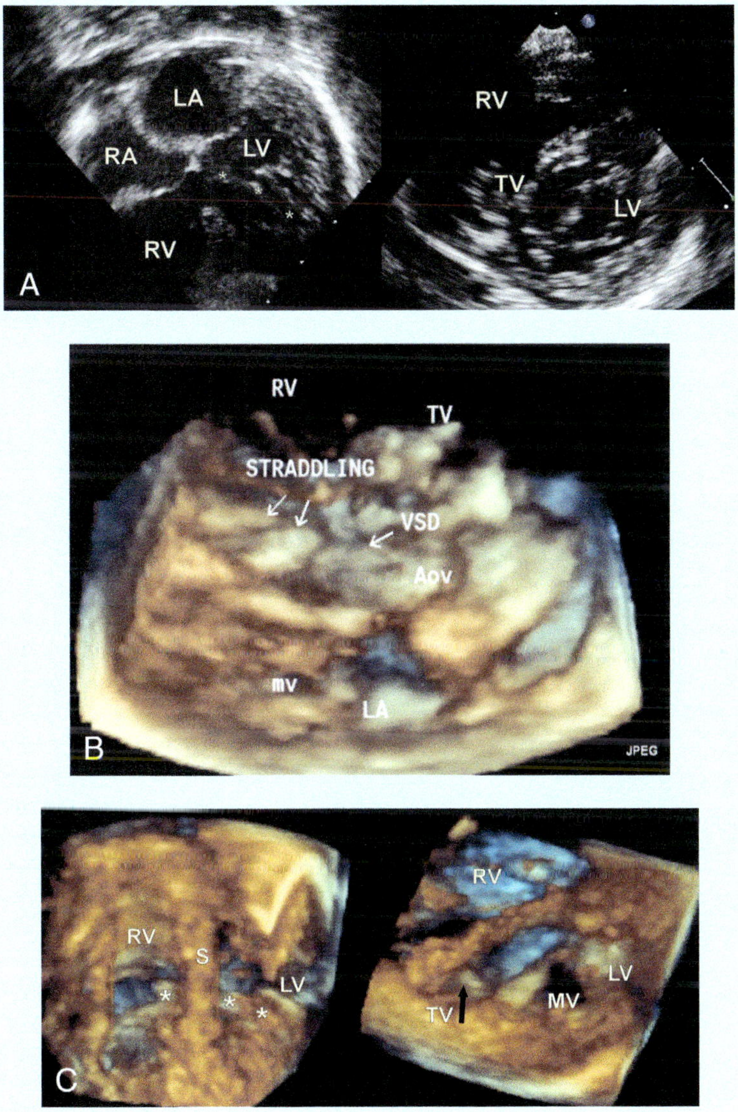

As well, this also provides optimal imaging in the smaller patient where the transesophageal probe is too large. The valve is best imaged from a four chamber position, and can be viewed from below or above, providing details of zones of coaptation, commissures, and sites of regurgitation. Quantitative techniques can be applied to assess degrees of tethering and prolapse, as well as annular shape and papillary muscle position.

- *Straddling tricuspid valve*: is seen more frequently in those hearts with varying degrees of hypoplasia of the right ventricle. In those hearts the posterior component of the interventricular septum is displaced such that the tricuspid annulus overrides the septum. As a result, it is the septal leaflet and posterior leaflets that straddle the ventricular septal defect. Two-dimensional echocardiography has been the main technique for diagnosing a straddling tricuspid valve and indeed due to the higher frame rates provides optimal imaging of thin structures. On the other hand 3DE has superb spatial resolution, providing superior definition of sites of chordal insertion, as well as leaflet detail (**Fig. 13-14**).

REFERENCES

1. Badano LP, Agricola E, Perez de Isla L, et al. Evaluation of the tricuspid valve morphology and function by transthoracic real-time three-dimensional echocardiography. Eur J Echocardiogr. 2009;10:477–484.
2. Sugeng L, Shernan SK, Salgo IS, et al. Live 3-dimensional transesophageal echocardiography initial experience using the fully-sampled matrix array probe. J Am Coll Cardiol. 2008;52:446–449.
3. Takehashi K, Mackie AS, Rebeyka IM, et al. Two-dimensional versus transthoracic real-time three-dimensional echocardiography in the evaluation of the mechanisms and sites of atrioventricular valve regurgitation in a congenital heart disease population. J Am Soc Echocardiogr. 2010;23:726–734.
4. Nii M, Roman KS, Macgowan CK, Smallhorn JF. Insight into normal mitral and tricuspid annular dynamics in pediatrics. A real-time three-dimensional echocardiographic study. J Am Soc Echo. 2005;18:805–814.
5. Nii M, Guerra V, Roman KS, et al. Three-dimensional tricuspid annular function provides insight into the mechanisms of tricuspid-valve regurgitation in classic hypoplastic left heart syndrome. *J Am Soc Echo.* 2006;19:391–402.
6. Takehashi K, Inage A, Rebeyka IM, et al. Real-time 3-dimensional echocardiography provides new insight into mechanisms of tricuspid valve regurgitation in patients with hypoplastic left heart syndrome. *Circulation.* 2009;120:1091–1098.
7. Fawzy H, Fukamachi K, Mazer CD, et al. Complete mapping of the tricuspid valve apparatus using three-dimensional sonomicrometry. *J Thorac Cardiovasc Surg.* 2011;141:1037–1043.
8. Fukuda S, Saracino G, Matsumura Y, et al. Three-dimensional geometry of the tricuspid annulus in healthy subjects and in patients with functional tricuspid regurgitation: A real-time 3-dimensional echocardiographic study. *Circulation.* 2006;114:492–498.
9. Sukmawan R, Watanabe N, Ogasawara Y, et al. Geometric changes of tricuspid valve tenting in tricuspid regurgitation secondary to pulmonary hypertension by novel system with transthoracic real-time 3-dimensional echocardiography. *J Am Soc Echocardiogr.* 2007;20:470–476.
10. Ton-Nu TT, Levine RA, Handschumacher MD, et al. Geometric determinants of functional tricuspid regurgitation insights from 3-dimensional echocardiography. *Circulation.* 2006;114:143–149.
11. Roshanali F, Saidi B, Mandegar MH, et al. Echocardiographic approach to the decision-making process for tricuspid valve repair. *J Thorac Cardiovasc Surg.* 2010;139:1483–1487.
12. Scherptong RWC, Vliegen HW, Winter MM, et al. Tricuspid valve surgery in adults with a dysfunctional systemic right ventricle repair or replace. *Circulation.* 2009;119:1467–1472.

CHAPTER 14

THREE-DIMENSIONAL AND FOUR-DIMENSIONAL FETAL ECHOCARDIOGRAPHY

Greggory R. DeVore, MD

ABSTRACT

This chapter covers fetal three-dimensional echocardiography (3DE) and four-dimensional echocardiography (3DE), including spatiotemporal image correlation, matrix-array technology, tomographic ultrasound imaging, B-mode phase inversion ultrasound, color and power Doppler imaging, and rendered blood flow imaging. Clinical applications of 3DE and 4DE screening examinations of the fetal heart are discussed as well as the guidelines published by the Pediatric Council of the American Society of Echocardiography for performance of a fetal echocardiogram. Methods of obtaining nine required four-dimensional views in the fetus are explained, including an apical four-chamber view, an apical five-chamber view; long-axis views of the left and right ventricular outflow tracts, short-axis views at the level of the great vessels and at the level of the ventricles, a caval long-axis view, a ductal arch view, and an aortic arch view.

INTRODUCTION

Unlike other organ systems in which B-mode real-time imaging is the primary technology used to identify normal and abnormal fetal anatomy, the fetal heart has been studied with a number of additional imaging modalities (M mode, pulsed Doppler, continuous Doppler, color Doppler, and tissue Doppler), each providing information that is important for a particular diagnosis.[1–49] During the past several years, three-dimensional (3D) and four-dimensional (4D) ultrasounds have become available for use in prenatal diagnosis of heart defects.[50–105] Because prenatal diagnosis of congenital heart defects is shared among physicians from various specialties (radiologists, obstetricians, maternal–fetal medicine specialists, and pediatric cardiologists), not all diagnosticians use the same equipment and approaches. This chapter focuses on the use of 3D and 4D fetal echocardiography prevalent in the nonpediatric cardiology community. We discuss the benefits and drawbacks of various imaging modalities to give the pediatric cardiologist an understanding of the commonly available imaging techniques that may be used by his or her colleagues in other specialties who may provide prenatal diagnostic services.

3D IMAGING

When 3D ultrasound was introduced, it consisted of multiple two-dimensional (2D) images that were stacked one behind the other during a manual or an automated sweep of the transducer beam through an area of interest (Fig. 14-1). The 3D data set is displayed on the screen as three perpendicular still-frame images representing the X, Y, and Z planes (Fig. 14-2). As the 2D images acquired during 3D volume acquisition are stacked one behind the other, a voxel is created that has an X, Y, and Z component (Fig. 14-2). The size of the voxel determines the resolution of the images in the X, Y, and Z planes (Fig. 14-2).

The X-plane image has the highest resolution and is equivalent to the 2D image displayed during the 3D volume acquisition. The X-plane image consists of pixels that have the properties of axial and lateral resolution, identical to a typical 2D image. Axial resolution provides the greatest detail for imaging structures in the plane of the ultrasound beam, whereas lateral resolution provides less detail because it displays structures lateral to the ultrasound beam (Fig. 14-2). The 3D Y plane displays an image perpendicular to the X plane in a vertical orientation (Fig. 14-2). This image has less detail than the X-plane image because it is reconstructed from voxels within the volume data set. Although the Y-plane image has less detail than the X-plane image, it has more detail than the Z-plane image. The Z-plane image is perpendicular and horizontal to the X plane (Fig. 14-2). Although the 3D static sweep can adequately identify cardiac anatomy, artifacts may occur in the Y- and Z-plane images if the sweep speed is too slow, resulting in the display of several cardiac cycles in the image (Fig. 14-3).

Figure 14-1

Multiple 2D images obtained during the sweep of the transducer beam through the fetal chest. These images are used to create a data set of voxels that are used to reconstruct 3D and 4D images of the fetal heart. This technique is used with mechanical transducers in nonpediatric 3D and 4D ultrasound machines.

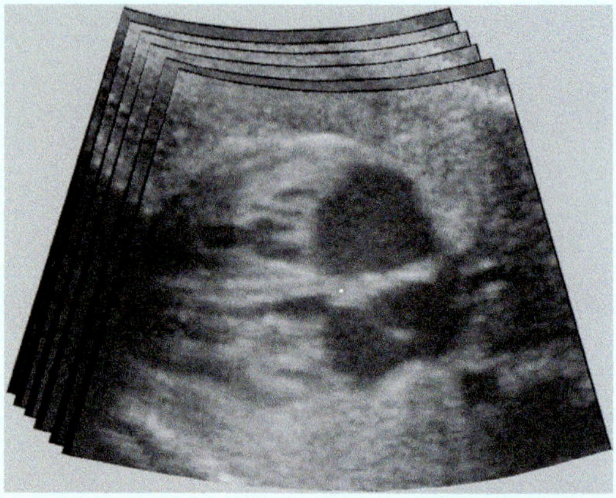

4D IMAGING

The following question is often asked: "what is 4D ultrasound?" The principles described in the previous section for 3D imaging apply to 4D ultrasound also. The only difference is that the fourth dimension is movement, that is, displaying the 3D data sets rapidly so that the structures viewed on the screen appear to be moving. One has the impression of motion such as a smiling face, movement of extremities, and contraction of the heart. 4D ultrasound is similar to real-time ultrasound in which static 2D images are displayed on the screen at a rapid frequency, giving the illusion of movement. The two 4D acquisition technologies that are commercially available are discussed in this chapter.

ACQUISITION TECHNOLOGY

Mechanical array transducer 4D spatiotemporal image correlation imaging

Spatiotemporal image correlation (STIC) was introduced in 2003.[50–52] STIC was a novel approach in which the examiner displays a cine loop of a single cardiac cycle, giving the appearance of a live 2D real-time examination from any angle within the volume data set. The STIC volume display consists of thousands of

Figure 14-2

Following the acquisition of sequential, parallel 2D images, voxels are created and entered in the volume data set. Each voxel consists of a volume of image pixels that have X, Y, and Z components. The X-plane image, obtained during the initial acquisition, comprises the axial (A) and lateral (L) resolution of the 2D image, which is a function of the characteristics of the transducer beam. The Y and Z planes also have axial and lateral resolution. However, the resolution in these planes is a function of the transducer beam as well as of the size of the voxel that is created from the original volume data set. For this reason, the images in the Y and Z planes are of lower resolution than the image in the X plane.

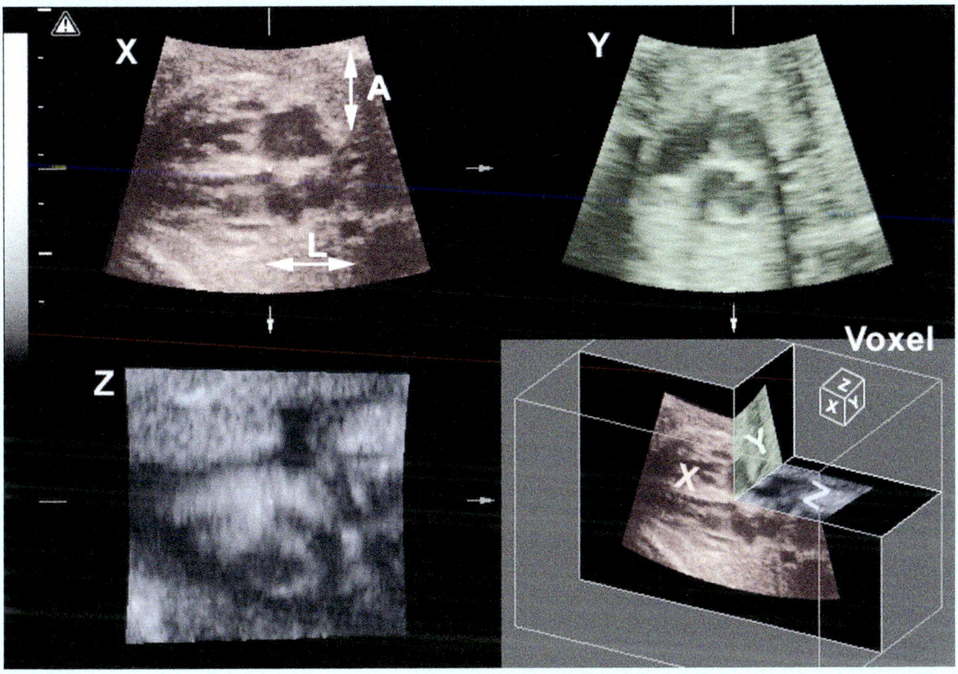

images acquired during a single sweep (7.5–15 seconds) through the area of interest. The images are analyzed, and multiple volumes are correlated with end-systole and end-diastole to create a cine loop of a single cardiac cycle from within the volume data set. This procedure allows the examiner to evaluate the volume data set in a manner identical to that accomplished with 3D static volume. The only differences are that the cardiac structures are viewed as a cine loop of a single cardiac cycle. STIC technology can display the data as a B-mode image, B mode with color Doppler, B mode with power Doppler, color Doppler, power Doppler, or M-mode image (Fig. 14-4).[50,54,60,61]

The only limitation of the STIC volume data set is the fact that fetal movement may occur during volume acquisition. Depending on the type of movement (fetal breathing, gross body movement, and maternal breathing), the images in the X, Y, and Z planes may be minimally altered or may become noninterpretable.

As with static 3D volume data acquisition, the resolution of the images in the X, Y, and Z planes is a function of how the user acquires the volume data set. The speed of the volume sweep can vary from 7.5 to 15 seconds, and the angle of the sweep can vary between 15° and 40°. The angle of the sweep is equivalent to the distance covered during the sweep; a short distance is equivalent to a small angle, and a large distance is equivalent to a large angle. For example, if the selected time is 7.5 seconds, a fixed number of images will be acquired whether the angle is 15° or 40°. Therefore, the image resolution would be higher if the angle is 15° than if it is 40° (Fig. 14-5).

Figure 14-3

Static 3D sweep through the fetal chest containing cardiac structures. This image acquisition is sagittal, from left to right. The Y plane illustrates the reconstructed four-chamber view of the heart. The upper panel shows the X and Y planes in which the sweep speed was set at a slow rate to acquire a greater number of 2D images to construct the 3D data set. Using this technique increases the image resolution in the X plane. However, because of the decreased sweep speed, the Y plane contains an artifact resulting from the contraction of the fetal heart during image acquisition. The lower panel demonstrates a similar sweep at a higher speed. The Y plane does not demonstrate the artifact; however, the image resolution of the four-chamber view is low.

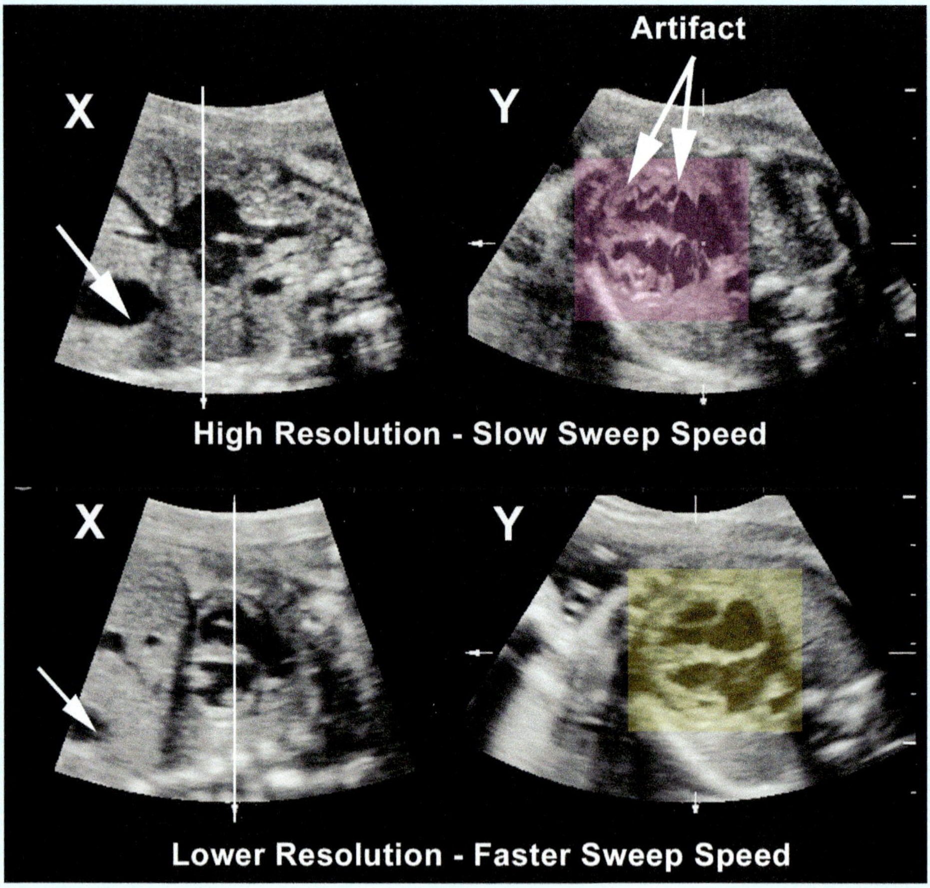

The reason for this result is that, although the same number of images is acquired during the 7.5 seconds, the distance between the images is greater when the angle is larger. Therefore, the images in the Y and Z planes in the 40° sweep are lower in resolution than those in the 15° sweep. Thus, the examiner should adjust the time and sweep angle to maximize the resolution (smaller angle, increased sweep time) for the size of the fetal heart being examined.

The advantages of STIC technology are as follows:

1. A looped cardiac cycle simultaneously displays cardiac anatomy in the X, Y, and Z planes.
2. Image resolution is improved compared with that from the 3D static volume sweep, depending on the settings selected (maximal time acquisition and minimal angle volume to image the cardiac structures).
3. The examiner can evaluate the cardiac anatomy frame by frame because a single cardiac cycle is displayed.
4. Color Doppler and power Doppler flow dynamics can be examined simultaneously in the X, Y, and Z planes (**Fig. 14-4**).

Figure 14-4

Multiplanar color Doppler STIC acquisition. The X illustrates the reference point. The green and yellow lines represent the cut-planes in the upper left image. The corresponding planes are outlined in green and yellow. IVC, inferior vena cava.

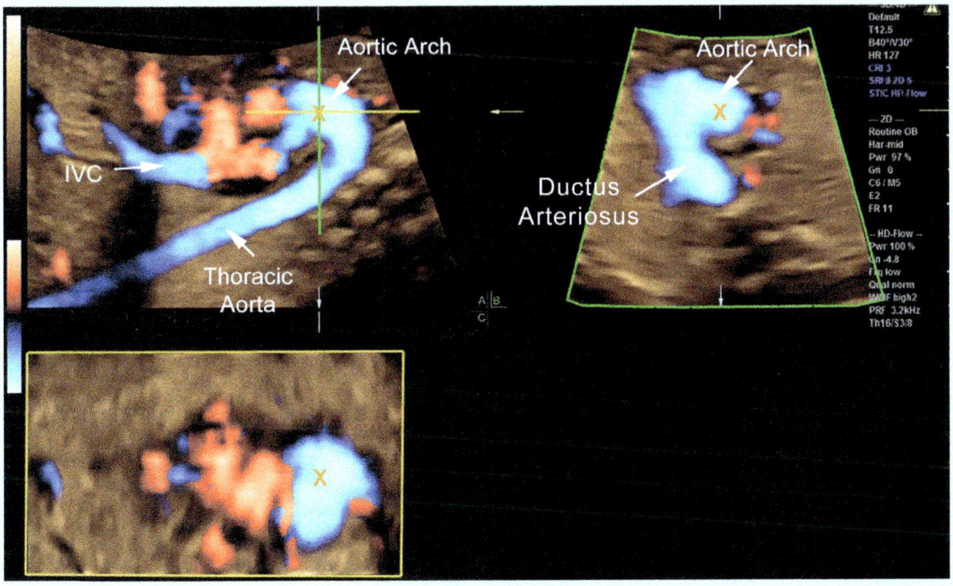

Figure 14-5

The number of frames acquired during image acquisition using STIC technology. When the sweep angle is 40°, the number of acquired frames increases when the duration of the acquisition is increased from 7.5 to 15 seconds. However, when the sweep angle is decreased to 15°, more frames are acquired for the same 15 seconds because the area examined is smaller. Adjusting these settings allows the examiner to optimize the volume data set for maximal resolution of the images in the Y and Z planes.

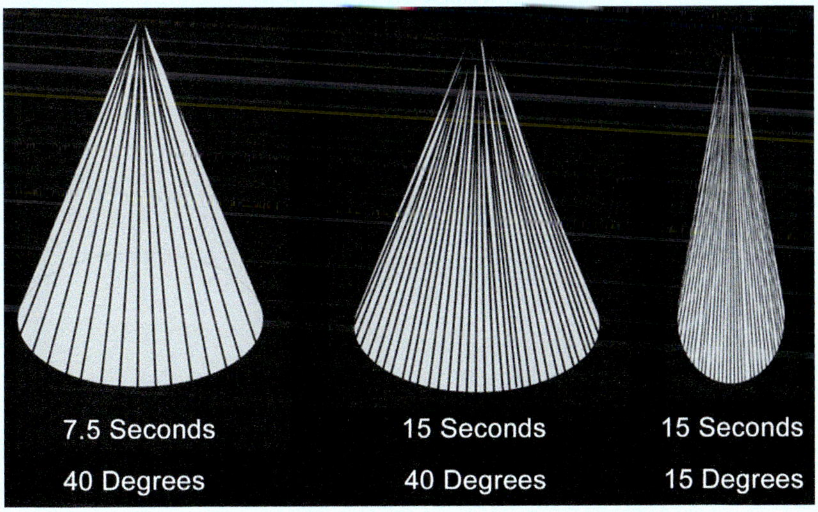

5. End-diastole and end-systole can be determined, and one can make cardiac measurements from images in the X, Y, and Z planes (**Fig. 14-6**).
6. M mode from any angle can be displayed for more precise measurement of cardiac structures at end-systole and end-diastole (**Fig. 14-7**).[106]

Matrix-array technology

In 2002, Philips Ultrasound (Bothell, Washington) introduced the matrix-array probe to adult cardiology in which all elements of the probe are fired simultaneously in a 3D matrix, generating a truncated pyramidal volume of ultrasound virtually instantaneously.[107] This modality operates differently from the 3D or 4D imaging described earlier, which reconstructs volumes from a series of 2D images acquired over time. For this reason, real-time 3D technology, unlike reconstructive 3D technology, does not require cardiac gating to capture cardiac motion. Because of the faster frame rate achieved with this technology than with the mechanical array probe, no movement artifact is introduced into the Y and Z planes of the volume data set (**Fig. 14-8**).[107]

Figure 14-6

Isolation of end-systole and end-diastole from a STIC volume from which measurements of atrial and ventricular chambers can be made from the four-chamber view (*A* and *C*). Using this approach facilitates cardiac measurements because the examiner can align the heart in the short-axis view (*B* and *D*) so that the widest and smallest dimensions of the ventricular or atrial chambers are measured accurately. LA, left atrium; LV, left ventricle; RA, right atrium; RV, right ventricle.

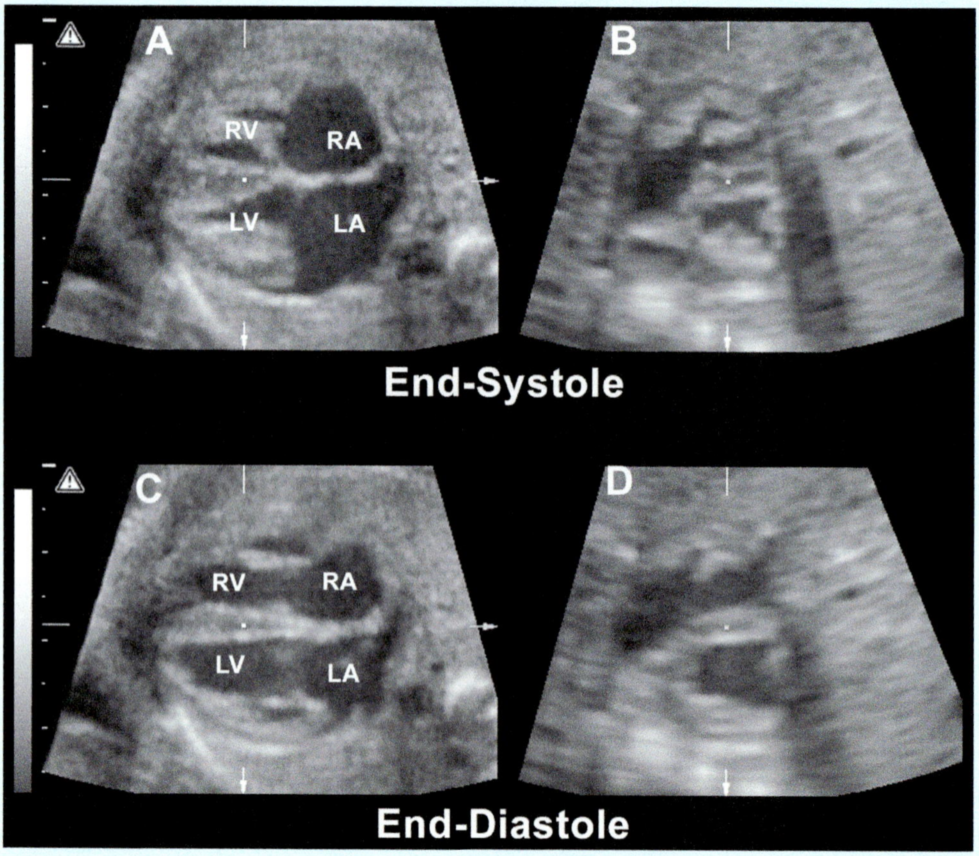

Figure 14-7

M-mode recordings obtained from a single STIC acquisition. The M-mode cursor can be placed anywhere within the volume and the M mode displayed. Measurements can be made of various cardiac structures from the M-mode display.

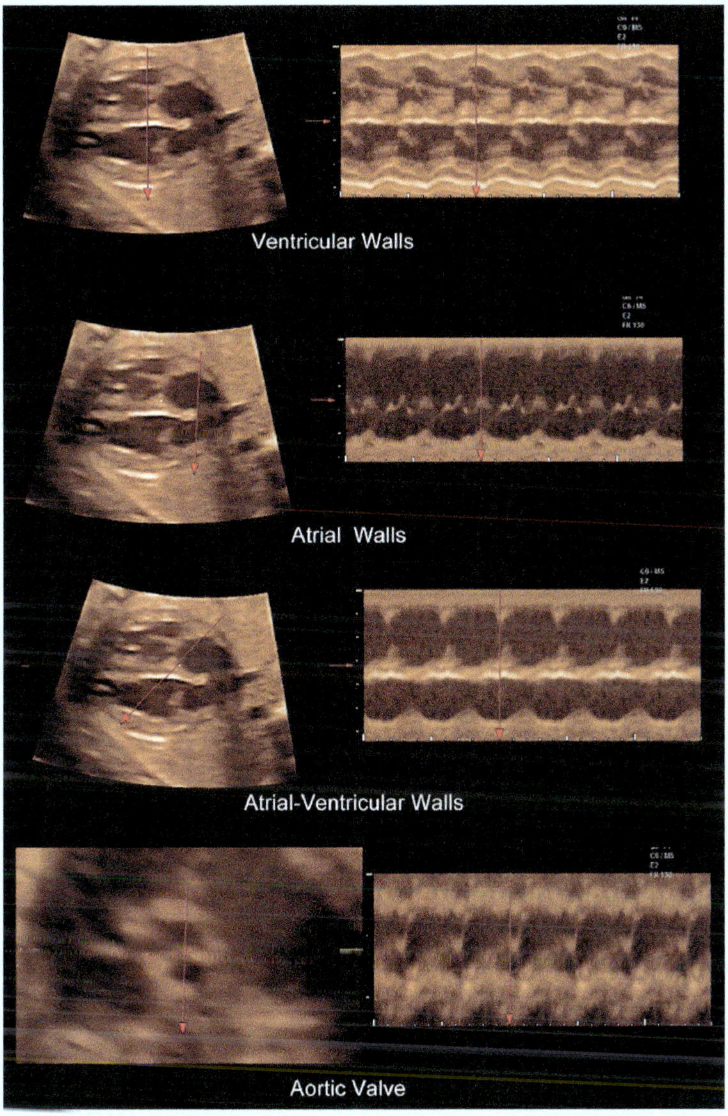

Image and rendering display of the acquired volumes

Once the volumes are acquired using either the mechanical array or the matrix-array transducer, the STIC volumes can be analyzed in multiple 2D image planes or rendered to display a 3D structure of the heart. These features are discussed in the following sections.

Image display of the acquired volumes

Simultaneous multiple image display. If the examiner directs the beam of the ultrasound probe in a transverse plane from the four-chamber view toward the fetal neck, the following views can be obtained: four-chamber view, five-chamber view, three-vessel view, and tracheal view.

Figure 14-8A, B, C, and D

A and *B*, Simultaneous B-mode image of the fetal heart obtained using a matrix array. The frame rate is 167/second. The vertical line in panel *A* demonstrates the location of the image displayed in panel *B*, which is perpendicular to the image in panel *A*. The cursor line can be moved throughout the image in panel *A* to display various perpendicular views in panel *B*. *C* and *D*, Real-time 4D volume examination of the fetal heart using the matrix-array 4D probe. The images of the fetal heart were taken using different orientations of the cut-plane as it passes through the four-chamber view. Because the ultrasound volume data set is acquired simultaneously in all planes (X, Y, and Z), the volume rate is higher (28 volumes/second) than when using the mechanical array probe (6 volumes/second).

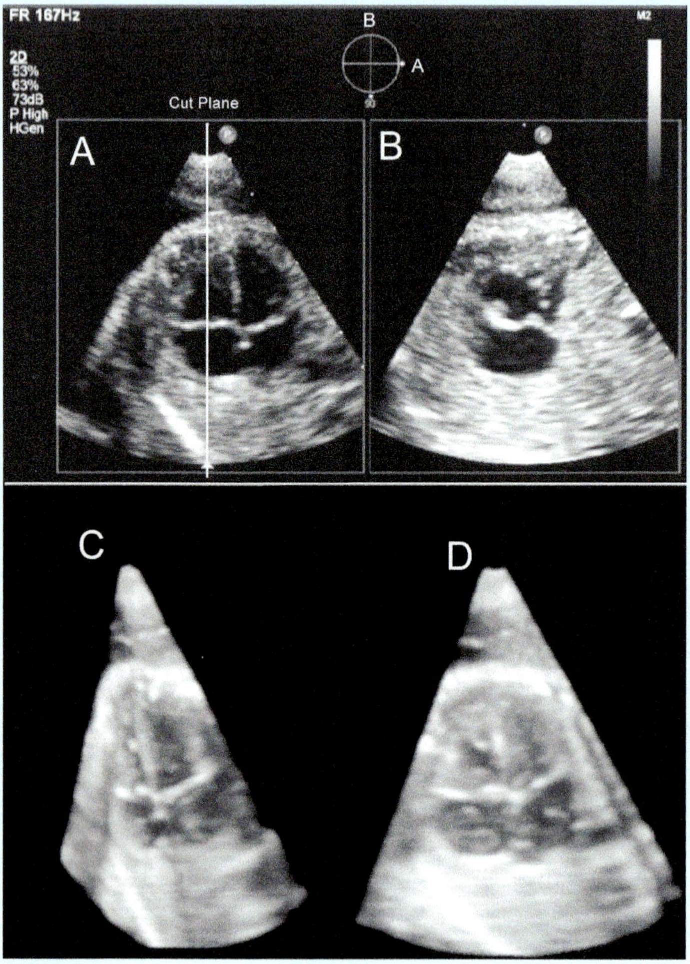

Several authors have described these views as important views for the identification of cardiac abnormalities (Fig. 14-9).[108–110]

When the examiner obtains a STIC acquisition in a transverse plane that includes the four-chamber, five-chamber, three-vessel, and tracheal views, multiple images can simultaneously be displayed on the screen. This type of display has several names, depending on the manufacturer of the ultrasound equipment. For purposes of discussion, we refer to this type of display as tomographic ultrasound imaging (TUI) (Fig. 14-10).[57,64,65,67]

Figure 14-9

Views obtained by directing the ultrasound beam from the four-chamber view to the upper thorax in a transverse plane. The views that are observed in sequential order are the four-chamber view, five-chamber view, three-vessel view, and tracheal view. If all of these views are normal, then major congenital heart defects can be eliminated. AA, ascending aorta; DA, ductus arteriosus; LA, left atrium; LV, left ventricle; PA, pulmonary artery; RA, right atrium; RV, right ventricle; SVC, superior vena cava; TA, transverse aortic arch.

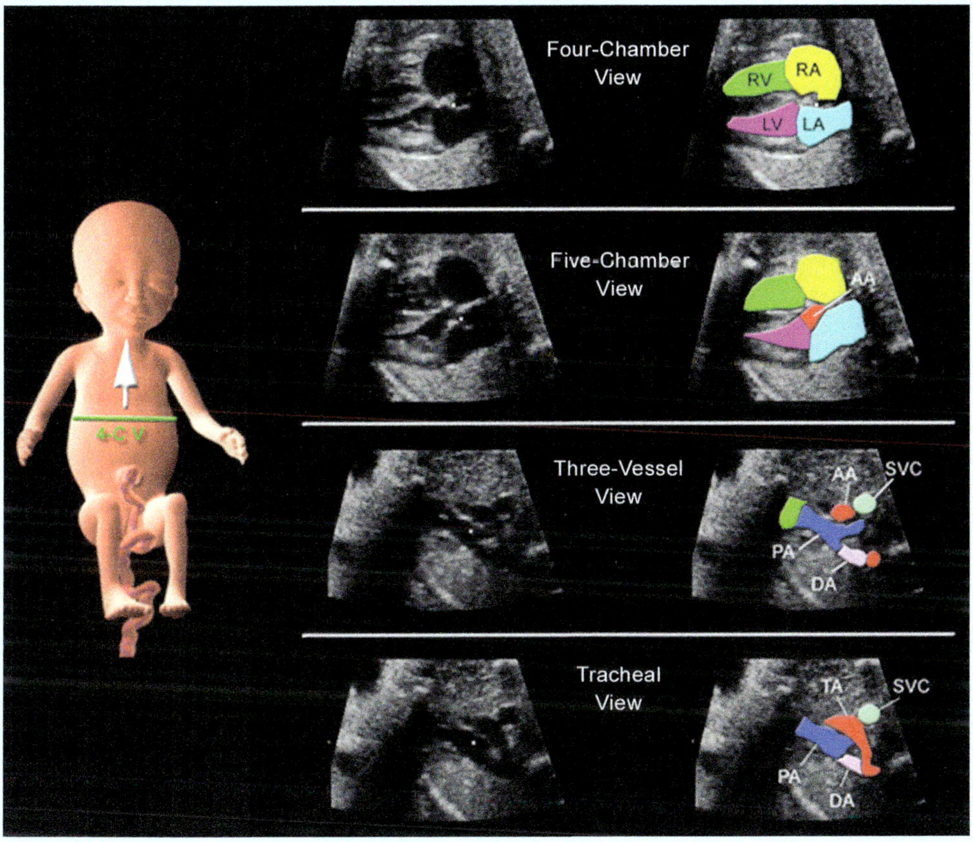

Rotation of the STIC volume to identify the outflow tracts and the aortic and ductal arches. Several investigators have published approaches for identifying the outflow tracts[55,104] and arch vessels by manipulating the STIC volume data set. The technique that we prefer is the "spin" technique.[55] With this approach, any vessel, observed in any view, can be identified by placing the reference dot within the vessel and rotating the volume in the Y-axis plane. In most cases, this process identifies the shape, length, and origin of the vessel being analyzed. Figure 14-11 illustrates this principle.

Rendering display of the acquired volumes

B-mode ultrasound. Another benefit of STIC volume acquisitions is that the 2D images contained within each volume can be compiled to create a 3D model of the heart anatomy and blood flow patterns. For example, the typical 2D four-chamber view can be rendered to provide a 3D structure that demonstrates

Figure 14-10

Images from a STIC acquisition. The images are displayed at exactly the same point in the cardiac cycle. The upper left image has parallel lines that represent the labeled images that are perpendicular to this image. The reference image is indicated by the asterisk (bottom left). From this point, images to the right are indicated by + mm and images to the left are indicated by − mm. The "+" and "−" millimeter indicators are not useful for purposes of identification, but the absolute value is. For example, the base of the four-chamber view is 6.1 mm below the reference image, the five-chamber view is 2.8 mm above the reference image, the bifurcation of the pulmonary artery is 8.4 mm above the reference image, and the transverse aortic arch is 12 mm above the reference image. AA, aortic arch; PA, pulmonary artery.

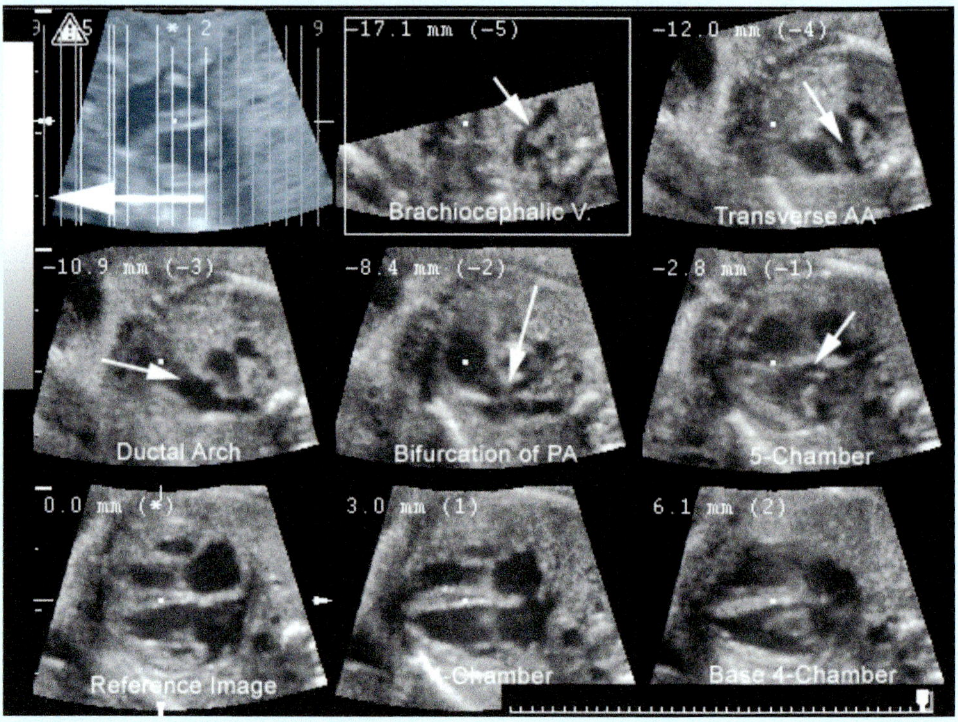

depth. Figure 14-12 illustrates a 3D rendered image that demonstrates an inferior vena cava in the back wall of the right atrium.

B-mode phase inversion ultrasound. Another method that is utilized for creating a 3D image of the heart is the inversion mode.[58] This technique requires the examiner to render the 3D heart (see earlier) and then invert the colors, thereby creating an image that has the appearance of a mold of the heart (Fig. 14-13).

Color and power Doppler imaging. When the STIC acquisition includes either color or power Doppler ultrasound, a rendered 3D image of the blood pool can be obtained.[54] The blood pool can be displayed as a static image or in real time (Fig. 14-14). This modality is useful when evaluating fetuses with complex outflow tract abnormalities.

Figure 14-11

Five-chamber view of the heart. *A*, A reference dot (white dot) is placed within the vessel inferior to the ascending aorta, which should be the right pulmonary artery (A). The volume data set is then turned around the Y axis (panels *B*, *C*, and *D*) until the right pulmonary artery is elongated and demonstrated to exit the main pulmonary artery (panel *D*). The spin technique can be used to identify any vessel in the cardiovascular system. A, aorta; AV, aortic valve; DA, ductus arteriosus; LA, left atrium; LV, left ventricle; MPA, main pulmonary artery; PV, pulmonary vein; RA, right atrium; RV, right ventricle; SVC, superior vena cava.

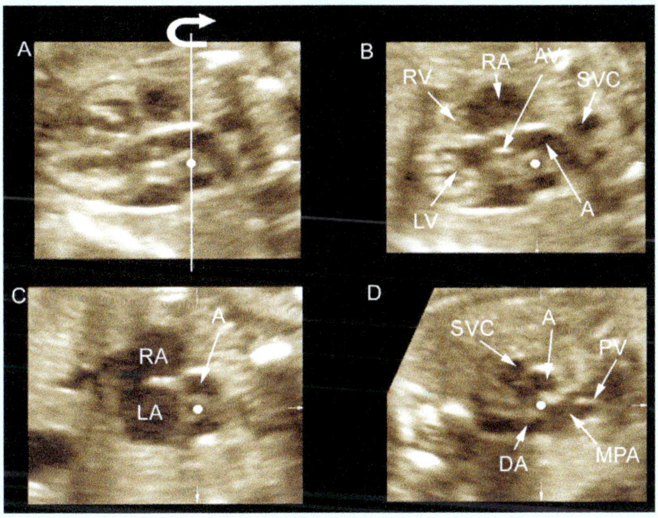

Figure 14-12

3D-rendered four-chamber view of the fetal heart. Although the image has the appearance of a 2D image, the rendering provides depth so that the back walls of the atrial and ventricular chambers can be identified. The right atrium (RA) demonstrates the opening of the inferior vena cava (IVC) and the left atrium (LA), the opening of one of the pulmonary veins. LV, left ventricle; PV, pulmonary vein; RV, right ventricle.

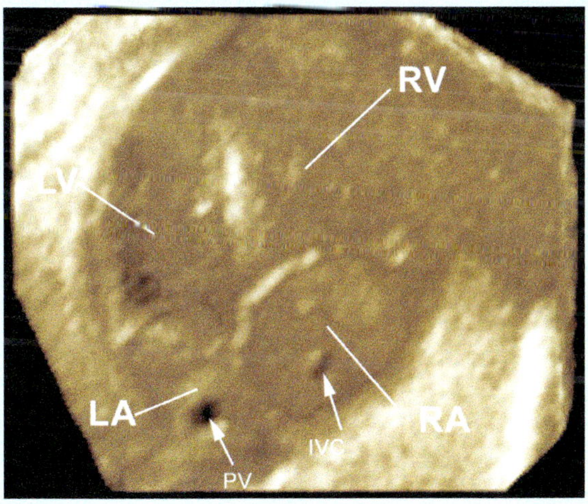

Figure 14-13

B-mode STIC image of the left outflow tract as it exits the left ventricle. The rendered inverted images demonstrate the crossing of the main pulmonary artery (P) and the aorta (A) as well as the ductus arteriosus (DA). AA, aortic arch; MPA, main pulmonary artery; SVC, superior vena cava.

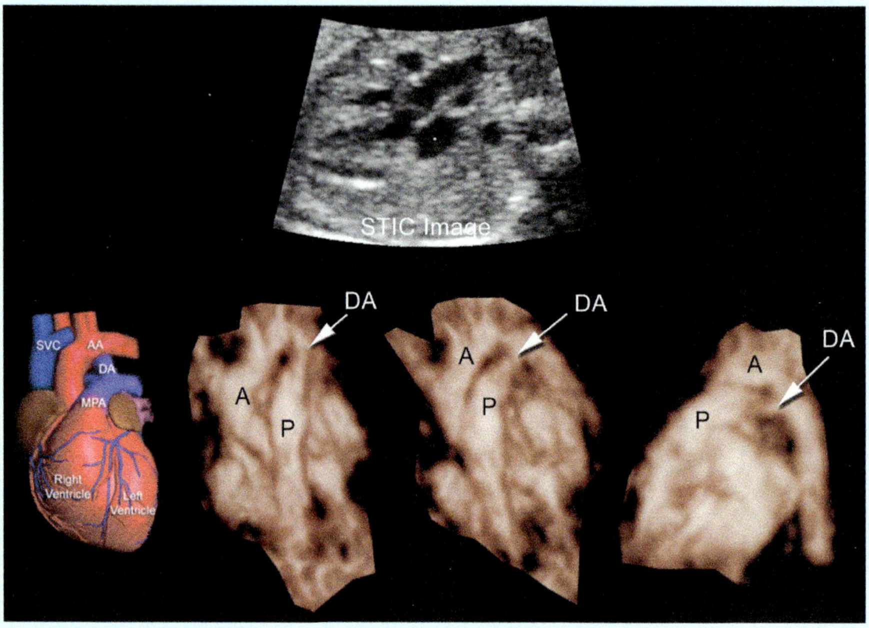

Rendered B flow. B-mode ultrasound identifies soft tissue and the blood pool when examining fetal cardiovascular structures. However, it does not identify the flow of blood. Most examiners use color Doppler or power Doppler to identify blood flow. One of the problems with the rendered color Doppler image is that the borders are not well defined between the blood pool and the chamber walls. However, B flow is a technique in which moving red blood cells are identified from the B-mode image.[69,74,77] This technology does not utilize Doppler principles to display blood flow. Once the B-flow image is acquired, it can be rendered to provide a 3D structure of the fetal cardiovascular system that resembles an angiogram (Fig. 14-15).

Figure 14-14

Rendered aorta using power Doppler.

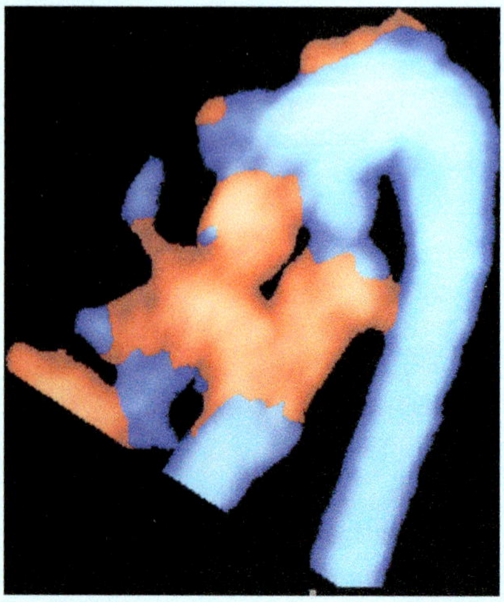

Clinical applications of 4D STIC echocardiographic screening examination of the fetal heart

Recent guidelines published by the American College of Radiology, American Institute of Medicine, and American College of Obstetricians and Gynecologists require that

Figure 14-15A, B, C, and D

B-flow image sequence from a 17-week-old fetus. *A*, Filling of the right ventricle (RV) and left ventricle (LV) chambers during diastole. *B*, Ventricular systole after the ventricles have emptied. This image demonstrates the relationships of the main pulmonary artery (MPA), right pulmonary artery (RPA) going beneath the aortic arch (AA), and the ductus arteriosus (DA) emptying into the thoracic aorta. *C*, Similar to image in panel *B* except later in the systolic cycle. *D*, Same image as in panel *C* except that the volume has been rotated to show the perpendicular relationship of MPA and AA.

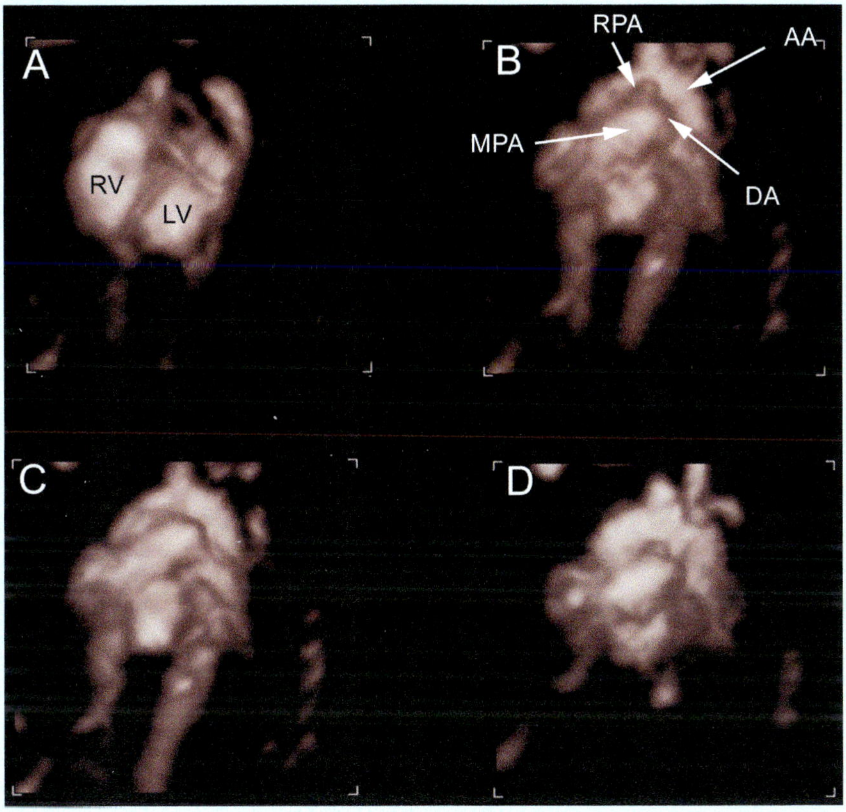

a physician sonographer who examines the fetus during the second and third trimesters of pregnancy must attempt to evaluate the four-chamber view and the outflow tracts of the fetal heart. Several studies have reported an approach for examining the outflow tracts that only requires the examiner to direct the ultrasound beam transversely from the level of the four-chamber view to the fetal neck.[108–112] The sequence of images that are required consists of the following: four-chamber, five-chamber, three-vessel, and tracheal views (Fig. 14-9). Using this approach, the location and size of the following structures can be identified: atrial and ventricular chambers, ascending aorta, main pulmonary artery, bifurcation of the main pulmonary artery, ductus arteriosus, and the transverse aortic arch.[108–112] Using STIC technology, the examiner can display these views either by scrolling through the volume or by simultaneously displaying multiple views using TUI (Fig. 14-10).[57,64,65,67] The distance between the sequential parallel views can be adjusted to be between 0.1 and 5 mm, providing the user with a precise determination of the distance between cardiac structures. The benefits of this approach are as follows:

- The normal relationships of the four-chamber view, five-chamber view, main pulmonary artery, bifurcation of the main pulmonary artery, ductus arteriosus, and transverse aortic arch can be quickly identified to screen for congenital heart defects.

Figure 14-16

Tomographic ultrasound images demonstrating pulmonary stenosis (PS). Image 4 (bottom right) demonstrates a dilated right ventricle (RV) with tricuspid regurgitation (TR). Image with an asterisk (center) demonstrates pulmonary artery regurgitation (PA Reg) and image 3 (top center) demonstrates the dilated main pulmonary artery. Although not present in this frame, the main pulmonary artery demonstrated aliasing. LV, left ventricle; RV, right ventricle.

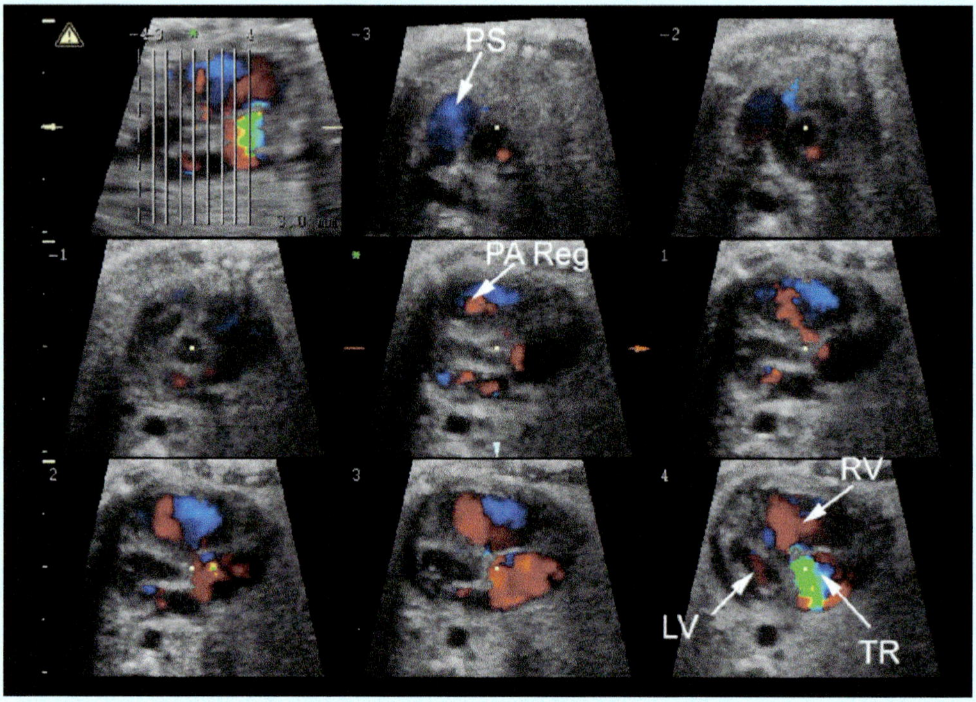

- This display technique can be used for B-mode as well as for color Doppler and power Doppler display modes (**Fig. 14-16**).
- Simultaneous display of multiple images may decrease the time required for analysis of the screening examination of the heart.

The limitation of the transverse sweep technique is that the examiner does not identify the aortic or ductal arches in their entirety. To address this problem, several investigators have described techniques for identifying these structures.[55,104] One approach is to use the spin technique at the level of the tracheal view.[55] One places a reference marker within the ductus arteriosus or the transverse aortic arch at the tracheal view level and then rotates the image until each vessel is vertical to the screen. When this process is completed, the respective ductal and aortic arches can be visualized in the B image (**Figs. 14-17** and **14-18**).

Clinical applications of 3D and 4D fetal echocardiography when performing the fetal echocardiogram

In 2004, the Pediatric Council of the American Society of Echocardiography published guidelines for the performance of a fetal echocardiogram.[113] The recommendations included nine 2D views of the fetal heart using nine different imaging planes (**Fig. 14-19**), Doppler measurements of specific intracardiac structures and extracardiac vessels, measurements of the ventricles and outflow tracts; examination of rhythm and rate, establishment of situs, and determination of gestational age by measuring the biparietal diameter or the femur length. STIC imaging may be useful for identifying the nine recommended 2D images, determining situs, and obtaining measurements from the 2D images.[113]

Figure 14-17

Upper panel illustrates a transverse plane through the upper fetal chest, demonstrating the ductus arteriosus (DA) and the transverse aortic arch (TA) in the X plane and a sagittal plane of the chest and upper abdomen in the Y plane. The straight arrow points to the reference point in the X plane. The lower panel demonstrates the effect of rotating the image (curved arrow in upper panel) in the X plane until the DA is vertical. Once this occurs, the ductal arch appears in the Y plane. SVC, superior vena cava.

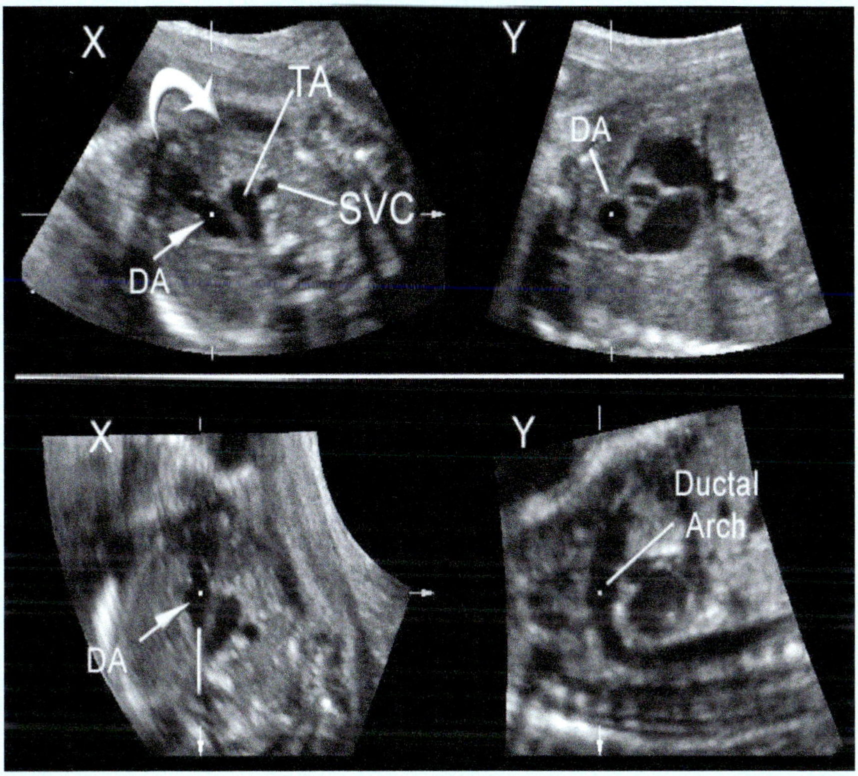

VIEWING THE NINE TOMOGRAPHIC IMAGING PLANES

Because the fetus may not always be in an ideal position to image the nine planes (Fig. 14-19) using conventional 2D imaging, 4D imaging technology may be of assistance using the approaches discussed in the following sections.

Transverse sweep

After obtaining a transverse sweep from the stomach to the fetal neck, the images are displayed in the TUI format. Identification of sequential transverse images allows the examiner to identify the following: position of the stomach in the abdomen, four-chamber view, five-chamber view, three-vessel view, and tracheal view (Fig. 14-9). This imaging sequence identifies two of the nine suggested imaging planes: (1) the apical four-chamber view and (2) the apical five-chamber view.

Sagittal short-axis sweep

After completing the transverse sweep as described in the previous section, the examiner obtains a 4D volume data set by directing the ultrasound sweep in a sagittal plane from either the right to left side or the left to right side of the fetus. When the interventricular septum is perpendicular to the ultrasound beam, the short axis of the ventricles is in proper alignment for their evaluation (image plane 6) (Fig. 14-20).

Figure 14-18

The upper panel shows the transverse plane through the upper fetal chest demonstrating the ductus arteriosus (DA) and the transverse aortic arch (TA) in the X plane and a sagittal view of the chest and upper abdomen in the Y plane. The straight arrow points to the reference point in the X plane. The lower panel demonstrates the effect of rotating the image (curved arrow in upper panel) in the X plane until the transverse aortic arch is vertical. Once this occurs, the aortic arch appears in the Y plane. AA, ascending aorta; SVC, superior vena cava.

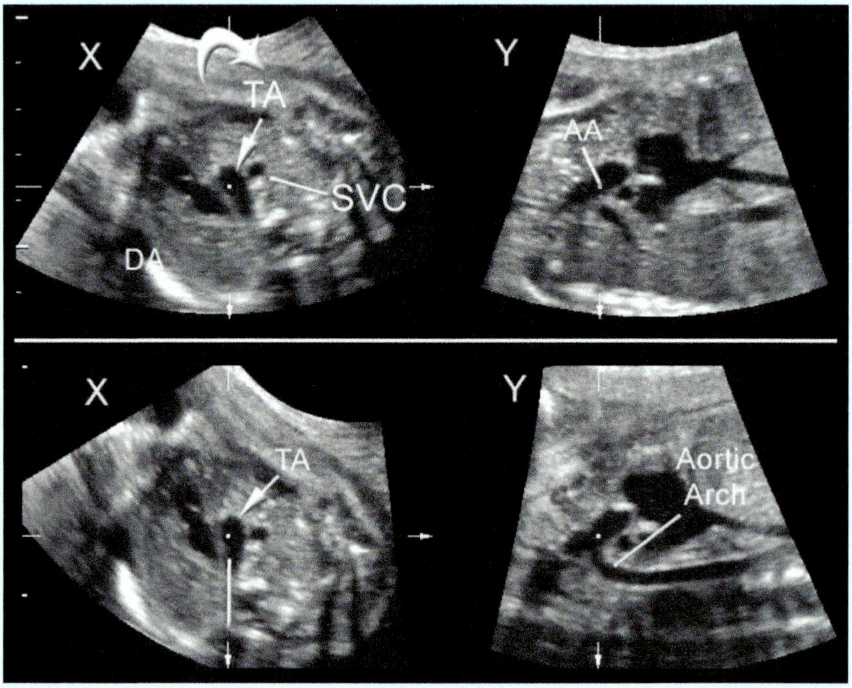

Sagittal sweep: caval long-axis view and aortic arch view

To identify the caval long-axis view and the aortic arch view (planes 7 and 9 of Fig. 14-19) using the sagittal sweep, the four-chamber view should be oriented so that the interventricular septum is 30° from the horizontal plane (Fig. 14-21). To accomplish this orientation, the examiner rotates the four-chamber view around the X axis. The TUI is then activated, displaying the caval long-axis and the aortic arch views (Fig. 14-21).

Sagittal sweep: short-axis view at the level of the great vessels and the ductal arch view

The five-chamber view is oriented so that the interventricular septum is 30° from the horizontal plane (Fig. 14-22). When TUI is activated, the short-axis view at the level of the great vessels and the ductal arch are identified (levels 5 and 8 of Fig. 14-19).

Examination of the interventricular septum

Evaluation of the interventricular septum is usually performed at the level of the four-chamber view. Unfortunately, this view represents only a portion of the septum. Using 4D STIC acquisitions, the entire septum can be examined for evidence of defects that are not in the plane of the four-chamber view Fig. 14-23).

Figure 14-19

Nine 2D views of the fetal heart using nine different imaging planes, recommended by the Pediatric Council of the American Society of Echocardiography. Ao, aorta; DA, ductus arteriosus; IVC, inferior vena cava; LA, left atrium; LV, left ventricle; LVOT, left ventricular outflow tract; MV, mitral valve; PA, pulmonary artery; RA, right atrium; RV, right ventricle; RVOT, right ventricular outflow tract; SVC, superior vena cava. Adapted with permission from Rychik et al.[113]

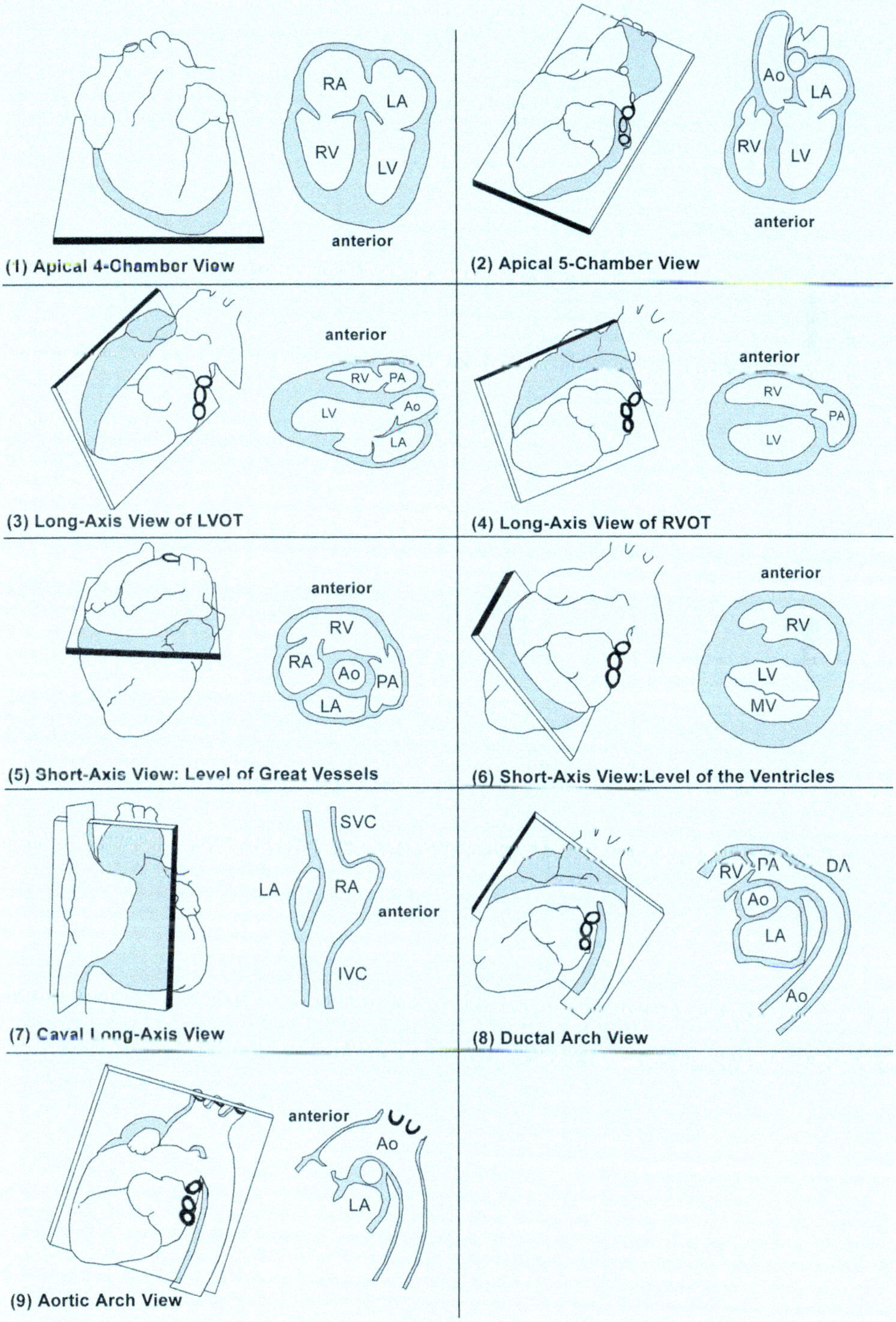

Figure 14-20

Sagittal sweep using either the static or the STIC technique. The image in P1 is the four-chamber view that would be displayed in the Y plane (Fig. 14-14). Using TUI, multiple simultaneous images of the short axis of the ventricles are displayed in frames P2–P6. P6 shows the size and shape of the tricuspid valve (TV) and mitral valve (MV). RV, right ventricle; LV, left ventricle. With permission from Rychik et al.[113]

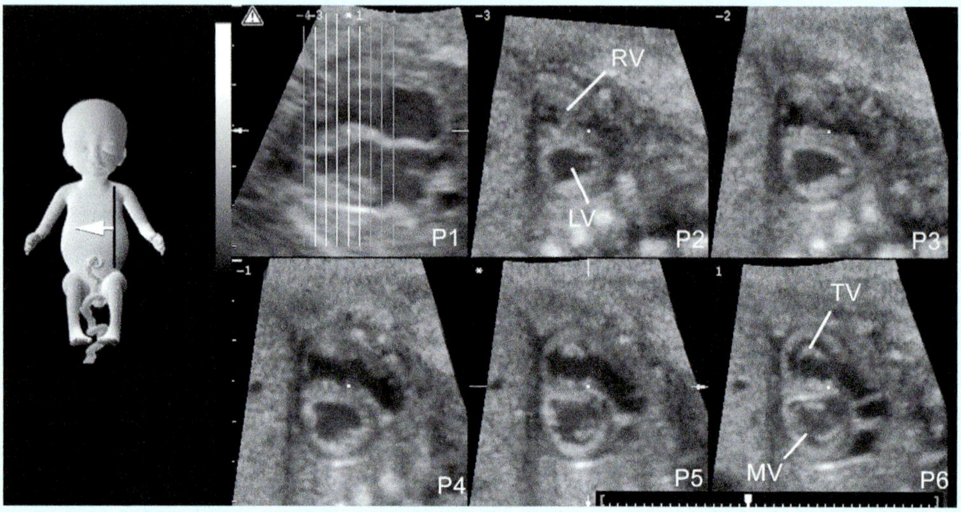

Figure 14-21

Sagittal sweep using either the static or the STIC technique. The image in P1 is the four-chamber view rotated 45°, which would be displayed in the Y plane (Fig. 14-14). Using TUI, multiple simultaneous images are displayed in frames P2–P4. P2 identified the aortic arch (AA) and P3 the caval long-axis view. IVC, inferior vena cava; LA, left atrium; LV, left ventricle; RA, right atrium; RV, right ventricle; SVC, superior vena cava.

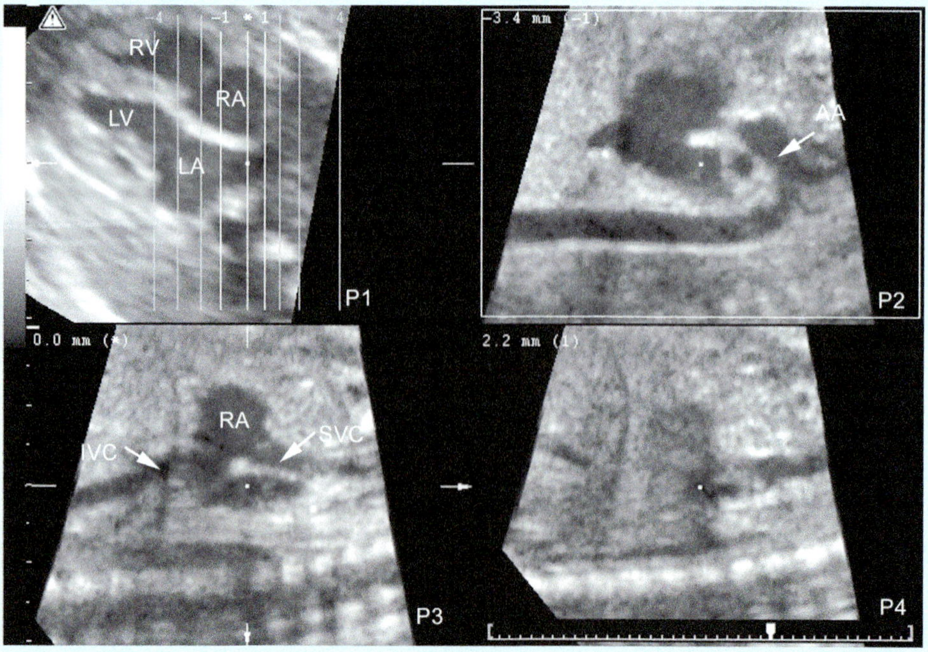

Figure 14-22

Sagittal sweep using either the static or the STIC technique. The image in P1 is the five-chamber view rotated 45°, which would be displayed in the Y plane (Fig. 14-14). Using TUI, multiple simultaneous images of the ductal arch are displayed in frames P2–P6. AV, aortic valve; DA, ductus arteriosus; PV, pulmonary valve.

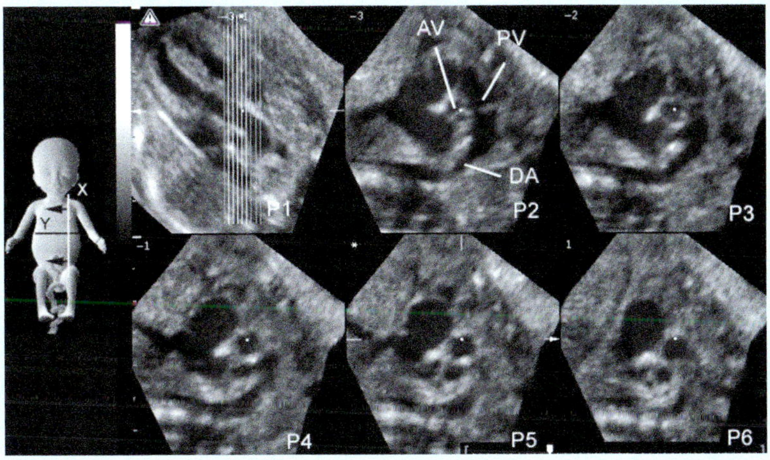

Figure 14-23

STIC acquisition of the four-chamber view. The upper and lower panels are identical images, except for the display of color Doppler in the lower panel. The upper panel demonstrates the four-chamber view in the X plane and an en face view (outlined by black line) of the ventricular septum in the Y plane. Careful examination does not suggest any pathological conditions of the interventricular septum. The lower panel, with color Doppler activated, demonstrates a shunting ventricular septal defect (VSD) near the apex in the X plane. The size and location of the septal defect are clearly identified in the en face view of the Y plane.

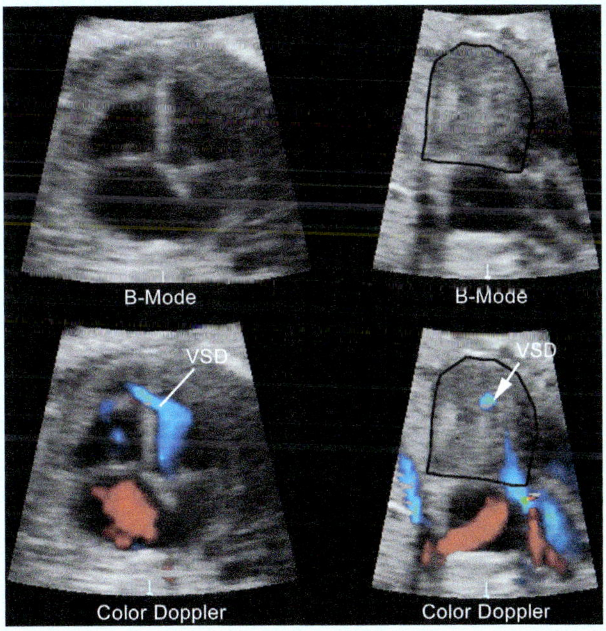

CARDIAC ABNORMALITIES AND ANOMALIES

Multicenter trials comparing STIC technology with traditional 2D imaging have found that STIC acquisition performs as well as traditional imaging.[85,93,97,103] In addition, researchers have reported the utility of transmitting STIC data sets over the Internet to distant tertiary referral centers for review by experts in fetal cardiology. They have found that this approach can facilitate long-distance consultation concerning suspected cardiac anomalies.[52,84] Examples of pathology identified with STIC technology using either TUI or rendered images from the STIC volume data set are illustrated: tetralogy of Fallot with an absent pulmonary valve (Fig. 14-24); rhabdomyoma, hypoplastic left ventricle, and D-transposition from a rendered matrix-array transducer (Fig. 14-25); D-transposition using the rendered inversion mode (Fig. 14-26); D-transposition of the arteries (Fig. 14-27); endocardial cushion defect (Fig. 14-28); truncus arteriosus (Fig. 14-29); ventricular septal defect (Fig. 14-30); and right-sided aortic arch (Fig. 14-31).

Figure 14-24

Tetralogy of Fallot with an absent pulmonary valve. Images from a STIC acquisition at 19 weeks. All four images are displayed at exactly the same point in the cardiac cycle. *A*, Image in the Y plane of the STIC acquisition demonstrating the level of cuts in panels *B*, *C*, and *D*. *D*, Four-chamber view. *C*, Five-chamber view with a ventricular septal defect (VSD) that overrides the aorta (A). *B*, What appears to be the pulmonary valve (PV) with a dilated main pulmonary artery (MPA). However, the pulmonary valve was absent, which resulted in blood moving in the MPA during both systole and diastole. This image also demonstrates a dilated aorta (DA). LA, left atrium; LV, left ventricle; RA, right atrium; RV, right ventricle.

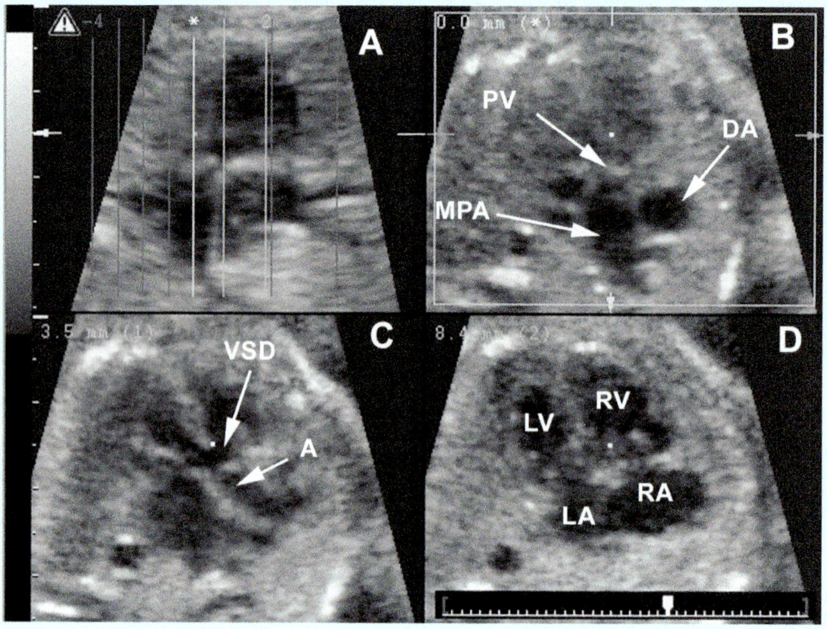

Figure 14-25

Examples of cardiac pathological conditions (rhabdomyoma, hypoplastic left ventricle, and D-transposition) imaged with the matrix-array transducer. All images are oriented in the same direction with the apex of the four-chamber view at 9 o'clock. The upper image demonstrates a rhabdomyoma (R) of the left ventricle, the image on the right shows a hypoplastic left ventricle, and the bottom image shows transposition of the great arteries. This image was obtained cephalad to the four-chamber view. LA, left atrium; LV, left ventricle; RA, right atrium; RV, right ventricle.

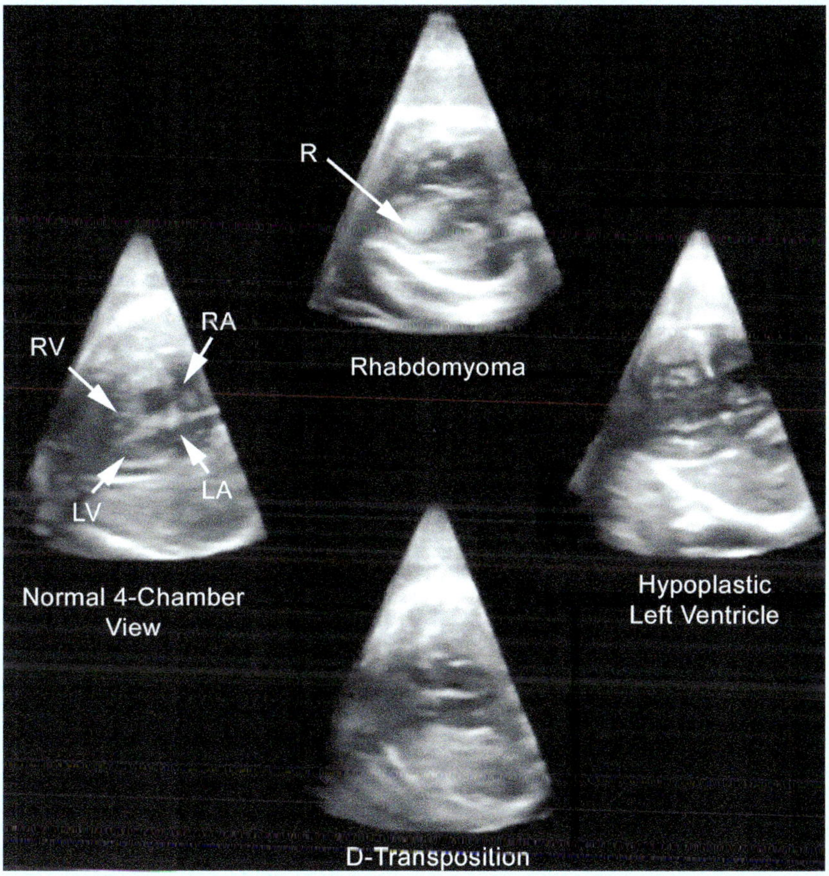

EVALUATION OF CARDIAC FUNCTION

Using the STIC volume data set, investigators have recently evaluated and computed ventricular stroke volumes.[73,78,88,92,98,100,101] Although these studies are promising, the computation of ventricular volumes is time consuming and has a potential for error because of the difficulty in identifying the borders of the chambers when performing the analysis.

Figure 14-26

Rendered image of the four chambers and the outflow tracts using the inversion mode in a fetus with transposition of the great arteries. The image on the left is a 3D model of a normal heart. AA, aortic arch; aorta, aorta exiting the right ventricle; DA, ductus arteriosus; LV, left ventricle; MPA, main pulmonary artery exiting the left ventricle; RV, right ventricle; SVC, superior vena cava.

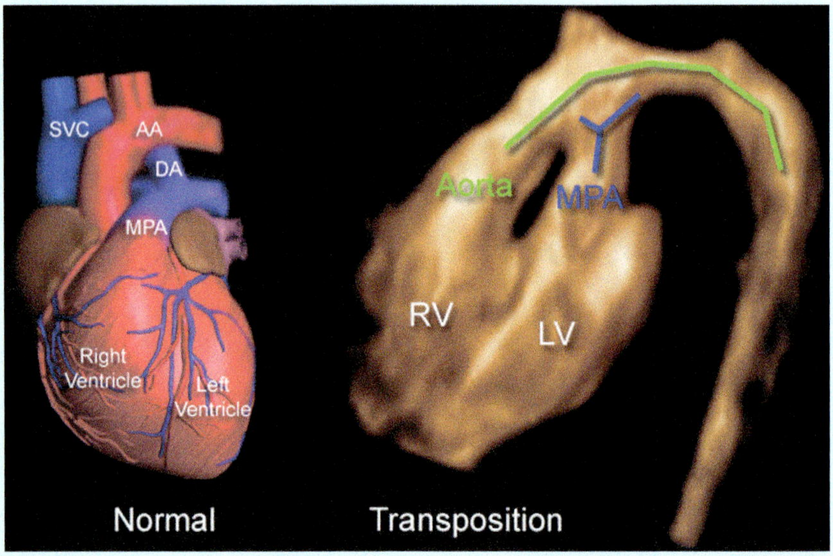

Figure 14-27

D-transposition of the arteries. TUI image demonstrating the parallel relationship of the outflow tracts with the main pulmonary artery (MPA) originating from the left ventricle (LV) and the aorta originating from the right ventricle (RV).

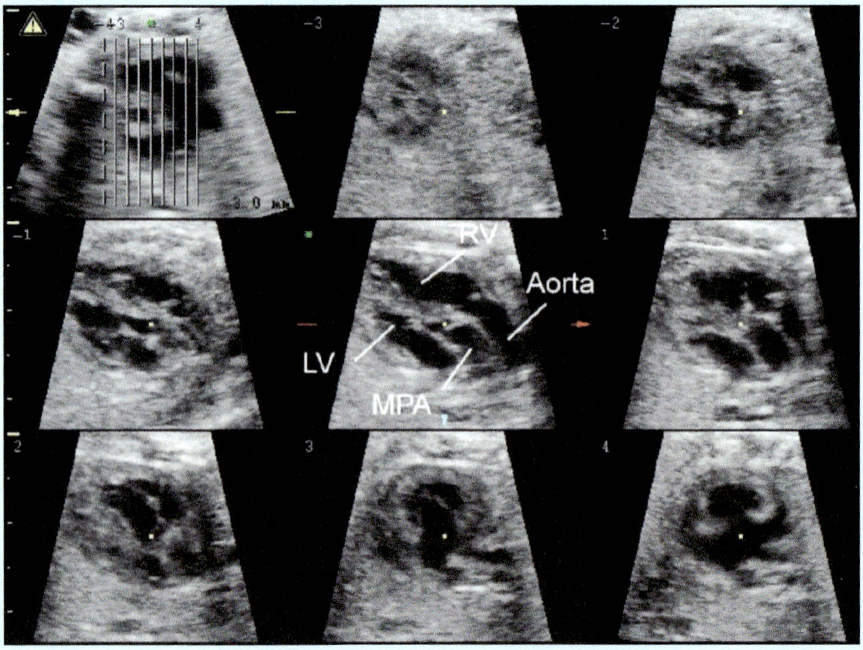

Figure 14-28

Endocardial cushion defect. TUI image through the four-chamber view of the heart. Image 4 (bottom right) is at the base of the heart. In image 1 (center right), the ventricular septum appears intact; just the plane superior to this (image) demonstrates the ventricular (VSD) and atrial (ASD) septal defects. LA, left atrium; LV, left ventricle; RA, right atrium; RV, right ventricle.

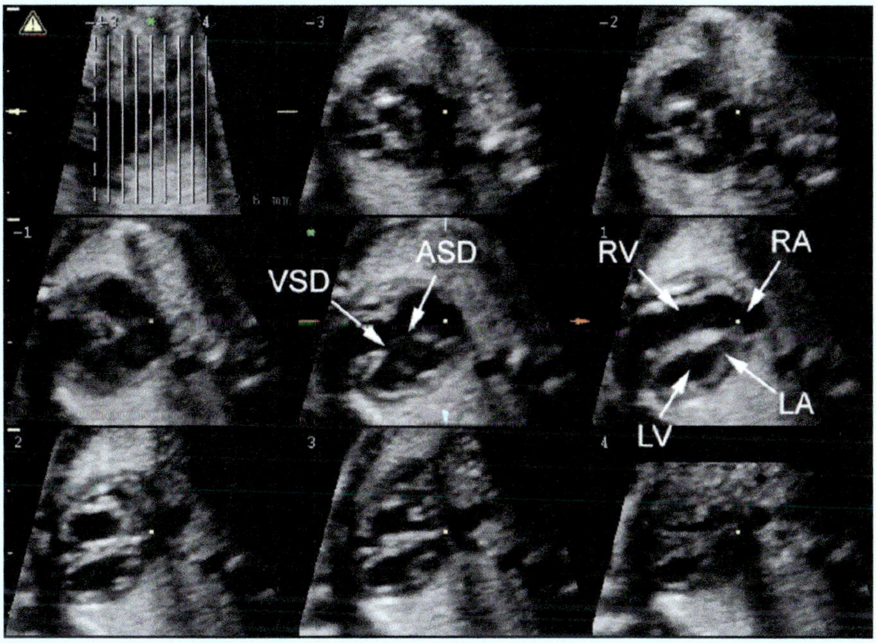

Figure 14-29

Rendered B-flow image of the heart demonstrating truncus arteriosus. The left image demonstrates the ventricles filling in diastole. The right image is the systolic phase of the cardiac cycle. The truncal vessels are outlined. LV, left ventricle; RV, right ventricle.

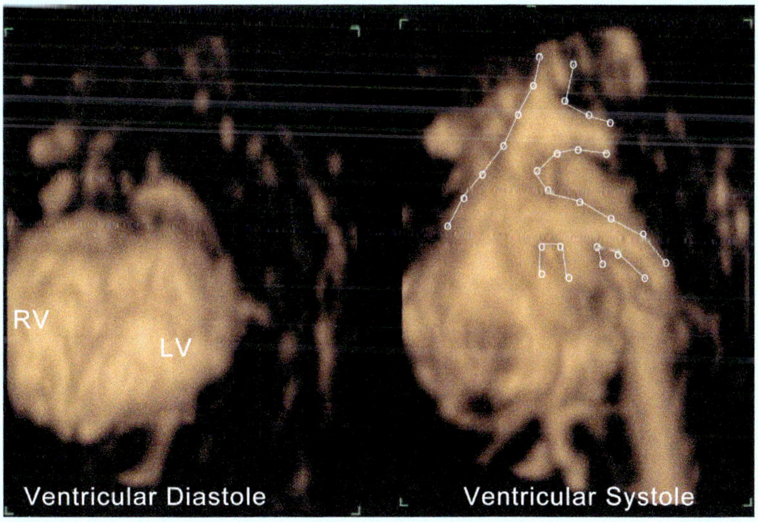

Figure 14-30

TUI image illustrating various levels from the four-chamber view demonstrating an apical ventricular septal defect (VSD). Image 3 (top center) does not show the apical VSD, whereas the other images do. LV, left ventricle; RV, right ventricle.

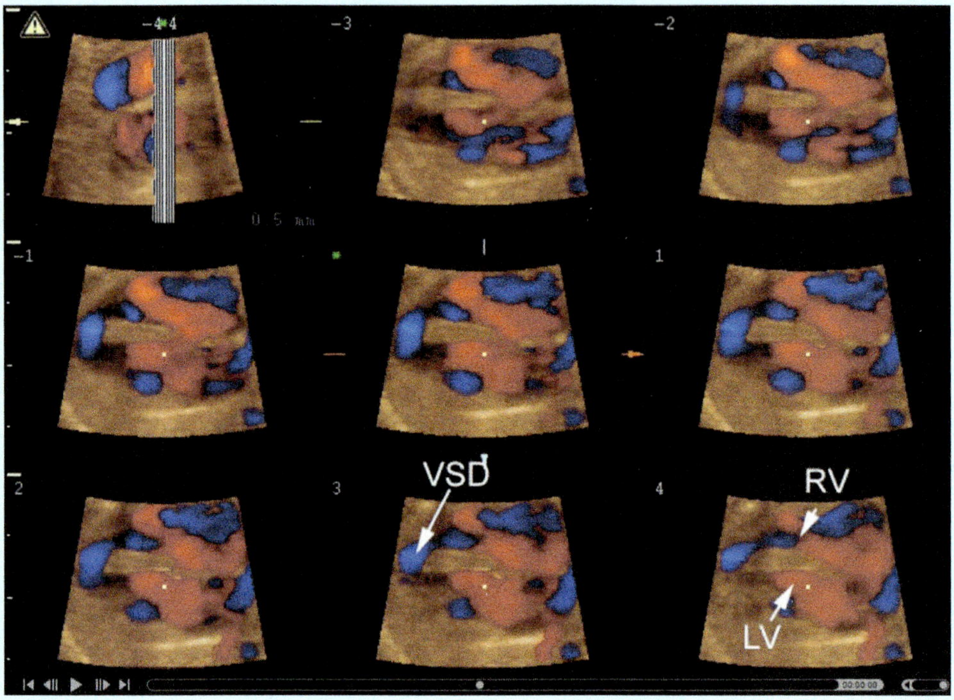

Figure 14-31

Rendered B-flow image of the ventricles and outflow tracts viewed from the anterior portion of the heart. The main pulmonary artery has been cut away, demonstrating the aorta coursing around and behind the trachea. The "ring" effect demonstrates the right-sided aortic arch. LV, left ventricle; RV, right ventricle.

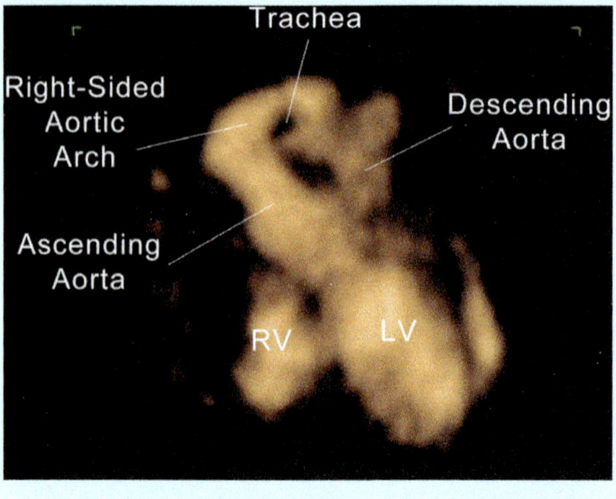

CONCLUSION

3D and 4D fetal echocardiography is an adjunct to traditional fetal echocardiography. Depending on the purpose of the examination and the findings, this new technology can aid in the diagnosis of cardiovascular defects, particularly of complex lesions. In some clinical settings, the technology can be used for screening, especially when the examiner desires to simultaneously identify views obtained in the transverse sweep of the chest. Although this technology is prevalent in the obstetric, radiological, and maternal–fetal medicine communities, it is relatively new to pediatric cardiologists. We recommend that pediatric cardiologists work closely with their colleagues in other disciplines to become familiar with 3D or 4D fetal echocardiography and use this technology to enhance their evaluation of fetuses at increased risk for congenital heart defects.

REFERENCES

1. Achiron R, Golan-Porat N, Gabbay U, et al. In utero ultrasonographic measurements of fetal aortic and pulmonary artery diameters during the first half of gestation. *Ultrasound Obstet Gynecol.* 1998;11(3):180–184.
2. Allan LD, Joseph MC, Boyd EG, et al. M-mode echocardiography in the developing human fetus. *Br Heart J.* 1982;47(6):573–583.
3. Allan LD, Chita SK, Al Ghazali W, et al. Doppler echocardiographic evaluation of the normal human fetal heart. *Br Heart J.* 1987;57(6):528–533.
4. Arduini D, Rizzo G, Romanini C. Fetal cardiac output measurements in normal and pathologic states. In: Copel JA, Reed KL, editors. *Doppler Ultrasound in Obstetrics and Gynecology*. New York: Raven Press; 1995. p. 271–290.
5. Cartier MS, Davidoff A, Warneke LA, et al. The normal diameter of the fetal aorta and pulmonary artery: echocardiographic evaluation in utero. *AJR Am J Roentgenol.* 1987;149(5):1003–1007.
6. Chang CH, Chang FM, Yu CH, et al. Systemic assessment of fetal hemodynamics by Doppler ultrasound. *Ultrasound Med Biol.* 2000;26(5):777–785.
7. Comstock CH, Riggs T, Lee W, et al. Pulmonary-to-aorta diameter ratio in the normal and abnormal fetal heart. *Am J Obstet Gynecol.* 1991;165(4 Pt 1):1038–1044.
8. De Smedt MC, Visser GH, Meijboom EJ. Fetal cardiac output estimated by Doppler echocardiography during mid- and late gestation. *Am J Cardiol.* 1987;60(4):338–342.
9. De Vore GR, Siassi B, Platt LD. Use of femur length as a means of assessing M-mode ventricular dimensions during second and third trimesters of pregnancy in normal fetus. *J Clin Ultrasound.* 1985;13(9):619–625.
10. Deng J, Cheng PX, Gao SY, et al. Echocardiographic evaluation of the valves and roots of the pulmonary artery and aorta in the developing fetus. *J Clin Ultrasound.* 1992;20(1):3–9.
11. DeVore GR, Siassi B, Platt LD. Fetal echocardiography. IV. M-mode assessment of ventricular size and contractility during the second and third trimesters of pregnancy in the normal fetus. *Am J Obstet Gynecol.* 1984;150(8):981–988.
12. DeVore GR, Siassi B, Platt LD. Fetal echocardiography. V. M-mode measurements of the aortic root and aortic valve in second- and third-trimester normal human fetuses. *Am J Obstet Gynecol.* 1985;152(5):543–550.
13. DeVore GR, Siassi B, Platt LD. The use of the abdominal circumference as a means of assessing M-mode ventricular dimensions during the second and third trimesters of pregnancy in the normal human fetus. *J Ultrasound Med.* 1985;4(4):175-182.
14. DeVore GR, Siassi B, Platt LD. Fetal echocardiography. VIII. Aortic root dilatation—a marker for tetralogy of Fallot. *Am J Obstet Gynecol.* 1988;159(1):129–136.
15. DeVore GR, Horenstein J. Color Doppler identification of a pericardial effusion in the fetus. *Ultrasound Obstet Gynecol.* 1994;4(2):115–120.
16. DeVore GR. Color Doppler examination of the outflow tracts of the fetal heart: a technique for identification of cardiovascular malformations. *Ultrasound Obstet Gynecol.* 1994;4(6):463–471.
17. DeVore GR, Alfi O. The use of color Doppler ultrasound to identify fetuses at increased risk for trisomy 21: an alternative for high-risk patients who decline genetic amniocentesis. *Obstet Gynecol.* 1995;85(3):378–386.
18. DeVore GR. Second trimester ultrasonography may identify 77 to 97% of fetuses with trisomy 18. *J Ultrasound Med.* 2000;19(8):565–576.
19. DeVore GR. Trisomy 21: 91% detection rate using second-trimester ultrasound markers. *Ultrasound Obstet Gynecol.* 2000;16(2):133–141.
20. DeVore GR. The genetic sonogram: its use in the detection of chromosomal abnormalities in fetuses of women of advanced maternal age. *Prenat Diagn.* 2001;21(1):40–45.

21. DeVore GR. The role of fetal echocardiography in genetic sonography. *Semin Perinatol.* 2003;27(2):160–172.
22. Di Renzo GC, Luzi G, Cucchia GC, et al. The role of Doppler technology in the evaluation of fetal hypoxia. *Early Hum Dev.* 1992;29(1-3):259–267.
23. Firpo C, Hoffman JI, Silverman NH. Evaluation of fetal heart dimensions from 12 weeks to term. *Am J Cardiol.* 2001;87(5):594–600.
24. Fouron JC, Proulx F, Miro J, et al. Doppler and M-mode ultrasonography to time fetal atrial and ventricular contractions. *Obstet Gynecol.* 2000;96(5 Pt 1):732–736.
25. Friedman DM, Rupel A, Glickstein J, et al. Congenital heart block in neonatal lupus: the pediatric cardiologist's perspective. *Indian J Pediatr.* 2002;69(6):517–522.
26. Gembruch U, Shi C, Smrcek JM. Biometry of the fetal heart between 10 and 17 weeks of gestation. *Fetal Diagn Ther* 2000;15(1):20–31.
27. Glickstein J, Buyon J, Kim M, et al; PRIDE Investigators. The fetal Doppler mechanical PR interval: a validation study. *Fetal Diagn Ther.* 2004;19(1):31–34.
28. Harada K, Rice MJ, Shiota T, et al. Gestational age- and growth-related alterations in fetal right and left ventricular diastolic filling patterns. *Am J Cardiol.* 1997;79(2):173–177.
29. Hornberger LK, Sanders SP, Rein AJ, et al. Left heart obstructive lesions and left ventricular growth in the midtrimester fetus. A longitudinal study. *Circulation.* 1995;92(6):1531–1538.
30. Hornberger LK, Sanders SP, Sahn DJ, et al. In utero pulmonary artery and aortic growth and potential for progression of pulmonary outflow tract obstruction in tetralogy of Fallot. *J Am Coll Cardiol.* 1995;25(3):739–745.
31. St. John Sutton MG, Gewitz MH, Shah B, et al. Quantitative assessment of growth and function of the cardiac chambers in the normal human fetus: a prospective longitudinal echocardiographic study. *Circulation.* 1984;69(4):645–654.
32. Kenny JF, Plappert T, Doubilet P, et al. Changes in intracardiac blood flow velocities and right and left ventricular stroke volumes with gestational age in the normal human fetus: a prospective Doppler echocardiographic study. *Circulation.* 1986;74(6):1208–1216.
33. Kiserud T, Rasmussen S. Ultrasound assessment of the fetal foramen ovale. *Ultrasound Obstet Gynecol.* 2001;17(2):119–124.
34. Mielke G, Benda N. Blood flow velocity waveforms of the fetal pulmonary artery and the ductus arteriosus: reference ranges from 13 weeks to term. *Ultrasound Obstet Gynecol.* 2000;15(3):213–218.
35. Mielke G, Benda N. Cardiac output and central distribution of blood flow in the human fetus. *Circulation.* 2001;103(12):1662–1668.
36. Rane HS, Purandare HM, Chakravarty A, et al. Fetal echocardiography--norms for M-mode measurements. *Indian Heart J.* 1990;42(5):351–355.
37. Reed KL, Meijboom EJ, Sahn DJ, et al. Cardiac Doppler flow velocities in human fetuses. *Circulation.* 1986;73(1):41–46.
38. Rizzo G, Arduini D. Fetal cardiac function in intrauterine growth retardation. *Am J Obstet Gynecol.* 1991;165 (4 Pt 1):876–882.
39. Romero R, Espinoza J, Gonçalves L, et al. Fetal cardiac dysfunction in preterm premature rupture of membranes. *J Matern Fetal Neonatal Med.* 2004;16(3):146–157.
40. Severi FM, Rizzo G, Bocchi C, et al. Intrauterine growth retardation and fetal cardiac function. *Fetal Diagn Ther.* 2000;15(1):8–19.
41. Shapiro I, Degani S, Leibovitz Z, et al. Fetal cardiac measurements derived by transvaginal and transabdominal cross-sectional echocardiography from 14 weeks of gestation to term. *Ultrasound Obstet Gynecol.* 1998;12(6):404–418.
42. Sharland GK, Allan LD. Normal fetal cardiac measurements derived by cross-sectional echocardiography. *Ultrasound Obstet Gynecol.* 1992;2(3):175–181.
43. Sharland GK, Chan KY, Allan LD. Coarctation of the aorta: difficulties in prenatal diagnosis. *Br Heart J.* 1994;71(1):70–75.
44. Tan J, Silverman NH, Hoffman JI, et al. Cardiac dimensions determined by cross-sectional echocardiography in the normal human fetus from 18 weeks to term. *Am J Cardiol.* 1992;70(18):1459–1467.
45. Ursell PC, Byrne JM, Fears TR, et al. Growth of the great vessels in the normal human fetus and in the fetus with cardiac defects. *Circulation.* 1991;84(5):2028–2033.
46. Van Bergen AH, Cuneo BF, Davis N. Prospective echocardiographic evaluation of atrioventricular conduction in fetuses with maternal Sjögren's antibodies. *Am J Obstet Gynecol.* 2004;191(3):1014–1018.
47. Yoo SJ, Lee YH, Cho KS, et al. Sequential segmental approach to fetal congenital heart disease. *Cardiol Young.* 1999;9(4):430–444.
48. Yoo SJ, Lee YH, Cho KS. Abnormal three-vessel view on sonography: a clue to the diagnosis of congenital heart disease in the fetus. *AJR Am J Roentgenol.* 1999;172(3):825–830.

49. Yoo SJ, Lee YH, Kim ES, et al. Tetralogy of Fallot in the fetus: findings at targeted sonography. *Ultrasound Obstet Gynecol.* 1999;14(1):29–37.
50. DeVore GR, Falkensammer P, Sklansky MS, et al. Spatio-temporal image correlation (STIC): new technology for evaluation of the fetal heart. *Ultrasound Obstet Gynecol.* 2003;22(4):380–387.
51. Gonçalves LF, Lee W, Chaiworapongsa T, et al. Four-dimensional ultrasonography of the fetal heart with spatiotemporal image correlation. *Am J Obstet Gynecol.* 2003;189(6):1792–1802.
52. Viñals F, Poblete P, Giuliano A. Spatio-temporal image correlation (STIC): a new tool for the prenatal screening of congenital heart defects. *Ultrasound Obstet Gynecol.* 2003;22(4):388–394.
53. Bhat AH, Corbett VN, Liu R, et al. Validation of volume and mass assessments for human fetal heart imaging by 4-dimensional spatiotemporal image correlation echocardiography: in vitro balloon model experiments. *J Ultrasound Med.* 2004;23(9):1151–1159.
54. Chaoui R, Hoffmann J, Heling KS. Three-dimensional (3D) and 4D color Doppler fetal echocardiography using spatio-temporal image correlation (STIC). *Ultrasound Obstet Gynecol.* 2004;23(6):535–545.
55. DeVore GR, Polanco B, Sklansky MS, et al. The 'spin' technique: a new method for examination of the fetal outflow tracts using three-dimensional ultrasound. *Ultrasound Obstet Gynecol.* 2004;24(1):72–82.
56. Chaoui R, Heling KS. New developments in fetal heart scanning: three- and four-dimensional fetal echocardiography. *Semin Fetal Neonatal Med.* 2005;10(6):567–577.
57. Devore GR, Polanko B. Tomographic ultrasound imaging of the fetal heart: a new technique for identifying normal and abnormal cardiac anatomy. *J Ultrasound Med.* 2005;24(12):1685–1696.
58. Ghi T, Cera E, Segata M, et al. Inversion mode spatio-temporal image correlation (STIC) echocardiography in three-dimensional rendering of fetal ventricular septal defects. *Ultrasound Obstet Gynecol.* 2005;26(6):679–680.
59. Gonçalves LF, Espinoza J, Romero R, et al. Four-dimensional fetal echocardiography with spatiotemporal image correlation (STIC): a systematic study of standard cardiac views assessed by different observers. *J Matern Fetal Neonatal Med.* 2005;17(5):323–331.
60. Messing B, Porat S, Imbar T, et al. Mild tricuspid regurgitation: a benign fetal finding at various stages of pregnancy. *Ultrasound Obstet Gynecol.* 2005;26(6):606–609; discussion 610.
61. Pooh RK, Korai A. B-flow and B-flow spatio-temporal image correlation in visualizing fetal cardiac blood flow. *Croat Med J.* 2005;46(5):808–811.
62. Shih JC, Chen CP. Spatio-temporal image correlation (STIC): innovative 3D/4D technique for illustrating unique and independent information and diagnosing complex congenital heart diseases. *Croat Med J.* 2005;46(5):812–820.
63. Viñals F, Mandujano L, Vargas G, et al. Prenatal diagnosis of congenital heart disease using four-dimensional spatio-temporal image correlation (STIC) telemedicine via an Internet link: a pilot study. *Ultrasound Obstet Gynecol.* 2005;25(1):25–31.
64. Devore G, Sklansky M. Three-dimensional imaging of the fetal heart: current applications and future directions. *Progress in Pediatric Cardiology.* 2006;22:9–29.
65. Gonçalves LF, Espinoza J, Romero R, et al. Four-dimensional ultrasonography of the fetal heart using a novel Tomographic Ultrasound Imaging display. *J Perinat Med.* 2006;34(1):39–55.
66. Gonçalves LF, Lee W, Espinoza J, et al. Examination of the fetal heart by four-dimensional (4D) ultrasound with spatio-temporal image correlation (STIC). *Ultrasound Obstet Gynecol.* 2006;27(3):336–348.
67. Paladini D, Vassallo M, Sglavo G, et al. The role of spatio-temporal image correlation (STIC) with tomographic ultrasound imaging (TUI) in the sequential analysis of fetal congenital heart disease. *Ultrasound Obstet Gynecol.* 2006;27(5):555–561.
68. Viñals F, Ascenzo R, Poblete P, et al. Simple approach to prenatal diagnosis of transposition of the great arteries. *Ultrasound Obstet Gynecol.* 2006;28(1):22–25.
69. Volpe P, Campobasso G, Stanziano A, et al. Novel application of 4D sonography with B-flow imaging and spatio-temporal image correlation (STIC) in the assessment of the anatomy of pulmonary arteries in fetuses with pulmonary atresia and ventricular septal defect. *Ultrasound Obstet Gynecol.* 2006;28(1):40–46.
70. Yagel S, Benachi A, Bonnet D, et al. Rendering in fetal cardiac scanning: the intracardiac septa and the coronal atrioventricular valve planes. *Ultrasound Obstet Gynecol.* 2006;28(3):266–274.
71. Messing B, Cohen SM, Valsky DV, et al. Fetal cardiac ventricle volumetry in the second half of gestation assessed by 4D ultrasound using STIC combined with inversion mode. *Ultrasound Obstet Gynecol.* 2007;30(2):142–151.
72. Paladini D. Standardization of on-screen fetal heart orientation prior to storage of spatio-temporal image correlation (STIC) volume datasets. *Ultrasound Obstet Gynecol.* 2007;29(6):605–611.
73. Rizzo G, Capponi A, Cavicchioni O, et al. Fetal cardiac stroke volume determination by four-dimensional ultrasound with spatio-temporal image correlation compared with two-dimensional and Doppler ultrasonography. *Prenat Diagn.* 2007;27(12):1147–1150.

74. Volpe P, Campobasso G, De Robertis V, et al. Two- and four-dimensional echocardiography with B-flow imaging and spatiotemporal image correlation in prenatal diagnosis of isolated total anomalous pulmonary venous connection. *Ultrasound Obstet Gynecol.* 2007;30(6):830–837.
75. Achiron R, Gindes L, Zalel Y, et al. Three- and four-dimensional ultrasound: new methods for evaluating fetal thoracic anomalies. *Ultrasound Obstet Gynecol.* 2008;32(1):36–43.
76. Araujo Junior E, de Bussamra LC, Barros FS, et al. Prenatal diagnosis of Ebstein's anomaly using spatio-temporal image correlation (STIC) and inversion mode. *Arch Gynecol Obstet.* 2008;278(4):387–391.
77. Hata T, Dai SY, Inubashiri E, et al. Four-dimensional sonography with B-flow imaging and spatiotemporal image correlation for visualization of the fetal heart. *J Clin Ultrasound.* 2008;36(4):204–207.
78. Molina FS, Faro C, Sotiriadis A, et al. Heart stroke volume and cardiac output by four-dimensional ultrasound in normal fetuses. *Ultrasound Obstet Gynecol.* 2008;32(2):181–187.
79. Paladini D, Sglavo G, Greco E, et al. Cardiac screening by STIC: can sonologists performing the 20-week anomaly scan pick up outflow tract abnormalities by scrolling the A-plane of STIC volumes? *Ultrasound Obstet Gynecol.* 2008;32(7):865–870.
80. Rizzo G, Capponi A, Muscatello A, et al. Examination of the fetal heart by four-dimensional ultrasound with spatiotemporal image correlation during routine second-trimester examination: the 'three-steps technique'. *Fetal Diagn Ther.* 2008;24(2):126–131.
81. Shih JC, Shyu MK, Su YN, et al. 'Big-eyed frog' sign on spatiotemporal image correlation (STIC) in the antenatal diagnosis of transposition of the great arteries. *Ultrasound Obstet Gynecol.* 2008;32(6):762–768.
82. Tutschek B, Sahn DJ. Semi-automatic segmentation of fetal cardiac cavities: progress towards an automated fetal echocardiogram. *Ultrasound Obstet Gynecol.* 2008;32(2):176–180.
83. Uittenbogaard LB, Haak MC, Spreeuwenberg MD, et al. A systematic analysis of the feasibility of four-dimensional ultrasound imaging using spatiotemporal image correlation in routine fetal echocardiography. *Ultrasound Obstet Gynecol.* 2008;31(6):625–632.
84. Viñals F, Ascenzo R, Naveas R, et al. Fetal echocardiography at 11 + 0 to 13 + 6 weeks using four-dimensional spatiotemporal image correlation telemedicine via an Internet link: a pilot study. *Ultrasound Obstet Gynecol.* 2008;31(6):633–638.
85. Wanitpongpan P, Kanagawa T, Kinugasa Y, et al. Spatio-temporal image correlation (STIC) used by general obstetricians is marginally clinically effective compared to 2D fetal echocardiography scanning by experts. *Prenat Diagn.* 2008;28(10):923–928.
86. Bennasar M, Martinez JM, Olivella A, et al. Feasibility and accuracy of fetal echocardiography using four-dimensional spatiotemporal image correlation technology before 16 weeks' gestation. *Ultrasound Obstet Gynecol.* 2009;33(6):645–651.
87. Gindes L, Hegesh J, Weisz B, et al. Three and four dimensional ultrasound: a novel method for evaluating fetal cardiac anomalies. *Prenat Diagn.* 2009;29(7):645–653.
88. Hamill N, Romero R, Hassan SS, et al. Repeatability and reproducibility of fetal cardiac ventricular volume calculations using spatiotemporal image correlation and virtual organ computer-aided analysis. *J Ultrasound Med.* 2009;28(10):1301–1311.
89. Tonni G, Centini G, Taddei F. Can 3D ultrasound and doppler angiography of great arteries be included in second trimester ecocardiographic examination? A prospective study on low-risk pregnancy population. *Echocardiography.* 2009;26(7):815–822.
90. Turan S, Turan OM, Maisel P, et al. Three-dimensional sonography in the prenatal diagnosis of aortic arch abnormalities. *J Clin Ultrasound.* 2009;37(5):253–257.
91. Turan S, Turan OM, Ty-Torredes K, et al. Standardization of the first-trimester fetal cardiac examination using spatiotemporal image correlation with tomographic ultrasound and color Doppler imaging. *Ultrasound Obstet Gynecol.* 2009;33(6):652–656.
92. Uittenbogaard LB, Haak MC, Spreeuwenberg MD, et al. Fetal cardiac function assessed with four-dimensional ultrasound imaging using spatiotemporal image correlation. *Ultrasound Obstet Gynecol.* 2009;33(3):272–281.
93. Bennasar M, Martinez JM, Gomez O, et al. Accuracy of four-dimensional spatiotemporal image correlation echocardiography in the prenatal diagnosis of congenital heart defects. *Ultrasound Obstet Gynecol.* 2010;36(4):458–464.
94. Bennasar M, Martinez JM, Gomez O, et al. Intra- and interobserver repeatability of fetal cardiac examination using four-dimensional spatiotemporal image correlation in each trimester of pregnancy. *Ultrasound Obstet Gynecol.* 2010;35(3):318–323.
95. Dan-Dan W, Xiao-Peng D, Wei C, et al. The value of spatiotemporal image correlation technique in the diagnosis of fetal ventricular septal defect. *Arch Gynecol Obstet.* 2011;283(5):965–969.

96. Espinoza J. Contemporary clinical applications of spatio-temporal image correlation in prenatal diagnosis. *Curr Opin Obstet Gynecol.* 2011;23(2):94–102.
97. Espinoza J, Lee W, Comstock C, et al. Collaborative study on 4-dimensional echocardiography for the diagnosis of fetal heart defects: the COFEHD study. *J Ultrasound Med.* 2010;29(11):1573–1580.
98. Hata T, Tanaka H, Noguchi J, et al. Four-dimensional volume-rendered imaging of the fetal ventricular outflow tracts and great arteries using inversion mode for detection of congenital heart disease. *J Obstet Gynaecol Res.* 2010;36(3):513–518.
99. Jantarasaengaram S, Vairojanavong K. Eleven fetal echocardiographic planes using 4-dimensional ultrasound with spatio-temporal image correlation (STIC): a logical approach to fetal heart volume analysis. *Cardiovasc Ultrasound.* 2010;8:41.
100. Rizzo G, Capponi A, Pietrolucci ME, et al. Role of sonographic automatic volume calculation in measuring fetal cardiac ventricular volumes using 4-dimensional sonography: comparison with virtual organ computer-aided analysis. *J Ultrasound Med.* 2010;29(2):261–270.
101. Uittenbogaard LB, Haak MC, Peters RJ, et al. Validation of volume measurements for fetal echocardiography using four-dimensional ultrasound imaging and spatiotemporal image correlation. *Ultrasound Obstet Gynecol.* 2010;35(3):324–331.
102. Volpe P, Tuo G, De Robertis V, et al. Fetal interrupted aortic arch: 2D-4D echocardiography, associations and outcome. *Ultrasound Obstet Gynecol.* 2010;35(3):302–309.
103. Yagel S, Cohen SM, Rosenak D, et al. Added value of 3D/4DUS in the offline analysis and diagnosis of congenital heart disease. *Ultrasound Obstet Gynecol.* 2011;37(4):432–437.
104. Yeo L, Romero R, Jodicke C, et al. Four-chamber view and 'swing technique' (FAST) echo: a novel and simple algorithm to visualize standard fetal echocardiographic planes. *Ultrasound Obstet Gynecol.* 2011;37(4):423–431.
105. Zhang M, Pu DR, Zhou QC, et al. Four-dimensional echocardiography with B-flow imaging and spatiotemporal image correlation in the assessment of congenital heart defects. *Prenat Diagn.* 2010;30(5):443–448.
106. Dawson D, Lygate CA, Saunders J, et al. Quantitative 3-dimensional echocardiography for accurate and rapid cardiac phenotype characterization in mice. *Circulation.* 2004;110(12):1632–1637.
107. Sklansky MS, DeVore GR, Wong PC. Real-time 3-dimensional fetal echocardiography with an instantaneous volume-rendered display: early description and pictorial essay. *J Ultrasound Med.* 2004;23(2):283–289.
108. Yoo SJ, Lee YH, Cho KS. Abnormal three-vessel view on sonography: a clue to the diagnosis of congenital heart disease in the fetus. *AJR Am J Roentgenol.* 1999;172(3):825–830.
109. Yoo SJ, Lee YH, Cho KS, et al. Sequential segmental approach to fetal congenital heart disease. *Cardiol Young.* 1999;9(4):430–444.
110. Yoo SJ, Lee YH, Kim ES, et al. Three-vessel view of the fetal upper mediastinum: an easy means of detecting abnormalities of the ventricular outflow tracts and great arteries during obstetric screening. *Ultrasound Obstet Gynecol.* 1997;9(3):173–182.
111. Yoo SJ, Lee YH, Kim ES, et al. Tetralogy of Fallot in the fetus: findings at targeted sonography. *Ultrasound Obstet Gynecol.* 1999;14(1):29–37.
112. Yagel S, Cohen SM, Achiron R. Examination of the fetal heart by five short-axis views: a proposed screening method for comprehensive cardiac evaluation. *Ultrasound Obstet Gynecol.* 2001;17(5):367–369.
113. Rychik J, Ayres N, Cuneo B, et al. American Society of Echocardiography guidelines and standards for performance of the fetal echocardiogram. *J Am Soc Echocardiogr.* 2004;17(7):803–810.

CHAPTER

15

ADULTS WITH CONGENITAL HEART DISEASE

Fadi G. Hage, MD; Navin C. Nanda, MD

ABSTRACT

With the increasing survival of patients who have congenital heart disease (CHD) that was surgically corrected during childhood, many adults with CHD will be under the care of clinical cardiologists in the coming years. Three-dimensional echocardiography (3DE) can provide incremental value to two-dimensional imaging for the accurate assessment of the morphology of atrial septal defects (ASDs) and the efficacy of percutaneous devices used for the closure of ASDs or patent foramen ovale, for the comprehensive evaluation of ostium primum ASDs, and for the assessment of isolated mitral valve cleft and papillary muscle abnormalities. 3DE is also valuable in assessing the size, shape, and location of ventricular septal defects and the anatomy of the surrounding tissue, measuring the size of a patent ductus arteriosus, and evaluating the complex geometry of coronary artery anomalies. It also aids in identifying quadricuspid aortic valves or the presence of subaortic stenosis and in evaluating patients with transposition of the great arteries corrected in childhood, Ebstein's anomaly, aortopulmonary window, Gerbode defect, eustachian valve, cor triatriatum sinister and dextra, and the Chiari network.

INTRODUCTION

Caring for patients with congenital heart disease (CHD) is one of the most difficult tasks that confront the adult cardiologist because of the complexity of the pathologies involved. CHD conditions in adults are often intricate, are occasionally difficult to diagnose, and always necessitate forming an elaborate plan of management. Treatment heavily depends on imaging modalities to guide its progress rather than on physical examination alone.[1–4] Two-dimensional transthoracic echocardiography (2DTTE) has been the most widely utilized imaging modality for the study of CHD, particularly in children, as emphasized in this book.[4] 2DTTE is especially attractive and has advantages over computed tomography and magnetic resonance imaging because it is entirely noninvasive, does not use harmful radiation, and does not require prolonged patient cooperation. Despite its widespread use and multiple advantages, 2DTTE suffers in comparison with the other imaging modalities in its limited ability to visualize three-dimensional (3D) complex structures. With the development of three-dimensional transthoracic echocardiography (3DTTE), echocardiography regained its edge for the evaluation of patients with CHD.[5] With the increasing survival of CHD patients who undergo surgical correction during childhood, clinical cardiologists will care for exponentially higher numbers of adults with CHD in the coming years and this field will likely benefit from current improvements in imaging technology.[6] This chapter summarizes the applicability of 3DTTE for the study of common CHD conditions encountered in adulthood.

ATRIAL SEPTAL DEFECTS

Atrial septal defects (ASDs) constitute about 10% of all CHD cases in adults.[7] In the presence of an ASD, blood can shunt from the left to the right side of the heart, resulting in volume overload.[7] ASDs can be divided into four types. Ostium secundum ASD, the most common type, occurs in the area of the fossa ovalis. Ostium primum ASDs are actually part of the spectrum of atrioventricular canals and are usually associated with a "cleft" mitral valve. Sinus venosus ASDs occur at the junction of the superior or inferior vena cava or the coronary sinus with the right atrium and are often associated with anomalous drainage of the pulmonary veins. Coronary sinus ASDs, the least common type, represent an unroofed coronary sinus.[7]

ASDs have traditionally been corrected surgically, but the recent development of percutaneous closure devices has introduced a practical alternative.[7] The indications for percutaneous or surgical ASD repair are the same; however, with percutaneous repair several attributes of ASDs must be evaluated in order to ensure candidacy for the procedure so that a closure device can be safely deployed with a catheter. These include the location of the defect, its shape and size, and the adequacy of its margins for the placement of such devices.[7,8] These features are best appreciated from an en face view similar to the view that the surgeon has access to intraoperatively. Thus, although two-dimensional transesophageal echocardiography (2DTEE) can supplement 2DTTE in diagnosing ASDs and complements its deficiencies in thisrespect,[8] it shares its limitations in defining the geometry of the defect and the characterization of the surrounding tissue because the defect is not visualized en face by either 2DTTE or 2DTEE. This is especially important because ASDs are known to have a complex geometry. Therefore, with 2DE one can measure one or two dimensions of the defect, but verifying that the maximum dimension has been measured is impossible because the ASD has not been seen in 3D.[9] It is now appreciated that an ASD is not always a single defect but can comprise multiple small defects (Swiss cheese pattern, Fig. 15-1).[10] Another relevant characteristic that can be detrimental to the percutaneous deployment of a closure device is the presence of small rims of tissue such that the device can encroach and damage other structures such as the aorta. However, two-dimensional (2D) technology does not permit definitive identification of the marginal rim and its size because the ASD is not directly en face visualized. With 3DTTE, the pyramidal 3D data set can be cropped in any direction and the defect can be seen en face from the right atrial and the left atrial perspective, thus giving 3DTTE a crucial advantage over 2DE (Fig. 15-2).[11]

Figure 15-1

Live real-time 3D right parasternal TTE examination of atrial septum and superior and inferior venae cavae. Color Doppler examination in a patient showing four separate secundum defects (numbered 1–4) at different levels of the atrial septum. In this 25-year-old woman, four ASDs at different levels of the atrial septum could be demonstrated by sequential cropping of the 3D data set. Only two of these defects could be visualized by 2DTTE. LA, left atrium; RA, right atrium. Reproduced with permission from Patel et al.[10]

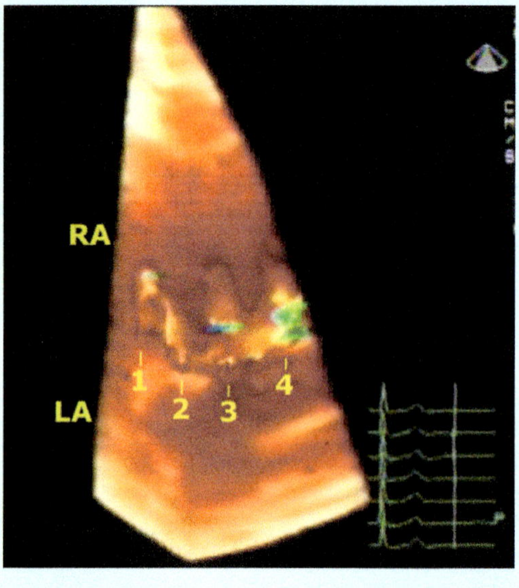

Figure 15-2A and B

Live real-time 3DTTE assessment of an ASD. Arrowheads point to a large secundum ASD visualized from both right (*A*) and left atrial (*B*) aspects. Note the large rim of tissue surrounding the defect. AS, atrial septum; LA, left atrium; RA, right atrium. Reproduced with permission from Mehmood et al.[11]

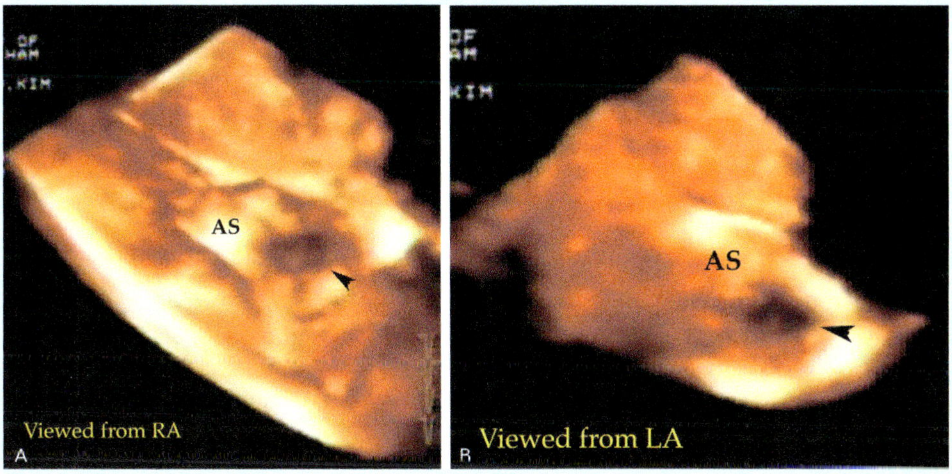

In 2004, our group established the accuracy, feasibility, and usefulness of 3DTTE for the assessment of ASDs.[11] 3DTTE was performed after completion of the 2DTTE standard examination in 12 patients with ASDs. Four of these patients eventually underwent surgical repair and had intraoperative 2DTEE with 3D reconstruction. Another seven patients had percutaneous repair using an Amplatzer Septal Occluder (AGA Medical Corp., Plymouth, Minnesota).[11] An en face view was possible in all 12 patients. The maximum dimension, circumference, and area measured by 3DTTE agreed well with those measured by 3D reconstruction of 2DTEE in patients treated surgically and with the sizing balloon in those treated percutaneously. Impressively, 3DTTE was able to characterize the tissue surrounding the defect and to measure the rim margin in order to evaluate the suitability of using an occluder device.[11] Interestingly, the size of the inferior rim seems to be more important than that of the superior rim for this purpose because the absence of atrial septal tissue in the atrial rim is considered a strong risk factor for device migration and embolization.[12] Rarely the occluder device can embolize into the pulmonary artery, and in such cases surgical extraction is necessary.[13] Thus, 3DTTE can provide the advantage of choosing the right-sized balloon in order to save time during percutaneous repair and can better characterize the size and proximity of as ASD to other structures, such as the aorta, in order to avoid damage, embolization, and residual leaks. A patent foramen ovale can also be visualized with the addition of an agitated saline contrast agent. Furthermore, 3DTTE (with and without color Doppler) can provide incremental value to 2DTTE and 2DTEE for the accurate assessment of the morphology and efficacy of percutaneous closure devices used for the closure of ASDs and patent foramen ovale.[14] 3DTTE was able to visualize well both the right atrial and left atrial disks of the transcatheter closure device in 3D and the waist of the device, that is, the part that connects the two disks together. The measurements of these devices obtained by 3DTTE correlate very well with those provided by the manufacturer.[14] Another important aspect of the 3D examination is its ability to verify the position of the device and to reveal whether there is any residual shunting.[14] 3DTTE can also be useful in imaging device migration, embolization, and fractures.[15]

3DTTE can also be used to provide a more comprehensive evaluation of ostium primum ASDs compared to 2DTTE.[16] This congenital defect results from incomplete fusion of the superior and inferior endocardial cushions during the first trimester of gestation. The spectrum of abnormalities ranges from partial to complete atrioventricular canal defects, with frequent abnormalities in the atrioventricular valves.[7] In order to accurately assess the size of all five individual leaflets of the common atrioventricular valve (three lateral leaflets: mural lateral on the left, mural inferior, and anterosuperior on the right; and two bridging leaflets: superior and inferior) and the ASD, extensive cropping of the 3D data set is required from multiple perspectives and angulations, but the data derived from this surpass any that can be obtained using 2DTTE (Fig. 15-3).[16,17] Because these five leaflets are not present in the same plane ensuring that all leaflets are accounted for is impossible in 2DTTE, and delineating the size and attachment of these valves with confidence is often not possible. Furthermore, with 3DTTE subclassification of these defects, as described by Rastelli et al.,[18] is possible with more confidence than with 2DTTE because the chordal and papillary muscle attachments of the common atrioventricular valve and the extension of the superior bridging leaflet into the right ventricle can be well delineated.[16,18] It is important to recognize that in atrioventricular septal defects anterior and superior displacement of the aorta results in elongation and narrowing of the left ventricular outflow tract and characteristic absence of wedging of the aorta between the mitral and tricuspid rings.[16] In addition, the papillary muscles can sometimes have abnormal arrangements that may result in subaortic obstruction of an already narrowed left ventricular outflow tract.[19] In partial atrioventricular septal defects, 3DTTE can reveal two scallops of the posterior leaflet of the left atrioventricular valve, compared with the usual three scallops, and the widened anteroseptal commissure of the right atrioventricular valve, which is often not possible with 2DTTE.[16] A cleft in the mitral valve can also be present without other associated findings. An isolated mitral valve cleft can be missed by 2DTTE. Whereas the mitral cleft points toward the right ventricle in atrioventricular canal defects, in an isolated mitral valve cleft it points toward the left ventricular outflow tract. With proper cropping and angulation, 3DTTE can provide quite useful views of the mitral valve (or the atrioventricular valve in ostium primum ASDs) cleft, enabling better assessment of its size and extent and interrogation of the surrounding tissue (Fig. 15-4).[20] While 3DTTE can verify the findings seen on 2DTTE and allow the echocardiographer more confidence in the diagnosis, it can also reveal new diagnoses not suspected on 2DE.[16] 3DTTE can reveal papillary muscle abnormalities, such as an anomalous papillary muscle projecting into the narrowed and elongated left ventricular outflow tract causing subaortic obstruction or abnormally closely attached papillary muscles (paired papillary muscles).[16] Better visualization of these complex structures can be invaluable for surgical planning.

The right parasternal view can be quite helpful for the evaluation of an ASD because such patients often have right ventricular enlargement, which opens an echocardiographic window with a perpendicular ultrasound path to the atrial septum (Fig. 15-1).[11] Therefore, although 3DTTE is not always useful for

Figure 15-3

Live real-time 3DTTE in complete atrioventricular septal defect in a 67-year-old woman. En face view of the common atrioventricular valve showing all five leaflets. 1, Superior bridging leaflet extending into right ventricle; 2, mural lateral leaflet; 3, inferior bridging leaflet; 4, mural inferior leaflet; 5, anterosuperior leaflet. AO, aorta. Reproduced with permission from Singh et al.[17]

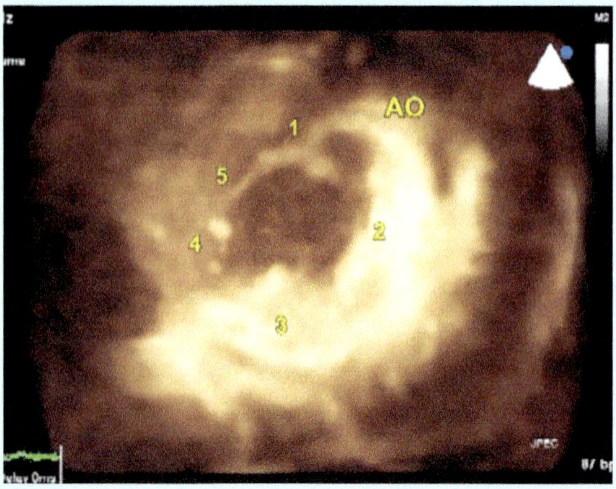

Figure 15-4

Live real-time 3DTTE assessment of isolated cleft mitral valve. The arrowhead points to the cleft in the anterior mitral valve leaflet seen in the open position. The cleft is directed toward the left ventricular outflow tract unlike the atrioventricular septal defect, where the cleft points medially. LV, left ventricle; PML, posterior mitral leaflet; RV, right ventricle. Reproduced with permission from Sinha et al.[20]

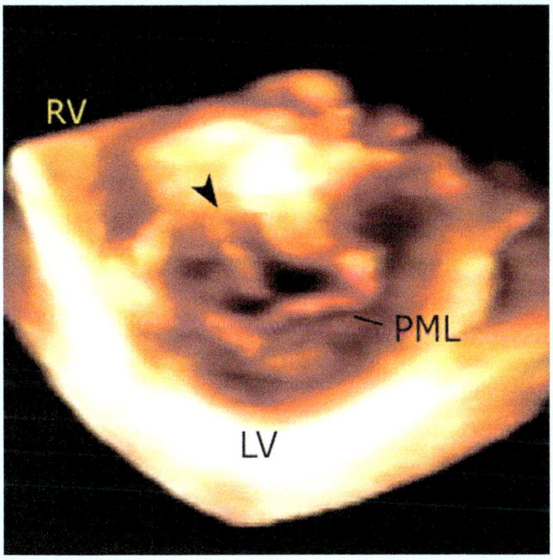

diagnosing small defects or patent foramen ovale because of its limited resolution, it is better than 2DTTE for the assessment of defect size, shape, and rim characterization and provides an advantage after device placement in assessing complications and residual shunts.

VENTRICULAR SEPTAL DEFECTS

Ventricular septal defects (VSDs) account for 20% of adult CHD cases.[21,22] Although surgical closure of VSDs was considered the norm for decades, percutaneous closure is now advocated as a less invasive alternative. Even perimembranous defects, which were once not amenable to percutaneous closure, are now candidates for this less invasive approach in some instances. However, when such an approach is contemplated careful patient selection and echocardiographic characteristics can be crucial for successful interventions.[22] In a manner very similar to that with ASDs, 2DTTE is limited in the assessment of VSDs because it is not able to appreciate the 3D complexity of these defects. With 2DTTE a cross-sectional plane through the defect can be viewed, but the echocardiographer is never certain that this plane is capturing the maximum dimension of the defect. With 3DTTE, conversely, the defect and the surrounding tissue can be entirely included in the data set. With proper cropping, the defect can be visualized en face and its circumference and area properly measured and the surrounding tissue better characterized (Fig. 15-5).[23] Because the size, shape, and location of the defect and the anatomy of the surrounding tissue are relevant for proper selection for percutaneous correction, 3DTTE can be considered the optimal imaging modality for preintervention assessment because it provides views that closely resemble intraoperative views.[24,25] Also important, 3DTTE, unlike 2DTTE, can measure the length of the VSD margin along the tricuspid valve, which is relevant for presurgical planning.[23] It can also show the spatial location of the tricuspid valve leaflet, right ventricular outflow tract, and aortic valve in relation to the VSD from the surgical perspective (Fig. 15-6).[25] Furthermore, better anatomic characterization of the defect size, the proximity of the defect to the tricuspid valve, and the suitability of the defect rim can improve the

Figure 15-5

Live real-time 3DTTE assessment of a VSD. The arrowhead points to a perimembranous ventricular septal (VS) defect viewed en face. LA, left atrium; LVOT, left ventricular outflow tract; MV, mitral valve; RV, right ventricle. Reproduced with permission from Mehmood et al.[23]

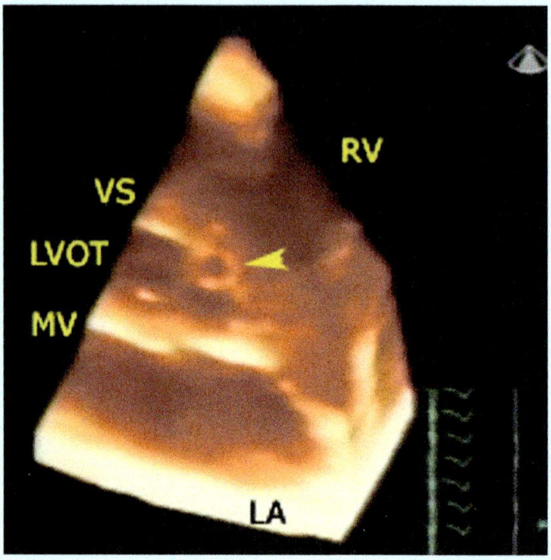

safety of percutaneous device deployment as well as decrease the complication rate.[23] The validity of these measurements by 3DTTE has been verified against the surgical and 3DTEE standards, showing very close correlations.[23,25]

PATENT DUCTUS ARTERIOSUS

While the ductus arteriosus is normally patent in fetal life and serves to shunt blood from the right ventricle to the systemic circulation by connecting the pulmonary artery to the descending thoracic aorta, it usually closes shortly after birth but occasionally remains patent into adult life.[26] Although 2DTTE can be helpful in establishing this diagnosis, it is not very reliable for measuring the size of the defect and identifying the exact location of the connection.[27] Magnetic resonance imaging and computed tomography can also be helpful in establishing the presence of patent ductus arteriosus (PDA) in adults.[28] With modern techniques, almost all PDAs can be safely and effectively closed using percutaneous techniques.[27] Using 3DTTE, the PDA and its surrounding structures can be visualized in 3D space. Careful cropping of the 3D data set can delineate the complex structure of a PDA and allow for the accurate measurement of its length and width. Because the data set includes the surrounding structures, meticulous assessment can reveal the connections of the PDA to the pulmonary artery and the descending thoracic aorta and allow for the measurement of these connections (Fig. 15-7).[29] The proximity of the PDA to the origin of the left pulmonary artery can also be accurately measured (an important consideration when planning closure). Applying color Doppler to the 3D examination can add confidence in differentiating vascular structures from artifacts and echo dropouts. This comprehensive evaluation of PDAs is essential for the proper selection of candidates for percutaneous correction and for the selection of the most appropriate approach for percutaneous closure. An adequate examination can also be helpful in determining procedural success and can identify complications faced during percutaneous treatment of PDAs.[30]

Figure 15-6A, B, C, and D

Live real-time 3DTTE assessment of a VSD. Perimembranous VSD (inlet, arrow). *A*, 3D volume-rendered image of the right ventricle displaying the right aspect of VSD. The location of the defect in relation to the tricuspid valve (TV) is shown. *B*, Surgical view of VSD from the right aspect. *C*, 3D volume-rendered image of the left ventricle displaying the left aspect of the VSD. The location of the defect in relation to the left ventricle outflow tract is shown. *D*, 2D parasternal long-axis view showing the VSD in relation to the aortic valve and the right ventricle. Ao, aorta; LA, left atrium; LV, left ventricle; RA, right atrium; RV, right ventricle. Reproduced with permission from Chen et al.[25]

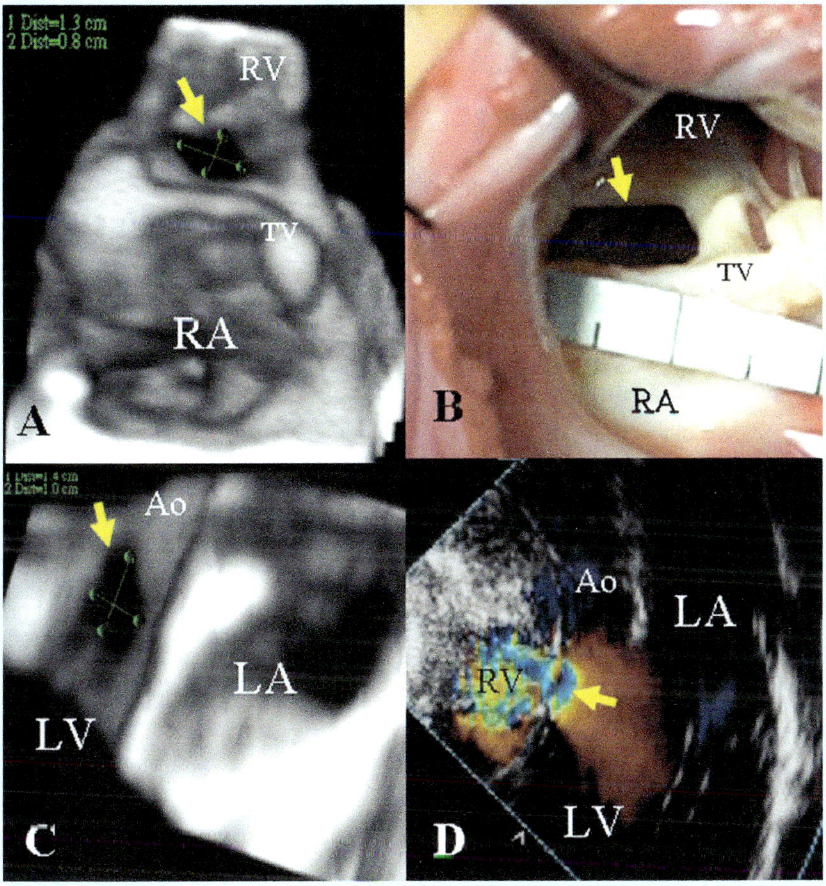

CORONARY ARTERY ANOMALIES

Anomalies of the coronary artery occur in more than 1% of the general population. Some of these anomalies are considered benign, whereas others can result in serious complications such as myocardial infarction and sudden death.[31] This prognostic differentiation, which is clinically very important, has been shown to be predictable from the anatomy of anomalous coronaries and their relationship to the great vessels.[31] A careful evaluation of the complex geometry can thus be useful for the assessment of prognosis and for guiding repair.

The left coronary artery can arise anomalously from the pulmonary artery, in which case blood can flow retrogradely from the coronary circulation into the low-pressure pulmonary circulation, resulting in myocardial ischemia and left ventricular dysfunction. This condition is fatal unless corrected surgically. 3DTTE can clearly delineate the orifice of the anomalous coronary artery and determine its exact location, but this is not possible with 2DTTE (Fig. 15-8).[32] In addition, the orifice of the anomalous artery can be

Figure 15-7

Live real-time 3DTTE in an adult with PDA. The pyramidal section has been cropped to show the full extent of the PDA (arrowhead) connecting the main pulmonary artery (PA) to the descending thoracic aorta (DA). The arrow points to the left atrial appendage. LPA, left pulmonary artery; LV, left ventricle; PV, pulmonary valve. Reproduced with permission from Sinha et al.[29]

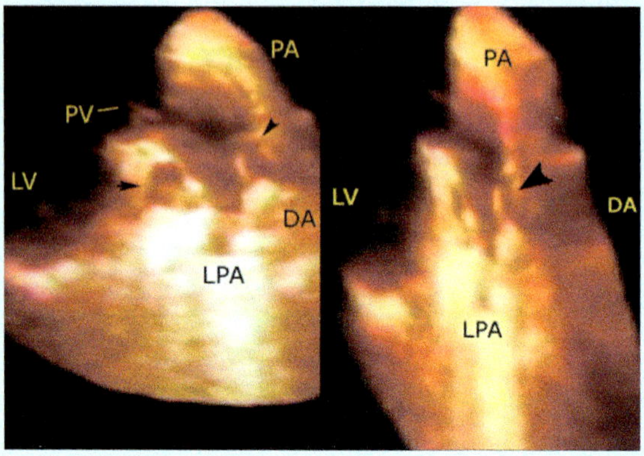

Figure 15-8

Live 3DTTE demonstration of anomalous origin of left coronary artery from the pulmonary artery. The arrow points to the orifice of the anomalous coronary artery, and the arrowhead shows the defect in the tunnel. AO, aorta; RPA, right pulmonary artery; RVOT, right ventricular outflow tract. Reproduced with permission from Ilgenli et al.[32]

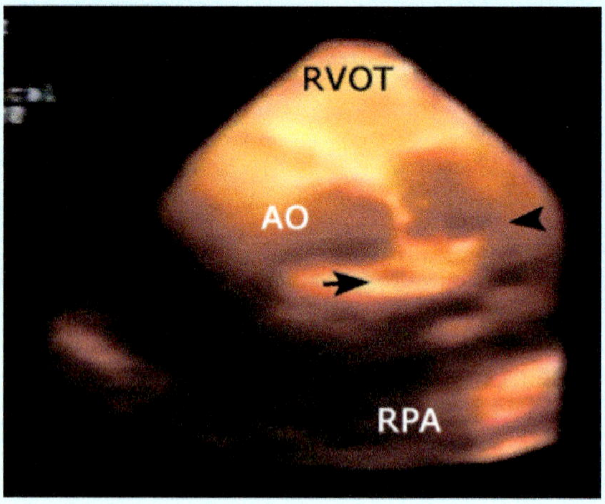

visualized en face, its size measured, and its surrounding tissue characterized. In patients who underwent surgical correction, visualization of the tunnel connecting the aorta to the pulmonary artery can also be clearly made. In these cases, 3D color Doppler imaging can be very helpful in establishing with confidence the orifice of the coronary artery.[32] With careful measurements of the orifice area and the time–velocity integral, the left-to-right shunt volume can be estimated. Similarly, 3DTTE can be helpful in the assessment of coronary artery to pulmonary artery fistulas and other coronary artery anomalies (Fig. 15-9).[33,34]

Figure 15-9

Live real-time 3DTTE detection of left main coronary artery fistula into the left ventricle. The entrance of the enlarged left main coronary artery into the left ventricle is denoted by an arrowhead. LV, left ventricle. Reproduced with permission from Nanda et al.[33]

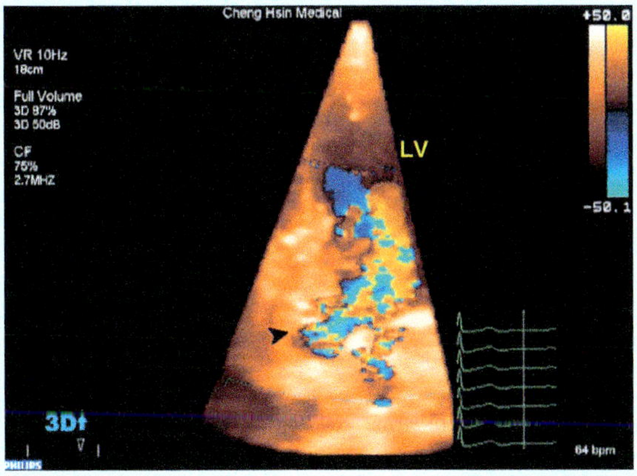

AORTIC AND SUBAORTIC STENOSES

Left ventricular outflow tract obstruction has been described at multiple levels.[35] Congenital aortic stenosis secondary to a bicuspid aortic valve is the most common cardiac congenital disease seen in adults.[36] The symptoms are similar to those seen with acquired aortic stenosis secondary to the calcification of leaflets but usually present earlier in life, around the fifth decade. Although a bicuspid aortic valve can result in aortic stenosis, aortic regurgitation, or both, when a bicuspid aortic valve is recognized on echocardiography in the absence of significant aortic stenosis, this is usually accompanied by redundancy in the aortic valve leaflets. This is because for the valve leaflets to have midline closure, the length of the opposing surfaces of the valve cusps would be smaller than the aortic circumference, resulting in severe aortic stenosis. However, if the leaflets are redundant, this will increase the surface length of the leaflets and prevent the development of significant aortic stenosis.[37] These redundancies in the leaflets can be well seen on 3DTTE (Figs. 15-10 and 15-11).[37] Another rare cause of aortic stenosis is a quadricuspid aortic valve, which can be easily missed on 2DTTE or misdiagnosed as a bicuspid aortic valve. All four leaflets can be well visualized on 3DTTE, and a more comprehensive evaluation of the severity of aortic stenosis and regurgitation can be performed (Fig. 15-12).[37,38]

Subvalvular obstruction is often dynamic, as seen in hypertrophic cardiomyopathy, but it can be a fixed anatomic obstruction as well. Fixed subaortic stenosis is most often secondary to a focal membranous structure that obstructs flow in the left ventricular outflow tract, but occasionally it is due to a diffuse tunnel-type lesion.[35,39] A high level of suspicion should be maintained for the presence of subaortic stenosis whenever high velocities are detected in the left ventricular outflow tract by flow but the valve anatomy appears normal, because discrete subaortic stenosis can often be missed and the patient can be misdiagnosed as having hypertrophic cardiomyopathy.[40] Indeed, even invasive hemodynamic assessment can occasionally miss the presence of this lesion.[41] Traditionally, 2DTEE has been advocated for full assessment of this lesion.[42,43] 3DTTE can complement 2DTTE examination by showing the exact site and the full extent of the membrane. Furthermore, the plane of the orifice can be visualized en face and, using appropriate software, the orifice can be planimetered to calculate its area and directly determine the severity of stenosis rather than depend on indirect measurement of Doppler gradients, which have been shown to be grossly unreliable.[43–47] Thus, 2DTTE may indicate the presence of significant subaortic obstruction due to the presence of a high Doppler gradient despite the absence of severe obstruction, whereas 3DTTE can provide the correct

Figure 15-10

Live real-time 3DTTE. Note the presence of several folds in the bicuspid aortic valve in the closed position viewed from the ventricular side. AV, aortic valve; LA, left atrium; RV, right ventricle. Reproduced with permission from Singh et al.[37]

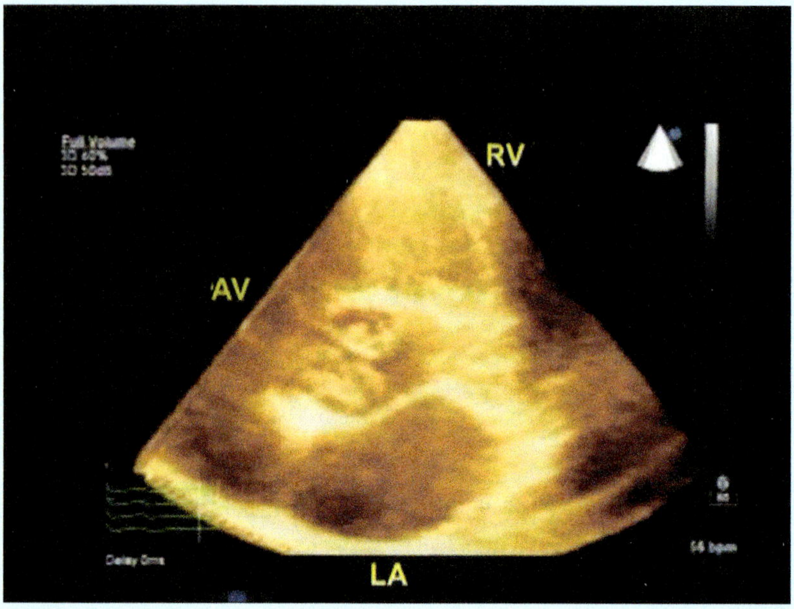

Figure 15-11

Bicuspid aortic valve. *A*, Bicuspid aortic valve with equal-sized cusps and midline closure. Because the length of the free margins of the aortic cusps equals the diameter of the aortic root and the aortic lumen circumference is more than three times the diameter, this will result in markedly restricted opening of the valve leaflets in systole, leading to severe stenosis. *B*, Same valve as in panel *A* but with multiple folds. The presence of these folds serves to substantially increase the length of the free margins of the leaflets, resulting in a fully opened aortic valve in systole. AV, aortic valve. Reproduced with permission from Singh et al.[37]

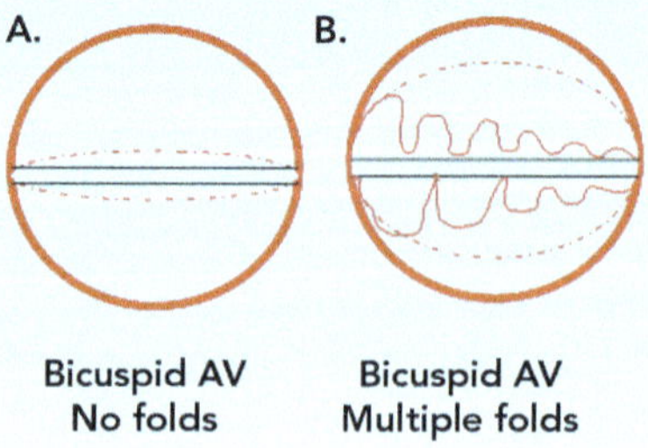

diagnosis because it relies on an anatomic assessment of obstruction severity (Fig. 15-13).[48] Therefore, 3DTTE can avoid many of the pitfalls traditionally associated with the inaccuracy of Doppler evaluation of obstructive lesions, such as the pressure-recovery phenomenon as well as the local variation of velocities. Also, the exact anatomic location of the membrane can be determined in relation to adjacent structures and

Figure 15-12

Live real-time 3DTTE. A quadricuspid aortic valve with four numbered leaflets clearly visualized. AV, aortic valve; LA, left atrium; RV, right ventricle; TV, tricuspid valve. Reproduced with permission from Burri et al.[38]

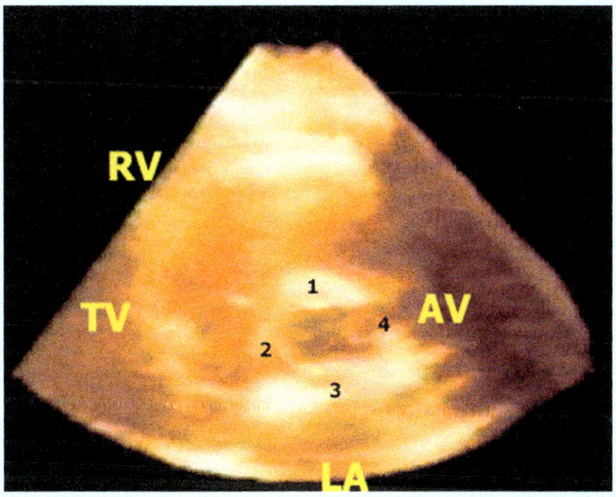

Figure 15-13

Live real-time 3DTTE. Discrete subaortic membrane. Subaortic membrane (arrowhead) and orifice viewed en face. The orifice measured 2.29 cm^2 by planimetry. LA, left atrium; RA, right atrium; RV, right ventricle. Reproduced with permission from Bandarupalli et al.[48]

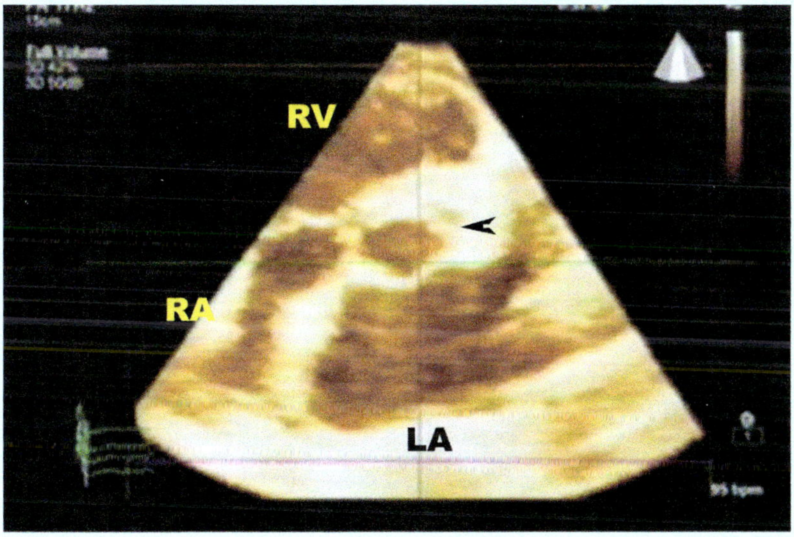

its attachments to the ventricular septum and the anterior mitral leaflet can be directly visualized. When the data set is cropped in order to visualize the orifice en face, it gives the appearance of a small circular opening in the middle of the membrane, or what has been dubbed the "hole in a hole" appearance characteristic of subaortic stenosis.

TRANSPOSITION OF THE GREAT ARTERIES

Transposition of the great arteries (TGA) occurs in two forms, dextro and levo (D-TGA and L-TGA, respectively). In D-TGA, there is ventriculoarterial discordance in that the aorta arises from the morphologic right ventricle while the pulmonary artery arises from the morphologic left ventricle.[49] For D-TGA to be compatible with life, mixing of blood between the pulmonary and systemic circulations must occur at some level and, therefore, D-TGA is always accompanied by other lesions such as an ASD, a VSD, or a PDA; otherwise, other shunt lesions must be created for survival to occur. Multiple corrective surgeries have been developed for this lesion including the Senning and the Mustard procedures, which consist of redirecting deoxygenated blood from the venae cavae to the morphologic left ventricle via an intra-atrial baffle. Because many long-term complications are associated with these procedures, including baffle leaks and obstructions, tricuspid valve regurgitation, arrhythmias, systemic right ventricular failure, and sudden death in adult life, arterial switch operations are now increasingly used for correcting D-TGA.[50] Adult cardiologists, however, continue to evaluate adult patients who underwent a Mustard repair during childhood. In evaluating patients with TGA, therefore, cardiologists must be cognizant of all these corrective techniques and recognize the complications associated with each of them.

L-TGA can be better perceived as a double switch in that it consists of atrioventricular as well as ventriculoatrial discordance. In these patients, the right atrium is connected to the morphologic left ventricle, which in turn is connected to the pulmonary artery, thus preserving the flow of deoxygenated blood from the right atrium to the pulmonary circulation. Similarly, the left atrium is connected to the morphologic right ventricle, which is in turn connected to the aorta; thereby, oxygenated blood from the lungs is delivered to the systemic circulation.[49] It is therefore not surprising that often patients with L-TGA do not require corrective surgery. The condition usually remains undiagnosed until adulthood when the right ventricle fails because it is not designed to withstand the high pressure of the systemic circulation.

Recently, an incremental value of 3DTTE has been demonstrated in patients with TGA over the conventionally used 2DTTE. It has been shown that 3DTTE can be used to provide a more comprehensive evaluation of these patients than 2DTTE and there is no need for more invasive, less convenient imaging modalities such as computed tomography or magnetic resonance imaging.[51] A major advantage of 3DTTE is its ability to fully interrogate the tricuspid valve. Unlike 2DTTE, which often is not able to visualize the posterior tricuspid leaflet, 3DTTE can clearly visualize all three tricuspid leaflets (Fig. 15-14). In addition, 3DTTE can reveal areas of leaflet noncoaptation that can cause regurgitation. The severity of regurgitation can be quantitated better with 3DTTE than with 2DTTE by measuring the vena contracta without making geometric assumptions regarding its shape, as is done with 2DTTE. When the valve is visualized from the atrial aspect, valve prolapse can be directly visualized and the prolapse localized to a specific leaflet segment.[52] 3DTTE can reveal a bicuspid pulmonary valve that can be easily missed by 2DTTE. 3DTTE can also fully examine the pulmonic valve and the left ventricular outflow tract by sequential cropping of these structures to evaluate for left ventricular outflow obstruction from various perspectives.

Figure 15-14

Live real-time 3DTTE. D-TGA. Multiple anatomic defects are present in the tricuspid valve (TV), which is viewed en face in the closed position in systole. Reproduced with permission from Enar et al.[51]

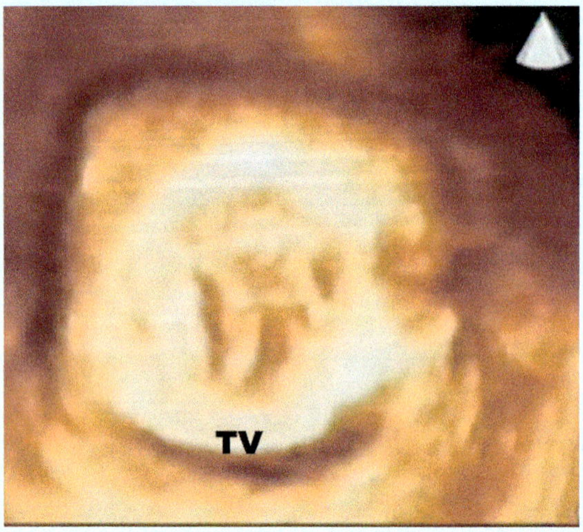

Evaluating the atrial baffle itself is also important in order to detect baffle leaks and obstructions. With 3DTTE, the baffle can be visualized well en face as a shelf. Baffle leaks and obstructions that are missed on 2DTTE can be directly visualized (Fig. 15-15).[51] Thus, 3DTTE can be invaluable for surgical planning in these patients by providing a comprehensive evaluation that is not possible with 2DTTE.

EBSTEIN'S ANOMALY

The classic appearance of Ebstein's anomaly as apical displacement of the tricuspid valve is now recognized to be secondary to the tethering of the tricuspid leaflet to the right ventricular wall.[53] Because 2DTTE provides only limited visualization of the tricuspid valve and is often unable to visualize all three leaflets, 3DTTE has shown value on top of the standard 2DTTE examination in evaluating patients with Ebstein's anomaly.[54,55] 3DTTE is able to assess the distribution and extent of the tethering in all three tricuspid leaflets.[56] With 3DTTE, the bulging of the nontethered areas of the tricuspid valve leaflets produces a characteristic "bubble-like" appearance that can be measured to estimate the free segments of the three leaflets of the tricuspid valve by sequential cropping from multiple views (Fig. 15-16).[56] A full evaluation of the extent of leaflet tethering can provide information that can be important for surgical planning because the availability of nontethered tricuspid valve tissue may facilitate tricuspid valve repair rather than replacement.[55,57] Also, with the use of color Doppler 3DTTE can assess the severity of tricuspid regurgitation by measuring the area of the vena contracta. Although this method relies on the same principles for the quantification of tricuspid regurgitation used by 2DTTE, it has been shown to be superior because the vena contracta can be visualized in three dimensions and its true area measured (the assumption that it has a spherical or elliptical shape is often invalid).[58]

Figure 15-15

Live real-time 3DTTE. D-TGA. Color Doppler examination. The arrow points to a defect in the intra-atrial baffle (B). PVA, pulmonary venous atrium; SVA, systemic venous atrium. Reproduced with permission from Enar et al.[51]

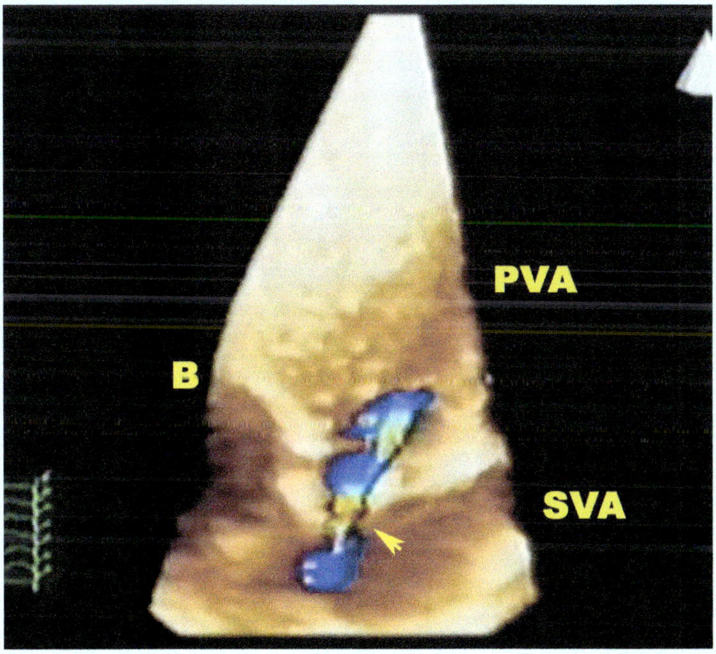

Figure 15-16

Live real-time 3DTTE in isolated Ebstein's anomaly. Transverse section taken at the apex of the tricuspid valve shows a large area of noncoaptation (N) as well as tethering and bubble-like appearance of anterior (yellow arrows) and posterior (black arrowhead) tricuspid valve leaflets. AV, aortic valve; RV, right ventricle. Reproduced with permission from Patel et al.[56]

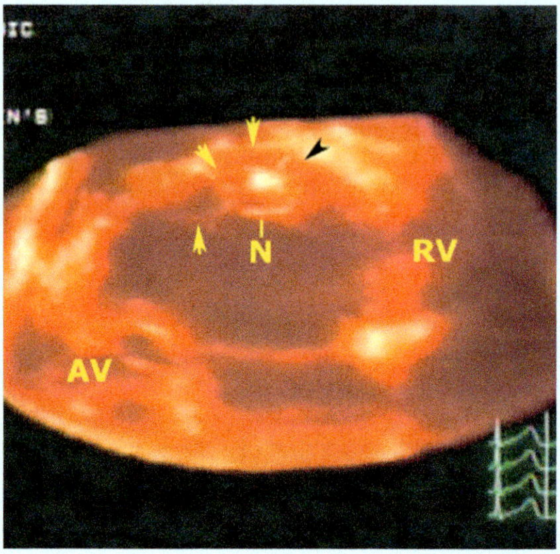

Figure 15-17

Live real-time 3DTTE in cor triatriatum sinister. Arrowhead points to a large opening in the cor triatriatum membrane (M) visualized en face. The dimensions were 3.06 cm × 1.03 cm, and the area was 2.3 cm^2. LV, left ventricle; LVO, left ventricular outflow tract; RV, right ventricle. Reproduced with permission from Patel et al.[62]

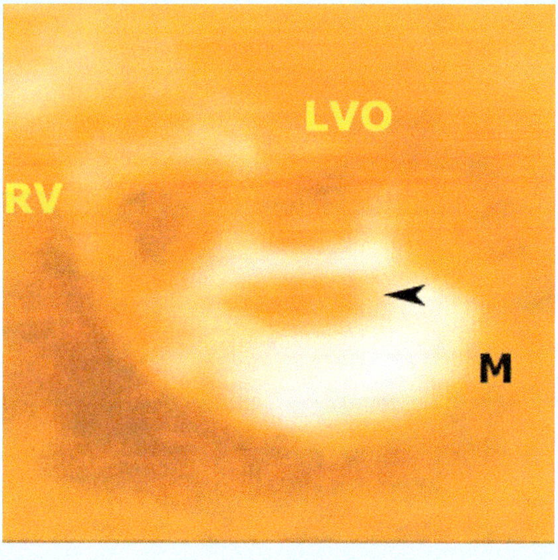

Figure 15-18

Live real-time 3DTTE of the Chiari network. Arrowheads point to some of the multiple openings in the large membrane, outlined by red dots. IVC, inferior vena cava; MV, mitral valve; RA, right atrium. Reproduced with permission from Pothineni et al.[61]

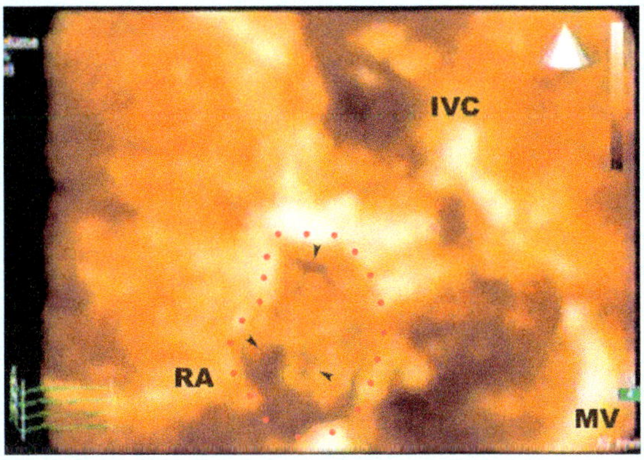

OTHER CHDS

3DTTE can be used for the visualization of multiple CHD lesions and has been shown to supplement 2DTTE examinations and provide incremental value in many of these conditions. It has also been used to aid in the diagnosis of an aortopulmonary window (a communication between the ascending aorta and the pulmonary artery),[59] a Gerbode defect (left ventricular–right atrial communication),[60] a eustachian valve and its differentiation from other lesions,[61] cor triatriatum sinister and dextra (Fig. 15-17),[62] and the Chiari network (Fig. 15-18).[61]

REFERENCES

1. Gutierrez FR, Ho ML, Siegel MJ. Practical applications of magnetic resonance in congenital heart disease. *Magn Reson Imaging Clin N Am*. 2008;16(3):403–435, v.
2. Valente AM, Powell AJ. Clinical applications of cardiovascular magnetic resonance in congenital heart disease. *Cardiol Clin*. 2007;25(1):97–110, vi.
3. Nicol ED, Gatzoulis M, Padley SP, et al. Assessment of adult congenital heart disease with multi-detector computed tomography: beyond coronary lumenography. *Clin Radiol*. 2007;62(6):518–527.
4. Pacileo G, Di Salvo G, Limongelli G, et al. Echocardiography in congenital heart disease: usefulness, limits and new techniques. *J Cardiovasc Med (Hagerstown)*. 2007;8(1):17–22.
5. Hage FG, Nanda NC. Real-time three-dimensional echocardiography: a current view of what echocardiography can provide? *Indian Heart J*. 2009;61(2):146–155.
6. Warnes CA, Williams RG, Bashore TM, et al. ACC/AHA 2008 Guidelines for the management of adults with congenital heart disease: executive summary. A report of the American College of Cardiology/American Heart Association task force on practice guidelines (writing committee to develop guidelines for the management of adults with congenital heart disease) developed in collaboration with the American Society of Echocardiography, Heart Rhythm Society, International Society for Adult Congenital Heart Disease, Society for Cardiovascular Angiography and Interventions, and Society of Thoracic Surgeons. *J Am Coll Cardiol*. 2008;52(23):1890–1947.
7. Moake L, Ramaciotti C. Atrial septal defect treatment options. *AACN Clin Issues*. 2005;16(2):252–266.
8. Chau AK, Leung MP, Yung T, et al. Surgical validation and implications for transcatheter closure of quantitative echocardiographic evaluation of atrial septal defect. *Am J Cardiol*. 2000;85(9):1124–1130.
9. Nanda NC, Abd El-Rahman SM, Khatri GK, et al. Incremental value of three-dimensional echocardiography over transesophageal multiplane two-dimensional echocardiography in qualitative and quantitative assessment of cardiac masses and defects. *Echocardiography*. 1995;12(6):619–628.

10. Patel V, Nanda NC, Upendram S, et al. Live three-dimensional right parasternal and supraclavicular transthoracic echocardiographic examination. *Echocardiography*. 2005;22(4):349–360.
11. Mehmood F, Vengala S, Nanda NC, et al. Usefulness of live three-dimensional transthoracic echocardiography in the characterization of atrial septal defects in adults. *Echocardiography*. 2004;21(8):707–713.
12. Dod HS, Reddy VK, Bhardwaj R, et al. Embolization of atrial septal occluder device into the pulmonary artery: a rare complication and usefulness of live/real time three-dimensional transthoracic echocardiography. *Echocardiography*. 2009;26(6):739–741.
13. Dod H, Reddy VK, Bhardwaj R, et al. Embolization of atrial septal occluder device into the pulmonary artery: a rare complication and usefulness of live/real time three-dimensional transthoracic echocardiography. *Echocardiography*. 2009;26(6):739–741.
14. Sinha A, Nanda NC, Misra V, et al. Live three-dimensional transthoracic echocardiographic assessment of transcatheter closure of atrial septal defect and patent foramen ovale. *Echocardiography*. 2004;21(8):749–753.
15. Berdat PA, Chatterjee T, Pfammatter JP, et al. Surgical management of complications after transcatheter closure of an atrial septal defect or patent foramen ovale. *J Thorac Cardiovasc Surg*. 2000;120(6):1034–1039.
16. Singh A, Romp RL, Nanda NC, et al. Usefulness of live/real time three-dimensional transthoracic echocardiography in the assessment of atrioventricular septal defects. *Echocardiography*. 2006;23(7):598–608.
17. Singh P, Mehta A, Nanda NC. Live/real time three-dimensional transthoracic echocardiographic findings in an adult with complete atrioventricular septal defect. *Echocardiography*. 2010;27(1):87–90.
18. Rastelli G, Kirklin JW, Titus JL. Anatomic observations on complete form of persistent common atrioventricular canal with special reference to atrioventricular valves. *Mayo Clin Proc*. 1966;41(5):296–308.
19. Reeder GS, Danielson GK, Seward JB, et al. Fixed subaortic stenosis in atrioventricular canal defect: a Doppler echocardiographic study. *J Am Coll Cardiol*. 1992;20(2):386–394.
20. Sinha A, Kasliwal RR, Nanda NC, et al. Live three-dimensional transthoracic echocardiographic assessment of isolated cleft mitral valve. *Echocardiography*. 2004;21(7):657–661.
21. Hoffman JI, Kaplan S. The incidence of congenital heart disease. *J Am Coll Cardiol*. 2002;39(12):1890–1900.
22. Butera G, Chessa M, Carminati M. Percutaneous closure of ventricular septal defects. State of the art. *J Cardiovasc Med (Hagerstown)*. 2007;8(1):39–45.
23. Mehmood F, Miller AP, Nanda NC, et al. Usefulness of live/real time three-dimensional transthoracic echocardiography in the characterization of ventricular septal defects in adults. *Echocardiography*. 2006;23(5):421–427.
24. Pedra CA, Pedra SR, Esteves CA, et al. Percutaneous closure of perimembranous ventricular septal defects with the Amplatzer device: technical and morphological considerations. *Catheter Cardiovasc Interv*. 2004;61(3):403–410.
25. Chen FL, Hsiung MC, Nanda N, et al. Real time three-dimensional echocardiography in assessing ventricular septal defects: an echocardiographic-surgical correlative study. *Echocardiography*. 2006;23(7):562–568.
26. Campbell M. Natural history of persistent ductus arteriosus. *Br Heart J*. 1968;30(1):4–13.
27. Grifka RG. Transcatheter closure of the patent ductus arteriosus. *Catheter Cardiovasc Interv*. 2004;61(4):554–570.
28. Sharma S, Mehta AC, O'Donovan PB. Computed tomography and magnetic resonance findings in long-standing patent ductus. Case reports. *Angiology*. 1996;47(4):393–398.
29. Sinha A, Nanda NC, Khanna D, et al. Live three-dimensional transthoracic echocardiographic delineation of patent ductus arteriosus. *Echocardiography*. 2004;21(5):443–448.
30. Hlavacek A, Lucas J, Baker H, et al. Feasibility and utility of three-dimensional color flow echocardiography of the aortic arch: The "echocardiographic angiogram". *Echocardiography*. 2006;23(10):860–864.
31. Patel S. Normal and anomalous anatomy of the coronary arteries. *Semin Roentgenol*. 2008;43(2):100–112.
32. Ilgenli TF, Nanda NC, Sinha A, et al. Live three-dimensional transthoracic echocardiographic assessment of anomalous origin of left coronary artery from the pulmonary artery. *Echocardiography*. 2004;21(6):559–562.
33. Nanda NC, Hsiung MC, Miller AP, et al. *Live/Real Time 3D Echocardiography*. Oxford, UK: Wiley-Blackwell; 2010.
34. Mehta D, Nanda NC, Vengala S, et al. Live three-dimensional transthoracic echocardiographic demonstration of coronary artery to pulmonary artery fistula. *Am J Geriatr Cardiol*. 2005;14(1):42–44.
35. Aboulhosn J, Child JS. Left ventricular outflow obstruction: subaortic stenosis, bicuspid aortic valve, supravalvar aortic stenosis, and coarctation of the aorta. *Circulation*. 2006;114(22):2412–2422.
36. Friedman T, Mani A, Elefteriades JA. Bicuspid aortic valve: clinical approach and scientific review of a common clinical entity. *Expert Rev Cardiovasc Ther*. 2008;6(2):235–248.
37. Singh P, Dutta R, Nanda NC. Live/real time three-dimensional transthoracic echocardiographic assessment of bicuspid aortic valve morphology. *Echocardiography*. 2009;26(4):478–480.
38. Burri MV, Nanda NC, Singh A, et al. Live/real time three-dimensional transthoracic echocardiographic identification of quadricuspid aortic valve. *Echocardiography*. 2007;24(6):653–655.
39. Tentolouris K, Kontozoglou T, Trikas A, et al. Fixed subaortic stenosis revisited. Congenital abnormalities in 72 new cases and review of the literature. *Cardiology*. 1999;92(1):4–10.

40. Bruce CJ, Nishimura RA, Tajik AJ, et al. Fixed left ventricular outflow tract obstruction in presumed hypertrophic obstructive cardiomyopathy: implications for therapy. *Ann Thorac Surg*. 1999;68(1):100–104.
41. Hage FG, Zoghbi G, Aqel R, et al. Subaortic stenosis missed by invasive hemodynamic assessment. *Echocardiography*. 2008;5(9):1007–1010.
42. Alboliras ET, Gotteiner NL, Berdusis K, et al. Transesophageal echocardiographic imaging for congenital lesions of the left ventricular outflow tract and the aorta. *Echocardiography*. 1996;13(4):439–446.
43. Agrawal GG, Nanda NC, Htay T, et al. Live three-dimensional transthoracic echocardiographic identification of discrete subaortic membranous stenosis. *Echocardiography*. 2003;20(7):617–619.
44. Baumgartner H, Stefenelli T, Niederberger J, et al. "Overestimation" of catheter gradients by Doppler ultrasound in patients with aortic stenosis: a predictable manifestation of pressure recovery. *J Am Coll Cardiol*. 1999;33(6):1655–1661.
45. Sakthi C, Yee H, Kotlewski A. Overestimation of aortic valve gradient measured by Doppler echocardiography in patients with aortic stenosis. *Catheter Cardiovasc Interv*. 2005;65(2):176–179.
46. Garcia D, Dumesnil JG, Durand LG, et al. Discrepancies between catheter and Doppler estimates of valve effective orifice area can be predicted from the pressure recovery phenomenon: practical implications with regard to quantification of aortic stenosis severity. *J Am Coll Cardiol*. 2003;41(3):435–442.
47. Aghassi P, Aurigemma GP, Folland ED, et al. Catheterization-Doppler discrepancies in nonsimultaneous evaluations of aortic stenosis. *Echocardiography*. 2005;22(5):367–373.
48. Bandarupalli N, Faulkner M, Nanda NC, et al. Erroneous diagnosis of significant obstruction by Doppler in a patient with discrete subaortic membrane: correct diagnosis by 3D-transthoracic echocardiography. *Echocardiography*. 2008;25(9):1004–1006.
49. Warnes CA. Transposition of the great arteries. *Circulation*. 2006;114(24):2699–2709.
50. Skinner J, Hornung T, Rumball E. Transposition of the great arteries: from fetus to adult. *Heart*. 2008; 94(9):1227–1235.
51. Enar S, Singh P, Douglas C, et al. Live/real time three-dimensional transthoracic echocardiographic assessment of transposition of the great arteries in the adult. *Echocardiography*. 2009;26(9):1095–1104.
52. Pothineni KR, Duncan K, Yelamanchili P, et al. Live/real time three-dimensional transthoracic echocardiographic assessment of tricuspid valve pathology: incremental value over the two-dimensional technique. *Echocardiography*. 2007;24(5):541–552.
53. Anderson KR, Zuberbuhler JR, Anderson RH, et al. Morphologic spectrum of Ebstein's anomaly of the heart: a review. *Mayo Clin Proc*. 1979;54(3):174–180.
54. Ports TA, Silverman NH, Schiller NB. Two-dimensional echocardiographic assessment of Ebstein's anomaly. *Circulation*. 1978;58(2):336–343.
55. Shiina A, Seward JB, Edwards WD, et al. Two-dimensional echocardiographic spectrum of Ebstein's anomaly: detailed anatomic assessment. *J Am Coll Cardiol*. 1984;3(2 Pt 1):356–370.
56. Patel V, Nanda NC, Rajdev S, et al. Live/real time three-dimensional transthoracic echocardiographic assessment of Ebstein's anomaly. *Echocardiography*. 2005;22(10):847–854.
57. Danielson GK, Driscoll DJ, Mair DD, et al. Operative treatment of Ebstein's anomaly. *J Thorac Cardiovasc Surg*. 1992;104(5):1195–1202.
58. Velayudhan DE, Brown TM, Nanda NC, et al. Quantification of tricuspid regurgitation by live three-dimensional transthoracic echocardiographic measurements of vena contracta area. *Echocardiography*. 2006;23(9):793–800.
59. Singh A, Mehmood F, Romp RL, et al. Live/real time three-dimensional transthoracic echocardiographic assessment of aortopulmonary window. *Echocardiography*. 2008;25(1):96–99.
60. Hansalia S, Manda J, Pothineni KR, et al. Usefulness of live/real time three-dimensional transthoracic echocardiography in diagnosing acquired left ventricular-right atrial communication misdiagnosed as severe pulmonary hypertension by two-dimensional transthoracic echocardiography. *Echocardiography*. 2009; 26(2):224–227.
61. Pothineni KR, Nanda NC, Burri MV, et al. Live/real time three-dimensional transthoracic echocardiographic visualization of Chiari network. *Echocardiography*. 2007;24(9):995–997.
62. Patel V, Nanda NC, Arellano I, et al. Cor triatriatum sinister: assessment by live/real time three-dimensional transthoracic echocardiography. *Echocardiography*. 2006;23(9):801–802.

CHAPTER

16

3D MATRIX TRANSESOPHAGEAL ECHOCARDIOGRAPHY

Lissa Sugeng, MD, MPH; and Sonal Chandra, MD

ABSTRACT

Transesophageal echocardiography (TEE) plays an integral role in the diagnosis of cardiovascular disease, perioperative evaluation, and guidance of interventional procedures. Three-dimensional TEE provides a unique anatomical visualization of mitral valve lesions and can aid in assessing disease severity, progression, complexity of repair, and postsurgical success. Real-time 3DE (RT3DE) can aid in gauging suitability of surgical strategy and in timing of surgery in repair of mitral regurgitation. In mitral stenosis, 3D TEE serves as an accurate means of quantifying mitral orifice area and assessing MV morphologic and motion characteristics in patients who have had MV repairs. It also facilitates imaging of the aortic valve (AV) and plays a role in the investigational percutaneous closure of paraprosthetic AV leaks. Other roles include quantification of left ventricular and left ventricular size and function and in imaging of congenital heart disease, including atrial and ventricular septal defects.

INTRODUCTION

Transesophageal echocardiography (TEE) plays an integral role in the diagnosis of cardiovascular disease, perioperative evaluation, and guidance of interventional procedures. As a result of its cardiac proximity, TEE provides clinicians with superior resolution, and with the addition of three-dimensional echocardiography (3DE), visualization of cardiac structures by TEE is further enhanced, facilitating better understanding of spatial relationships and enabling volumetric measurements of valvular and ventricular function.[1] Over decades, the technology has evolved from a single rotating element to now a fully sampled 3D matrix array TEE (3D MTEE) capable of volume-rendered imaging and simultaneous biplane two-dimensional (2D) display in addition to basic function typical of a multiplane TEE probe. Use of 3D TEE is now widespread, including in perioperative and percutaneous practice, especially in transcatheter procedures such as atrial septal closure, mitral valve (MV) repair, and aortic valve (AV) replacement. Although 2D TEE remains the mainstay of cardiac imaging, 3D visualization has acknowledged benefits. Herein, we discuss the incremental use of 3D MTEE in current practice.

MITRAL VALVE

The MV is a complex saddle-shaped structure with a fibromuscular annulus, anterior and posterior leaflets, an anterolateral and posteromedial commissure, chordae, and papillary muscles. The posterior leaflet is composed of three scallops—lateral (P1), middle (P2), and medial (P3)—with corresponding virtual anterior segments (A1, A2, A3) as seen in Figure 16-1. This leaflet segmentation, based on the Carpentier nomenclature, is widely used when localizing specific MV lesions. Routine 2D imaging of the MV requires a systematic acquisition of the valve from a midesophageal position with slight retroflexion. Sequential views obtained starting from the four-chamber view (0°), bicommissural (60°), two-chamber (90°–100°), and long-axis views (120°–150°) subsequently necessitate mental reconstruction of images to understand the pathology involved (Fig. 16-2A–D); however, 3DE of the MV eases visualization of all these scallops from a left atrial (LA) and left ventricular (LV) perspective. The location of these 2D slice planes on a 3D image is demonstrated in Figure 16-2. There are three modes of 3D acquisition, including narrow-angled, zoom mode, and wide-angled acquisition (Fig. 16-3A–C). A 3D image of the MV is best obtained utilizing the zoom mode of acquisition, which minimizes motion artifacts due to translational motion, respiration, and esophageal peristalsis or arrhythmias. In contrast, the full-volume or wide-angled modes have higher frame rates but are more prone to these artifacts. Once the image acquisition is complete, the MV can be viewed from both an LA or a "surgeon's view" and a ventricular perspective. Although there is no official consensus on the orientation of the MV, the surgical view is the favored perspective contributing to a shared terminology in the dialogue

Figure 16-1A, B, C, and D

The MV is seen in a four-chamber view, *A*, and a simultaneous 90° view, *B*, using x-plane imaging. Rotating the second plane allows evaluation of the mitral valve in a bicommissural view at 60°, *C*, and a long axis view at 145°, *D*. A, anterior; LA, left atrium; P, posterior.

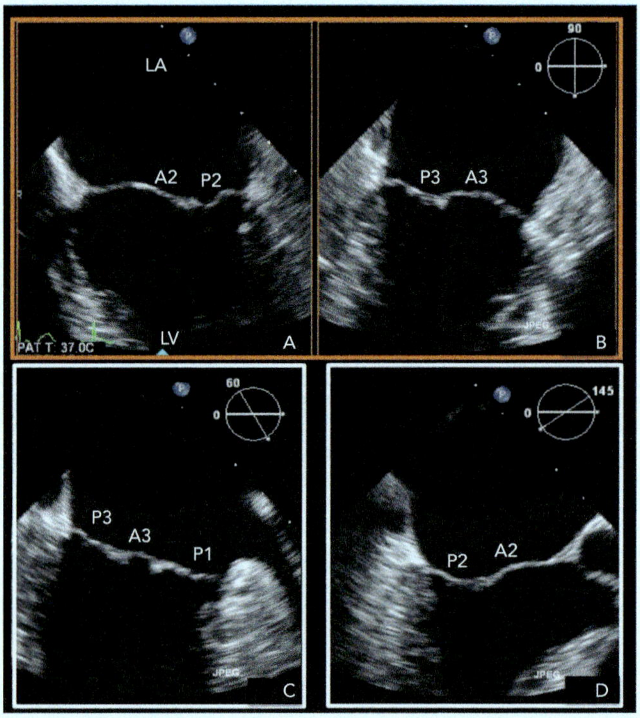

Figure 16-2A and B

A, Two-dimensional images of the MV (**1–4**) correspond to the location seen on the 3D image of the MV viewed from a left atrial perspective (*A*). In panel *B*, the MV scallops are visualized from an LV perspective.

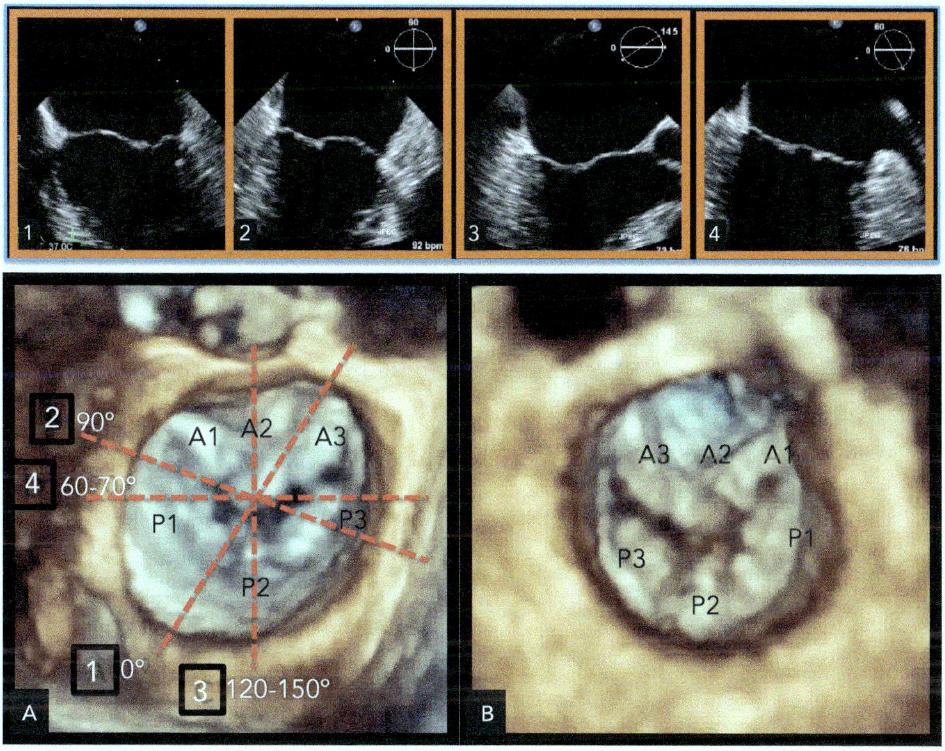

Figure 16-3A, B, and C

Three modes of acquisition: narrow angled, *A*, zoom, *B*, and wide angled, *C*.

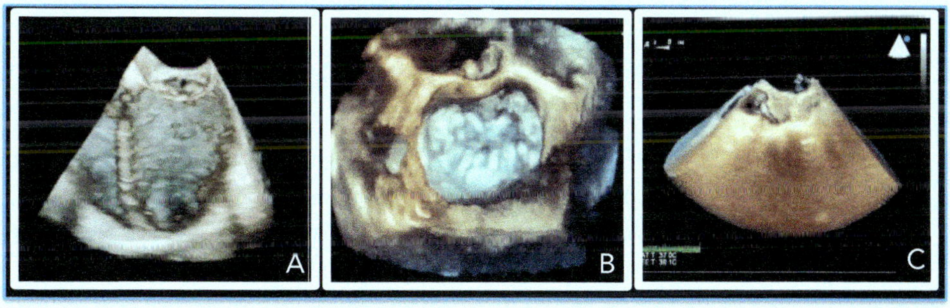

between the echocardiographer and the surgeon. This view is acquired by using the 3D zoom mode on the midesophageal four-chamber view and then by rotating the MV to display the AV at the 12 o'clock position. Abnormalities in any of the components of the MV apparatus including the annulus, leaflets, tendinous chordae, and papillary muscles can contribute to a regurgitant or stenotic orifice. A thorough visualization of anatomic derangements is feasible by 3DE and improves diagnostic accuracy when assessing pathophysiology of mitral regurgitation (MR) in patients with ischemic, degenerative, or stenotic MV disease.

Degenerative MV disease is a spectrum of phenotypic manifestations from a single scallop to multisegmental involvement with resultant Carpentier's type II MR. Degenerative MV disease includes Barlow's disease and fibroelastic deficiency, with the former characterized by presence of excessive leaflet tissue, chordal elongation or rupture, annular dilatation, chordal thickening, and possible calcification of papillary muscle and annulus. In contrast, in fibroelastic deficiency, chordae can be thin with mildly dilated annulus with one or more prolapsing segments, usually the P2 segment. Identification of abnormal scallops has always been feasible with 2D TEE; however, with 3D TEE's dynamic LA or surgical views, a specific etiologic differentiation between Barlow's disease and fibroelastic deficiency is now possible irrespective of operator experience (Figs. 16-4A and 16-4B). Specifically, 3D TEE provides enhanced visualization of the pathomorphology of the MV, allowing reproducible delineation of abnormal segments or scallops and facilitating objective assessment of regurgitant mechanism and etiology. Although 2D TEE is able to identify the lesion from multiple views, 3D TEE has proven to be superior in segmental prolapse or billowing analysis, particularly in patients with commissural involvement, and importantly, in determining the overall complexity of lesions at any expertise level.[2–5] The complexity of a lesion depends on its location, number of segments, and bileaflet involvement.[6] Presurgical planning is integral in determining whether a valve is suitable for repair or whether referral is needed to a center with expertise in MV repair. The lack of reliable preoperative assessment can lead to a mismatch between the complexity of disease and the surgical expertise, resulting in either unsuccessful repair or conversion to replacement and thus to poor outcomes in patients with complex valvular disease.[7,8]

In addition to providing a unique anatomical visualization of the MV scallops and annulus and pathologic changes, using commercially available software, a multitude of MV parameters can be derived from an MV volumetric dataset, including annular area, anterior-posterior to intercommissural diameter ratio (circularization of annulus), planarity index, annular dynamics and extent of leaflet area, billowing, or prolapse volume (Fig. 16-5). These objective metrics can be used to assess disease severity, progression, complexity of repair, and postsurgical success.[9,10] Postrepair systolic anterior motion can be problematic, and although no single parameter exists that can reliably predict its occurrence, 3D TEE–derived measurements of abnormal mitral–aortic angle, presence of excess tissue, integrity of subvalvular geometry, billowing volume, and displacement of mitral coaptation line can alert the clinician to its future likelihood.[11]

The shape of the MV annulus is well known based on the landmark study by Levine et al.[12] describing the specific "saddle" shape and also clarifying the diagnosis of MV prolapse. Obviating cumbersome and invasive fluoroscopic marker tracking or sonomicrometry, 3DE has been instrumental in emphasizing the role of annular nonplanarity and continues to play a role in assessing suitability of customized prostheses or other repair strategies aimed at restoring or maintaining the saddle shape of the annulus.[13–15] Theoretically, maintenance of this saddle shape should lead to a reduction in leaflet stress and therefore to improved durability of repair. The geometric changes resulting from annuloplasty can be assessed in the operating department postoperatively using 3D TEE.[16]

Ischemic MR results from geometric alterations of the MV, especially the subvalvular apparatus, which is susceptible to underlying LV remodeling. Displacement of the papillary muscles is common, resulting in tethered chords and consequently in leaflet malcoaptation and therefore MR. The exact mechanisms to which MR is attributed vary in the literature, with some studies emphasizing abnormal LV remodeling while others stress the importance of papillary muscle positioning as the reasons behind abnormal MV kinematics.[17–19] However, despite dissimilar mechanisms, annular reduction has been the primary surgical solution to the reduction of MR. Real-time 3DE (RT3DE) allows dynamic volumetric measurements of the mitral apparatus, offering a possible means to gauge suitability of one surgical strategy over another, whether annuloplasty, reduction in LV size, or approaches that limit tethering.[20] Superior views of the subvalvular apparatus using 3D TEE, along with volumetric quantification of tenting volume and coaptation depth, are instrumental in guiding surgical interventions.

An accurate assessment of MR severity is essential in optimizing the timing of surgery, which in turn has survival implications. Grading the severity of MR based on 2D quantitative approaches such as flow

Figure 16-4A and B

In panel *A*, there is single-scallop myxomatous degeneration with a ruptured chord, typically referred to as fibroelastic degeneration. The *white arrow* indicates the ruptured chord. Multisegmental myxomatous degeneration involving both anterior and posterior leaflet is shown in panel *B*.

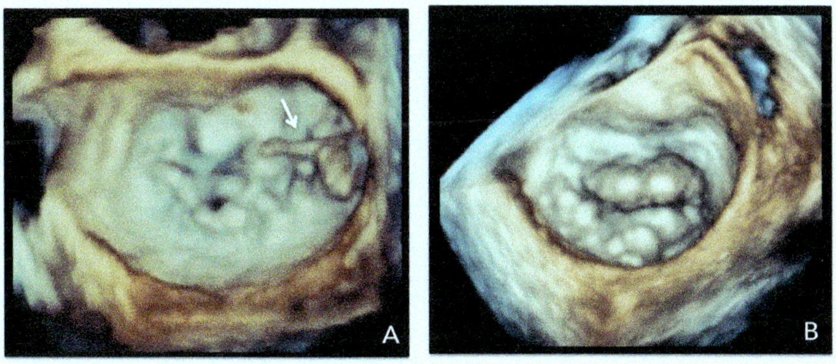

Figure 16-5

Mitral valve parameters derived from a 3D MV dataset. A, anterior; AL, anterior lateral papillary muscle; Ao, aortic valve; P, posterior; PM, posterior medial papillary muscle.

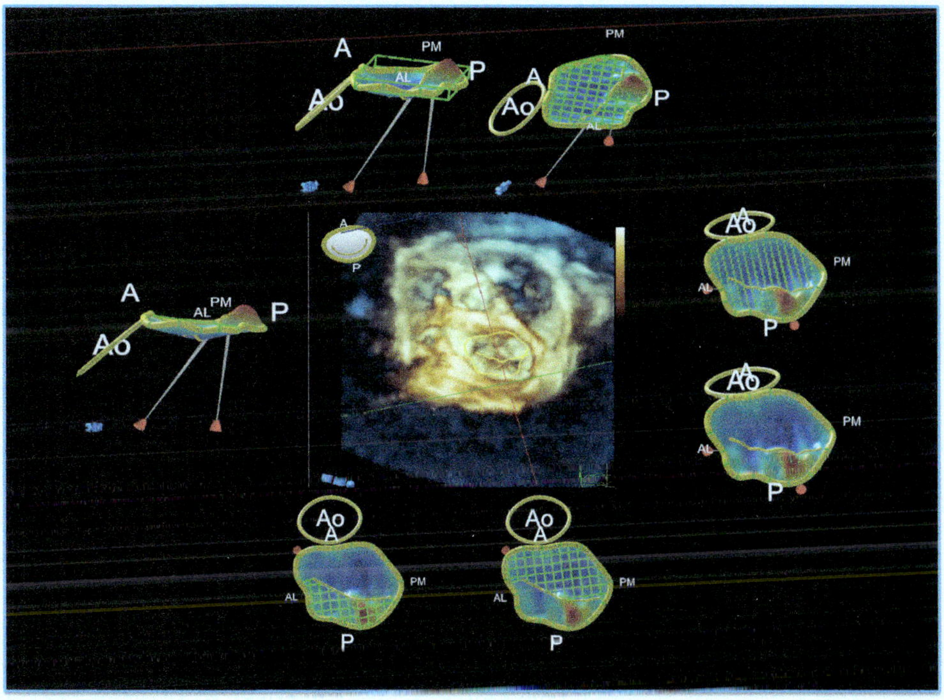

convergence is limited by geometric assumptions about the regurgitant orifice. 3D TEE has enabled a new approach for MR quantification involving direct measurement of regurgitant orifice area (Fig. 16-6).[21] The anatomic regurgitant orifice area demonstrated better correlation with the flow convergence technique when the orifice was round or less complex, thereby providing insight into the limitations of conventional 2D measurements of the vena contracta and proximal isovelocity area.[22] This method avoids some of the geometric

Figure 16-6A, B, and C

Severe eccentric MR is seen in a patient with multisegmental degeneration of the posterior leaflet in panel *A*. In panel *B*, a left atrial view demonstrates severe prolapse of the P3 scallop, easily seen on the parametric model, *C*. The regurgitant orifice is also easily delineated during MV analysis (*arrows*). A, anterior; AL, anterior lateral papillary muscle; Ao, aortic valve; P, posterior; PM, posterior medial papillary muscle.

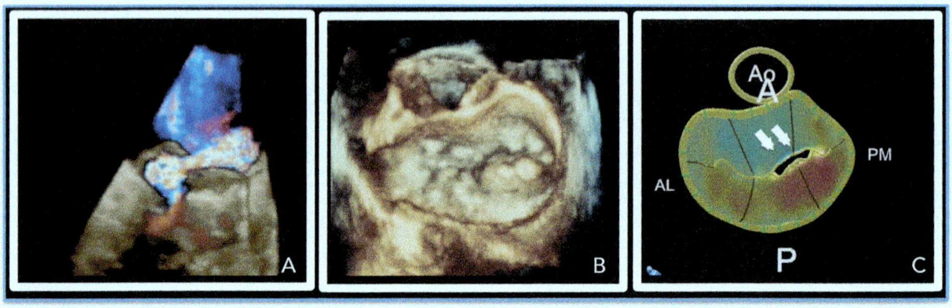

Figure 16-7A and B

A, Left atrial view of a stenotic MV. *B*, From a unique ventricular perspective doming of the anterior leaflet, the MV orifice and equal commissural fusion are easily appreciated.

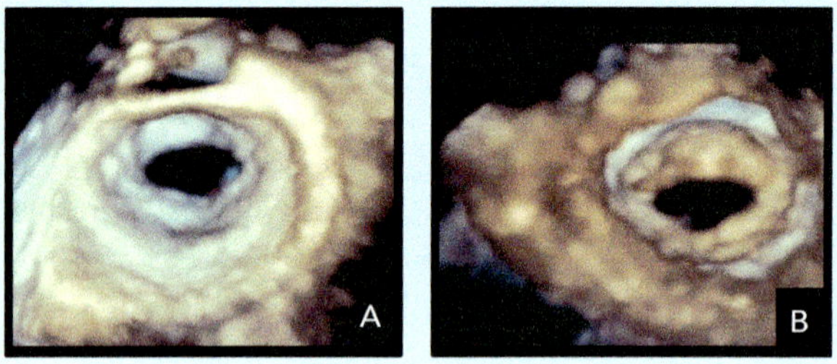

and flow assumptions plaguing the 2D flow convergence techniques. 3D TEE may prove to be useful in quantifying severity in instances of multiple or highly eccentric jets stemming from complex orifice geometry. 3D TEE–derived measurements of severity are highly reproducible, thus supporting its use when image quality or spatial resolution is an issue with transthoracic echocardiography (TTE). An in-depth discussion of the quantification of congenital and acquired heart diseases using 3D Doppler echocardiography can be found in Chapter 4.

Mitral stenosis

In mitral stenosis, 3D TEE serves as an accurate means of quantifying mitral orifice area when evaluation by TTE is hampered in patients with poor sonographic windows. The symmetry of commissural fusion is also easily viewed from a ventricular orientation, which is not always achieved from a 2D transgastric window (Fig. 16-7). 3D TEE is instrumental during percutaneous balloon mitral valvuloplasty in guiding balloon placement and in assessing postprocedural extent of commissural splitting, a good predictor of outcome.[23,24] In addition, the spatial relationships between the MV, the LA appendage, the LA, the interatrial septum, and the chords are easily evident on 3D TEE. Color Doppler imaging provides instant feedback on the presence and severity of postvalvuloplasty MR.

Prosthetic mitral valve

The higher spatial resolution of 3D TEE facilitates a realistic assessment of MV morphologic and motion characteristics in patients who have had MV repairs. Measurement and visualization of mechanical MV orifice area by 3D TEE is feasible from the atrial and ventricular perspectives, although the latter can be more challenging owing to reverberations from the highly reflective components of the prosthesis. 3D TEE correlates well with orifice area as measured by the manufacturer.[25] It is particularly superior as a diagnostic tool in determining the anatomic characteristics, such as location and size, of prosthetic paravalvular regurgitant orifices.[26–28] The areas of dehiscence following repair is usually present on 3DE as a well-demarcated area of missing tissue with smoothed edges and with a clear dynamic separation of the MV ring from the adjoining tissue during the cardiac cycle. RT3DE combined with TEE color flow Doppler has demonstrated with high accuracy the presence and severity of regurgitant flow through the dehisced segments, thereby preventing the misdiagnosis of areas of echo dropout as paravalvular defects. Volumetric datasets acquired using 3D TEE can be further manipulated to measure the width and circumferential length of defects, which have implications not only for type of device but also for choice of a percutaneous versus a surgical approach.[29] Visualization of the catheter course and tip using RT3D TEE is especially useful in guiding and eventually placing the occluder against a moving prosthesis. The intra- or postprocedural en face view of the defect makes 3D TEE a desirable imaging modality for operators performing surgical or percutaneous repair on these lesions.[30] However, although visual assessment is readily performed online, at present detailed measurements of the orifice dimensions do require offline processing.

Percutaneous mitral valve repair or replacement

Intraoperative guidance of MV clip repair by 3D TEE facilitates better visualization of catheter trajectory, optimal clip positioning (zoom imaging of the en face view: A2-P2), and orientation of clip arms, thereby reducing procedural time.[31] Postprocedurally, the presence of mitral stenosis can be excluded by assessing the double orifice using 3D TEE by planimetry.

Real-time 3D TEE is also very useful to the interventionist performing transcatheter valve-in-valve procedures in the MV position. From catheter positioning of the prosthesis to assessing differences between pre- and postballoon dilation, 3D TEE has guided successful deployment of the bioprosthesis. 3D TEE is instrumental in maneuvering the guidewire across the valve orifice rather than through a leaflet perforation, which could lead to an embolism after the balloon inflation.[32]

AORTIC VALVE

The AV is part of a dynamic aortic root complex spanning from the basal attachments of the valvular leaflets in the ventricle to the sinotubular junction. A normal AV consists of three leaflets: the left, right, and noncoronary, which are based on their relationship to the coronary artery origin. The leaflets attach just below the sinus of Valsalva. Detailed 3D analysis of the AV has demonstrated that this clinically defined region does not have a truly circular or discrete annular structure but is frequently elliptical with an appearance resembling a three-pronged coronet. The aortic root complex appears simple but is intricate in its anatomic and mechanical relationship with other adjoining structures, specifically the MV.

Imaging of the AV should be comprehensive encompassing all components of the aortic root complex, especially their spatial and geometric interrelationships. A zoom mode or wide-angled acquisition with 3D TEE permits precise measurement of the aortic root at any desired level or plane and plays an integral role in planning for surgical and percutaneous interventions in the aortic position. A biplane and aortic view of the AV in a normal subject and in a patient with severe aortic stenosis are compared in Figures 16-8A and 16-8B. Accurate preoperative assessment of the dimensions of the aortic root complex is critical for surgical planning and patient selection and to ensure a successful procedure in patients undergoing transcatheter AV implantation for severe aortic stenosis. In contrast to 2D-derived aortic annular measurements from sagittal views, which provide underestimated values, 3D TEE–derived measurements from both sagittal and coronal views correlate strongly with dual-source computed tomographic aortic measurements.[33] Measurements of the coronal diameters using 3DE have been reported to be significantly larger than measurements obtained using 2D TTE or 2D TEE.[33] Inherent to 2D measurements is the assumption that the aortic annulus is circular rather than ellipsoidal as demonstrated by computed tomography and magnetic resonance imaging.[34–36] 3D TEE is useful in reproducibly assessing the distance between the aortic annulus and the coronary ostia in order to prevent ostial coronary occlusion by prostheses. However, significant calcification may affect image quality when using 3D TEE, limiting the accuracy of some of these measurements. Transcutaneous AV implantation (TAVI) is easily viewed using biplane imaging; however, visualization of the valve from an aortic orientation demonstrates the stent with blooming artifact and poor visualization of the aortic leaflets (Fig. 16-8C). Although 3D TEE may aid in assessing the aortic annular diameter and in guiding the TAVI procedure, assessment of paravalvular leaks remains challenging and is primarily qualitative.

The investigational percutaneous closure of paraprosthetic AV leaks is gaining traction in the treatment of patients who are not deemed to be suitable surgical candidates. Small or clinically insignificant leaks are not infrequent, but when they are significant they can be associated with hemolysis, arrhythmias, or congestive

Figure 16-8A, B, and C

Biplane imaging along with an aortic view of the AV in a normal subject, *A*, a patient with aortic stenosis, *B*, and a patient who has had a transcutaneous AV replacement, *C*.

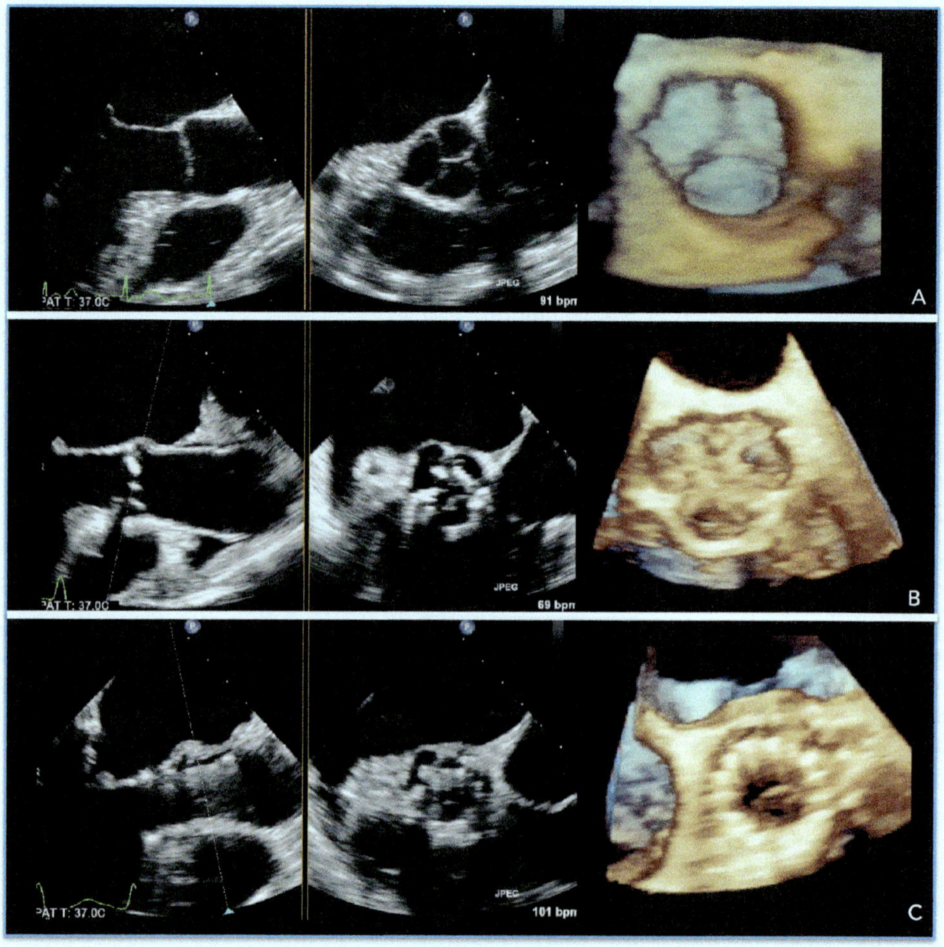

heart failure.[37] This is especially challenging in patients with high reoperative mortality rates. From guiding the course of guidewires to ultimate device positioning, 3D TEE can be instrumental in percutaneous closure of these regurgitant orifices with occluder devices.

Three-dimensional TEE is able to delineate the morphologic details of an AV despite its propensity for dropout artifacts. 3D TEE is superior to 2D TEE in detecting valve perforations by enabling en face anatomic views of the valve cusps and leaflets, thereby allowing precise localization of valve perforation.[38] In patients with bicuspid AV, 3D TEE morphologic designations strongly correlated with surgical anatomic findings, which is helpful not only in identifying the disease entity but also in determining contraindications to percutaneous valve therapy.[39] Severity of aortic stenosis can be assessed by planimetry of the AV orifice area. 3D TEE can play an adjunctive role in determining the optimal cross-sectional plane containing the smallest valve orifice for planimetry.[40] Similarly, 3D TEE can aid in planimetry of the valvular regurgitant orifice area in aortic regurgitation. Additionally, type and extent of obstruction in LV outflow and supra-aortic regions are easier to visualize and quantify using 3D TEE.[41]

LEFT VENTRICLE

Quantification of LV size and function and assessment of regional wall motion abnormalities are an essential aspect of TEE. LV function is a major determinant of morbidity and mortality and serves as a means of risk-stratifying patients irrespective of the cause of dysfunction.[42–46] Qualitative evaluation of LV ejection fraction is still commonplace despite inadequate interobserver variability. However, 2D quantitative techniques are limited by their reliance on geometric assumptions despite underlying cardiomyopathy, subjectivity in angulation, and difficulty with endocardial definitions.[47–49] The added dimension confers superiority over 2D technique by allowing volumetric quantification (Figs. 16-9A and 16-9B). Because it is not subject to the geometric assumptions of 2DE, 3DE permits accurate quantification, endocardial differentiation, and visualization of the apex. Therefore, 3DE is more suitable for performing volumetric measurements when the LV shape is distorted by ischemic insults resulting in regional wall motion abnormalities or aneurysms, or when there is asymmetry as a consequence of congenital heart disease or nonischemic cardiomyopathy.

Figure 16-9A and B

A, Biplane imaging of the LV shows a four-chamber view (top and bottom left) and simultaneous three-chamber (top right) and two-chamber (bottom right) views. *B*, 3D quantitation of the LV using a semiautomatic border tracking program (Q-Lab, Philips Healthcare, Andover, MA).

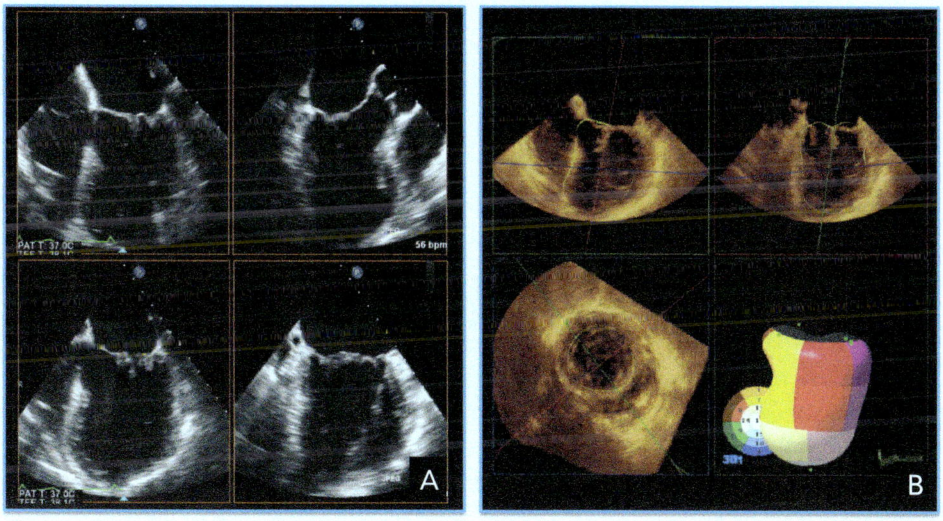

Volume measurements are performed in full-volume mode over three to four seconds, requiring subvolumes to be stitched together. The semiautomated system of quantification currently requires identification of reference points on the MV and apex, resulting in generation of a manually correctible endocardial border. 3D TEE is helpful perioperatively in quantifying ejection fraction, enabling surgical teams to risk stratify patients accordingly. It is incrementally helpful in the operating department in postventriculectomy patients. The use of a wide-angled LV volume acquisition facilitates characterization of global and regional function. Regional wall motion abnormalities can be confirmed in short-axis views in addition to the standard long-axis views. As online border detection software becomes fully integrated, it will significantly reduce time spent on offline analysis, further improving clinical workflow.

RIGHT VENTRICLE

Evaluation of right ventricular (RV) function and dimension is diagnostically challenging owing to complex structural geometry of the RV, which does not easily lend itself to quantification. 2D volumetric assessment relies on geometric assumptions and is prone to image plane-positioning errors.[50] The RV is crescentic with a convex-shaped free wall and a concavely contoured interventricular septum; it consists of an inlet and a muscular apical and outflow tract that lacks a straight axis.[51] Changes in RV function or size have prognostic implications and therefore require a diagnostic tool that can overcome the limitations of reduced accuracy and variability plaguing the conventional qualitative 2D evaluations.[52–55] This is particularly relevant during cardiac surgery when perioperative changes in RV function can be crucial and can influence medical management or surgical interventions accordingly.[56,57] Although magnetic resonance imaging is currently the gold standard for RV quantification, it is not suitable for perioperative evaluation in part because of its strong magnetic fields. 3D TTE utilizing custom software has demonstrated RV volumes comparable to those shown on magnetic resonance imaging in normal individuals; generated its own set of reference values; and confirmed utility in pathologic states including valvular heart disease, pulmonary hypertension, and congenital heart disease.[58–61] 3D TEE yields RV volumes comparable to TTE and has the potential to increase the endocardial border enhancement; thus it may become an indispensable tool for intraoperative evaluation of RV function during orthotopic heart transplantation or surgical correction for tetralogy of Fallot, tricuspid atresia, and Ebstein's anomaly.[52,62] RT3DE has the added potential for tracking beat-to-beat changes in ventricular volumes, which may provide the necessary insight into contractility of the RV and LV.[63]

CONGENITAL HEART DISEASE

Complicated surgical repairs combined with challenges posed by acoustic windows make 3D TEE a complementary imaging modality in patients with congenital heart disease. The en face views available using 3D TEE allow a comprehensive evaluation of atrioventricular valve leaflet defects. In addition to the valvular structures, the overall complexity and spatial relationships of the adjoining atrial and ventricular septal defects can be discerned using 3D TEE. Multiplanar reformations facilitate accurate sizing of these defects. Many congenital defects do not lend themselves easily to an evaluation by 2DE. 3DE facilitates these unobtainable views that potentially include all the components of the planned surgical repair.[51]

Atrial septal defect

Percutaneous device closure of interatrial communications has become widely accepted as a surgical alternative for prevention of paradoxical embolism or significant left-to-right shunting. 3D TEE has been employed successfully not only in the evaluation of the size, type, dynamic changes, location, and adjoining rims of atrial septal defects (ASDs) but also in selection of patients for percutaneous occlusion.[64–67] Intraoperatively, RT3DE plays an important role in the guidance and manipulation of catheters, as seen in Figure 16-10A–C.[68,69] Image projections can easily be manipulated to reveal the relationship between the catheter delivery system, including the occluder, and the defect.[70] RT3D TEE is also better at defining the complex shape and the spatial relations of the ASD and the surrounding structures such as the valves, pulmonary veins, and great vessels.[67,71] Offline

Figure 16-10A, B, C, D, E, F, and G

Biplane imaging of a secundum ASD during transcatheter closure visualizes crossing of the catheter thru the ASD, panels *A*, *D*, and *E*. Using 3DE the catheter is seen from a left atrial perspective, *D*, and a right atrial viewpoint, *E*. Placement of the device guided by biplane imaging shows malalignment of the device, *B*, and final implantation, *C*. This closure device encompasses the entire interatrial septum and approaches the MV annulus as seen from the left atrium, *F*, and can be viewed from the right atrial orientation, *G*. LA, left atrium; RA, right atrium.

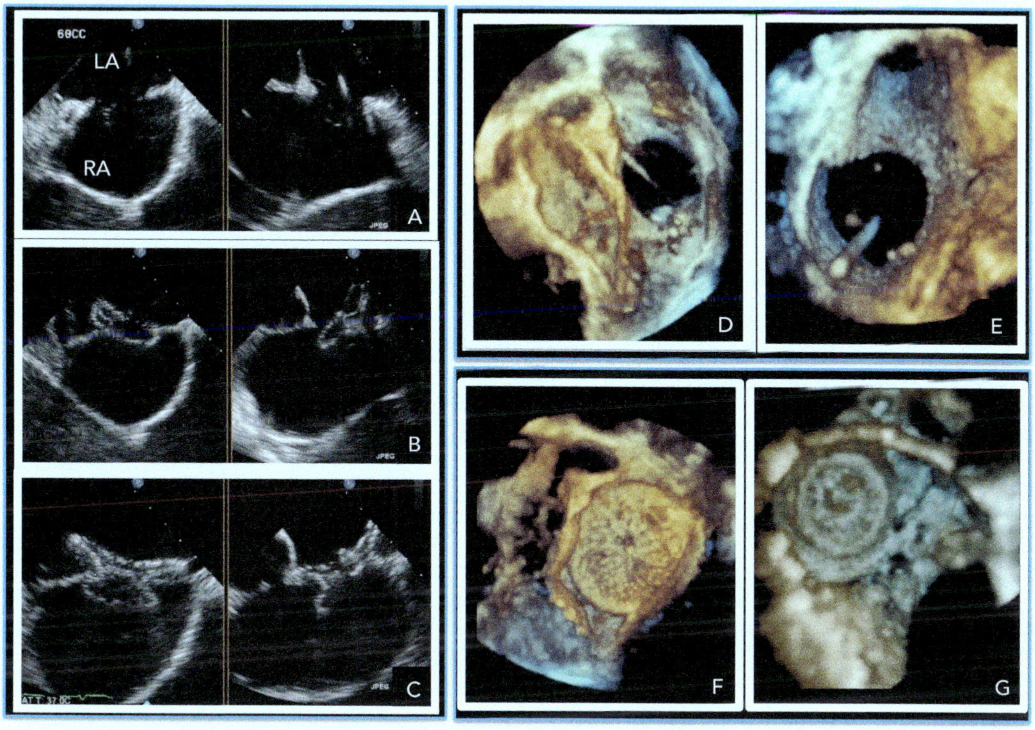

3D TEE correlates well with an invasive balloon technique in the measurement of the diameter of the ASD and provides a precise localization of multiple ASDs.[72,73] The use of RT3D TEE to guide placement of percutaneous device closure of ASDs has been well described.

Ventricular septal defect

The size, number, shape, and location of the ventricular septal defect can be visualized either as a guide to surgical planning or to guide percutaneous intervention for defects thought suitable for catheter closure. The ability of 3DE to assess complex shapes of ventricular septal defects makes it an ideal technique to monitor closure of ventricular septal defects

CONCLUSION

In summary, 3D TEE has become an indispensable part of routine echocardiography, especially in situations in which the image quality of TTE is impaired. 3D TEE technology is currently limited by spatial and temporal resolution and would benefit further from reduced footprints, higher frequencies, and automated quantitative software.

REFERENCES

1. Sugeng L, Shernan SK, Salgo IS, et al. Live 3-dimensional transesophageal echocardiography initial experience using the fully-sampled matrix array probe. *J Am Coll Cardiol.* 2008;52(6):446–449.
2. Chandra S, Salgo IS, Sugeng L, et al. Characterization of degenerative mitral valve disease using morphologic analysis of real-time three-dimensional echocardiographic images: objective insight into complexity and planning of mitral valve repair. *Circ Cardiovasc Imaging.* 2011;4(1):24–32.
3. Garcia-Orta R, Moreno E, Vidal M, et al. Three-dimensional versus two-dimensional transesophageal echocardiography in mitral valve repair. *J Am Soc Echocardiogr.* 2007;20(1):4–12.
4. Grewal J, Mankad S, Freeman WK, et al. Real-time three-dimensional transesophageal echocardiography in the intraoperative assessment of mitral valve disease. *J Am Soc Echocardiogr.* 2009;22(1):34–41.
5. Pepi M, Tamborini G, Maltagliati A, et al. Head-to-head comparison of two- and three-dimensional transthoracic and transesophageal echocardiography in the localization of mitral valve prolapse. *J Am Coll Cardiol.* 2006;48(12):2524–2530.
6. Omran AS, Woo A, David TE, et al. Intraoperative transesophageal echocardiography accurately predicts mitral valve anatomy and suitability for repair. *J Am Soc Echocardiogr.* 2002;15(9):950–957.
7. David TE. Outcomes of mitral valve repair for mitral regurgitation due to degenerative disease. *Semin Thorac Cardiovasc Surg.* 2007;19(2):116–120.
8. Lee EM, Shapiro LM, Wells FC. Superiority of mitral valve repair in surgery for degenerative mitral regurgitation. *Eur Heart J.* 1997;18(4):655–663.
9. Maffessanti F, Marsan NA, Tamborini G, et al. Quantitative analysis of mitral valve apparatus in mitral valve prolapse before and after annuloplasty: a three-dimensional intraoperative transesophageal study. *J Am Soc Echocardiogr.* 2011;24(4):405–413.
10. Grewal J, Suri R, Mankad S, et al. Mitral annular dynamics in myxomatous valve disease: new insights with real-time 3-dimensional echocardiography. *Circulation.* 2010;121(12):1423–1431.
11. Kim DH, Handschumacher MD, Levine RA, et al. In vivo measurement of mitral leaflet surface area and subvalvular geometry in patients with asymmetrical septal hypertrophy: insights into the mechanism of outflow tract obstruction. *Circulation.* 2010;122(13):1298–1307.
12. Levine RA, Triulzi MO, Harrigan P, Weyman AE. The relationship of mitral annular shape to the diagnosis of mitral valve prolapse. *Circulation.* 1987;75(4):756–767.
13. Watanabe N, Ogasawara Y, Yamaura Y, et al. Quantitation of mitral valve tenting in ischemic mitral regurgitation by transthoracic real-time three-dimensional echocardiography. *J Am Coll Cardiol.* 2005;45(5):763–769.
14. Kaplan SR, Bashein G, Sheehan FH, et al. Three-dimensional echocardiographic assessment of annular shape changes in the normal and regurgitant mitral valve. *Am Heart J.* 2000;139(3):378–387.
15. Kwan J, Shiota T, Agler DA, et al. Geometric differences of the mitral apparatus between ischemic and dilated cardiomyopathy with significant mitral regurgitation: real-time three-dimensional echocardiography study. *Circulation.* 2003;107(8):1135–1140.
16. Mahmood F, Subramaniam B, Gorman JH 3rd, et al. Three-dimensional echocardiographic assessment of changes in mitral valve geometry after valve repair. *Ann Thorac Surg.* 2009;88(6):1838–1844.
17. Otsuji Y, Handschumacher MD, Liel-Cohen N, et al. Mechanism of ischemic mitral regurgitation with segmental left ventricular dysfunction: three-dimensional echocardiographic studies in models of acute and chronic progressive regurgitation. *J Am Coll Cardiol.* 2001;37(2):641–648.
18. Kaul S, Spotnitz WD, Glasheen WP, Touchstone DA. Mechanism of ischemic mitral regurgitation. An experimental evaluation. *Circulation.* 1991;84(5):2167–2180.
19. Yosefy C, Beeri R, Guerrero JL, et al. Mitral regurgitation after anteroapical myocardial infarction: new mechanistic insights. *Circulation.* 2011;123(14):1529–1536.
20. Veronesi F, Corsi C, Sugeng L, et al. Quantification of mitral apparatus dynamics in functional and ischemic mitral regurgitation using real-time 3-dimensional echocardiography. *J Am Soc Echocardiogr.* 2008;21(4):347–354.
21. Chandra S, Salgo IS, Sugeng L, et al. A three-dimensional insight into the complexity of flow convergence in mitral regurgitation: adjunctive benefit of anatomic regurgitant orifice area. *Am J Physiol Heart Circ Physiol.* 2011;301(3):H1015–1024. Epub 2011 Jun 10.
22. Altiok E, Hamada S, van Hall S, et al. Comparison of direct planimetry of mitral valve regurgitation orifice area by three-dimensional transesophageal echocardiography to effective regurgitant orifice area obtained by proximal flow convergence method and vena contracta area determined by color Doppler echocardiography. *Am J Cardiol.* 2011;107(3):452–458.

23 Langerveld J, Valocik G, Plokker HW, et al. Additional value of three-dimensional transesophageal echocardiography for patients with mitral valve stenosis undergoing balloon valvuloplasty. *J Am Soc Echocardiogr.* 2003;16(8):841–849.
24. Fatkin D, Roy P, Morgan JJ, Feneley MP. Percutaneous balloon mitral valvotomy with the Inoue single-balloon catheter: commissural morphology as a determinant of outcome. *J Am Coll Cardiol.* 1993;21(2):390–397.
25. Mannaerts H, Li Y, Kamp O, et al. Quantitative assessment of mechanical prosthetic valve area by 3-dimensional transesophageal echocardiography. *J Am Soc Echocardiogr.* 2001;14(7):723–731.
26. Zamorano JL, Badano LP, Bruce C, et al. EAE/ASE recommendations for the use of echocardiography in new transcatheter interventions for valvular heart disease. *J Am Soc Echocardiogr.* 2011;24(9):937–965.
27. Perk G, Lang RM, Garcia-Fernandez MA, et al. Use of real time three-dimensional transesophageal echocardiography in intracardiac catheter based interventions. *J Am Soc Echocardiogr.* 2009;22(8):865–882.
28. Kronzon I, Sugeng L, Perk G, et al. Real-time 3-dimensional transesophageal echocardiography in the evaluation of post-operative mitral annuloplasty ring and prosthetic valve dehiscence. *J Am Coll Cardiol.* 2009;53(17):1543–1547.
29. Pate GE, Thompson CR, Munt BI, Webb JG. Techniques for percutaneous closure of prosthetic paravalvular leaks. *Catheter Cardiovasc Interv.* 2006;67(1):158–166.
30. Hamilton-Craig C, Boga T, Platts D, et al. The role of 3D transesophageal echocardiography during percutaneous closure of paravalvular mitral regurgitation. *JACC Cardiovasc Imaging.* 2009;2(6):771–773.
31. Biner S, Perk G, Kar S, et al. Utility of combined two-dimensional and three-dimensional transesophageal imaging for catheter-based mitral valve clip repair of mitral regurgitation. *J Am Soc Echocardiogr.* 2011;24(6):611–617.
32. Nunez-Gil IJ, Gonçalves A, Rodriguez E, et al. Transapical mitral valve-in-valve implantation: a novel approach guided by three-dimensional transoesophageal echocardiography. *Eur J Echocardiogr.* 2011;12(4):335–337.
33. Altiok E, Koos R, Schröder J, et al. Comparison of two-dimensional and three-dimensional imaging techniques for measurement of aortic annulus diameters before transcatheter aortic valve implantation. *Heart.* 2011;97(19):1578–1584. Epub 2011 Jun 23.
34. Tops LF, Wood DA, Delgado V, et al. Noninvasive evaluation of the aortic root with multislice computed tomography implications for transcatheter aortic valve replacement. *JACC Cardiovasc Imaging.* 2008;1(3):321–330.
35. Piazza N, de Jaegere P, Schultz C, et al. Anatomy of the aortic valvar complex and its implications for transcatheter implantation of the aortic valve. *Circ Cardiovasc Interv.* 2008;1(1):74–81.
36. Messika-Zeitoun D, Serfaty JM, Brochet E, et al. Multimodal assessment of the aortic annulus diameter: implications for transcatheter aortic valve implantation. *J Am Coll Cardiol.* 2010;55(3):186–194.
37. Pate GE, Al Zubaidi A, Chandavimol M, et al. Percutaneous closure of prosthetic paravalvular leaks: case series and review. *Catheter Cardiovasc Interv.* 2006;68(4):528–533.
38. Thompson KA, Shiota T, Tolstrup K, et al. Utility of three-dimensional transesophageal echocardiography in the diagnosis of valvular perforations. *Am J Cardiol.* 2011;107(1):100–102.
39. Espinola-Zavaleta N, Munoz-Castellanos L, Attie F, et al. Anatomic three-dimensional echocardiographic correlation of bicuspid aortic valve. *J Am Soc Echocardiogr.* 2003;16(1):46–53.
40. Nakai H, Takeuchi M, Yoshitani H, et al. Pitfalls of anatomical aortic valve area measurements using two-dimensional transoesophageal echocardiography and the potential of three-dimensional transoesophageal echocardiography. *Eur J Echocardiogr.* 2010;11(4):369–376.
41. Marechaux S, Juthier F, Banfi C, et al. Illustration of the echocardiographic diagnosis of subaortic membrane stenosis in adults: surgical and live three-dimensional transoesophageal findings. *Eur J Echocardiogr.* 2011;12(1):E2.
42. Dujardin KS, Enriquez-Sarano M, Schaff HV, et al. Mortality and morbidity of aortic regurgitation in clinical practice. A long-term follow-up study. *Circulation.* 1999;99(14):1851–1857.
43. Ling LH, Enriquez-Sarano M, Seward JB, et al. Clinical outcome of mitral regurgitation due to flail leaflet. *N Engl J Med.* 1996;335(19):1417–1423.
44. Moss AJ, Daubert J, Zareba W. MADIT-II: clinical implications. *Card Electrophysiol Rev.* 2002;6(4):463–465.
45. White HD, Norris RM, Brown MA, et al. Left ventricular end-systolic volume as the major determinant of survival after recovery from myocardial infarction. *Circulation.* 1987;76(1):44–51.
46. Wong M, Johnson G, Shabetai R, et al. Echocardiographic variables as prognostic indicators and therapeutic monitors in chronic congestive heart failure. Veterans Affairs cooperative studies V-HeFT I and II. V-HeFT VA Cooperative Studies Group. *Circulation.* 1993;87(suppl 6):VI65–VI70.
47. Malm S, Frigstad S, Sagberg E, et al. Accurate and reproducible measurement of left ventricular volume and ejection fraction by contrast echocardiography: a comparison with magnetic resonance imaging. *J Am Coll Cardiol.* 2004;44(5):1030–1035.

48. Thomson HL, Basmadjian AJ, Rainbird AJ, et al. Contrast echocardiography improves the accuracy and reproducibility of left ventricular remodeling measurements: a prospective, randomly assigned, blinded study. *J Am Coll Cardiol.* 2001;38(3):867–875.
49. Yu EH, Sloggett CE, Iwanochko RM, et al. Feasibility and accuracy of left ventricular volumes and ejection fraction determination by fundamental, tissue harmonic, and intravenous contrast imaging in difficult-to-image patients. *J Am Soc Echocardiogr.* 2000;13(3):216–224.
50. Aebischer NM, Czegledy F. Determination of right ventricular volume by two-dimensional echocardiography with a crescentic model. *J Am Soc Echocardiogr.* 1989;2(2):110–118.
51. Simpson JM, Miller O. Three-dimensional echocardiography in congenital heart disease. *Arch Cardiovasc Dis.* 2011;104(1):45–56.
52. Fusini L, Tamborini G, Gripari P, et al. Feasibility of intraoperative three-dimensional transesophageal echocardiography in the evaluation of right ventricular volumes and function in patients undergoing cardiac surgery. *J Am Soc Echocardiogr.* 2011;24(8):868–877.
53. Kaul TK, Fields BL. Postoperative acute refractory right ventricular failure: incidence, pathogenesis, management and prognosis. *Cardiovasc Surg.* 2000;8(1):1–9.
54. Sun JP, James KB, Yang XS, et al. Comparison of mortality rates and progression of left ventricular dysfunction in patients with idiopathic dilated cardiomyopathy and dilated versus nondilated right ventricular cavities. *Am J Cardiol.* 1997;80(12):1583–1587.
55. Salehian O, Schwerzmann M, Merchant N, et al. Assessment of systemic right ventricular function in patients with transposition of the great arteries using the myocardial performance index: comparison with cardiac magnetic resonance imaging. *Circulation.* 2004;110(20):3229–3233.
56. Rudski LG, Lai WW, Afilalo J, et al. Guidelines for the echocardiographic assessment of the right heart in adults: a report from the American Society of Echocardiography endorsed by the European Association of Echocardiography, a registered branch of the European Society of Cardiology, and the Canadian Society of Echocardiography. *J Am Soc Echocardiogr.* 2010;23(7):685–713; quiz 86–88.
57. Haddad F, Doyle R, Murphy DJ, Hunt SA. Right ventricular function in cardiovascular disease, part II: pathophysiology, clinical importance, and management of right ventricular failure. *Circulation.* 2008;117(13):1717–1731.
58. Tamborini G, Marsan NA, Gripari P, et al. Reference values for right ventricular volumes and ejection fraction with real-time three-dimensional echocardiography: evaluation in a large series of normal subjects. *J Am Soc Echocardiogr.* 2010;23(2):109–115.
59. Leibundgut G, Rohner A, Grize L, et al. Dynamic assessment of right ventricular volumes and function by real-time three-dimensional echocardiography: a comparison study with magnetic resonance imaging in 100 adult patients. *J Am Soc Echocardiogr.* 2010;23(2):116–126.
60. Grewal J, Majdalany D, Syed I, et al. Three-dimensional echocardiographic assessment of right ventricular volume and function in adult patients with congenital heart disease: comparison with magnetic resonance imaging. *J Am Soc Echocardiogr.* 2010;23(2):127–133.
61. Nesser HJ, Tkalec W, Patel AR, et al. Quantitation of right ventricular volumes and ejection fraction by three-dimensional echocardiography in patients: comparison with magnetic resonance imaging and radionuclide ventriculography. *Echocardiography.* 2006;23(8):666–680.
62. De Simone R, Wolf I, Mottl-Link S, et al. Intraoperative assessment of right ventricular volume and function. *Eur J Cardiothorac Surg.* 2005;27(6):988–993.
63. Jenkins C, Bricknell K, Hanekom L, Marwick TH. Reproducibility and accuracy of echocardiographic measurements of left ventricular parameters using real-time three-dimensional echocardiography. *J Am Coll Cardiol.* 2004;44(4):878–886.
64. Balzer J, Kuhl H, Franke A. Real-time three-dimensional transoesophageal echocardiography for guidance of atrial septal defect closures. *Eur Heart J.* 2008;29(18):2226.
65. Ge S. How can we best image congenital heart defects? Are two-dimensional and three-dimensional echocardiography competitive or complementary? *J Am Soc Echocardiogr.* 2010;23(7):722–725.
66. Belohlavek M, Foley DA, Gerber TC, et al. Three-dimensional ultrasound imaging of the atrial septum: normal and pathologic anatomy. *J Am Coll Cardiol.* 1993;22(6):1673–1678.
67. Marx GR, Fulton DR, Pandian NG, et al. Delineation of site, relative size and dynamic geometry of atrial septal defects by real-time three-dimensional echocardiography. *J Am Coll Cardiol.* 1995;25(2):482–490.
68. Lodato JA, Cao QL, Weinert L, et al. Feasibility of real-time three-dimensional transoesophageal echocardiography for guidance of percutaneous atrial septal defect closure. *Eur J Echocardiogr.* 2009;10(4):543–548.

69. Magni G, Hijazi ZM, Pandian NG, et al. Two- and three-dimensional transesophageal echocardiography in patient selection and assessment of atrial septal defect closure by the new DAS-Angel Wings device: initial clinical experience. *Circulation*. 1997;96(6):1722–1728.
70. Georgakis A, Radtke WA, Lopez C, et al. Complex atrial septal defect: percutaneous repair guided by three-dimensional echocardiography. *Echocardiography*. 2010;27(5):590–593.
71. Franke A, Kuhl HP, Rulands D, et al. Quantitative analysis of the morphology of secundum-type atrial septal defects and their dynamic change using transesophageal three-dimensional echocardiography. *Circulation*. 1997;96(suppl 9):II-323–II-327.
72. Zhu W, Cao QL, Rhodes J, Hijazi ZM. Measurement of atrial septal defect size: a comparative study between three-dimensional transesophageal echocardiography and the standard balloon sizing methods. *Pediatr Cardiol*. 2000;21(5):465–469.
73. Abdel-Massih T, Dulac Y, Taktak A, et al. Assessment of atrial septal defect size with 3D-transesophageal echocardiography: comparison with balloon method. *Echocardiography*. 2005;22(2):121–127.

Index

Note: Page numbers followed by f refer to figures; page numbers followed by t refer to tables.